New Insights into Suicide and Mental Health Conditions

New Insights into Suicide and Mental Health Conditions

Guest Editors

Cory R. Weissman
Zafiris Daskalakis

MDPI

Basel • Beijing • Wuhan • Barcelona • Belgrade • Novi Sad • Cluj • Manchester

Guest Editors
Cory R. Weissman
Department of Psychiatry
University of California
San Diego
La Jolla
USA

Zafiris Daskalakis
Department of Psychiatry
University of California
San Diego
La Jolla
USA

Editorial Office
MDPI AG
Grosspeteranlage 5
4052 Basel, Switzerland

This is a reprint of the Special Issue, published open access by the journal *Journal of Clinical Medicine* (ISSN 2077-0383), freely accessible at: https://www.mdpi.com/journal/jcm/special_issues/6L2SN9SUZM.

For citation purposes, cite each article independently as indicated on the article page online and as indicated below:

Lastname, A.A.; Lastname, B.B. Article Title. *Journal Name* **Year**, *Volume Number*, Page Range.

ISBN 978-3-7258-5795-1 (Hbk)
ISBN 978-3-7258-5796-8 (PDF)
https://doi.org/10.3390/books978-3-7258-5796-8

Contents

Journal of
Clinical Medicine

MDPI

Systematic Review

Psychedelics and Suicide-Related Outcomes: A Systematic Review

Shakila Meshkat [1], Taha Malik [1], Richard Zeifman [2,3], Jennifer Swainson [4,5], Yanbo Zhang [4,5], Lisa Burback [4,5], Olga Winkler [4], Andrew J. Greenshaw [4,5], Amy Claire Reichelt [6,7], Eric Vermetten [8], David Erritzoe [3], Manish K. Jha [9], Walter Dunn [10], Rakesh Jetly [11], Muhammad Ishrat Husain [12,13] and Venkat Bhat [1,13,*]

1. Interventional Psychiatry Program, St. Michael's Hospital, Toronto, ON M5B 1M8, Canada; shakila.meshkat@unityhealth.to (S.M.)
2. NYU Center for Psychedelic Medicine, NYU Grossman School of Medicine, New York, NY 10016, USA
3. Center for Psychedelic Research, Department of Brain Sciences, Imperial College London, London SW7 2AZ, UK
4. Department of Psychiatry, University of Alberta, Edmonton, AB T6G 2R3, Canada
5. Neuroscience and Mental Health Institute (NMHI), University of Alberta, Edmonton, AB T6G 2R3, Canada
6. Department of Physiology and Pharmacology, Western University, London, ON N6A 5C1, Canada
7. School of Biomedicine, University of Adelaide, Adelaide, SA 5005, Australia
8. Department of Psychiatry, Leiden University Medical Center, 2333 ZA Leiden, The Netherlands
9. Department of Psychiatry, UT Southwestern, Dallas, TX 75247, USA
10. The Department of Psychiatry, University of California, Los Angeles, CA 90095, USA
11. The Institute of Mental Health Research, University of Ottawa, Ottawa, ON K1Z 7K4, Canada
12. Campbell Family Mental Health Research Institute, Centre for Addiction and Mental Health, Toronto, ON M6J 1H4, Canada
13. Department of Psychiatry, University of Toronto, Toronto, ON M5S 3E5, Canada

* Correspondence: venkat.bhat@utoronto.ca; Tel.: +1-(416)-360-4000-x76404; Fax: +1-(416)-864-5996

Abstract: Background/Objectives: Suicide accounts for 1.4% of global deaths, and the slow-acting nature of traditional treatments for suicide risk underscores the need for alternatives. Psychedelic therapies may rapidly reduce suicide risk. This systematic review evaluates impact of psychedelic therapies on suicide-related outcomes. **Methods:** A systematic search of MEDLINE, Embase, PsycINFO, and ClinicalTrials.gov was conducted up to November 2024. **Results**: Four randomized controlled trials (RCTs) evaluated suicidality as a secondary outcome or safety measure, showing significant reductions in suicidal ideation with psilocybin (three studies) and MDMA-assisted therapy (MDMA-AT; one study). Effect sizes, measured by Cohen's d, ranged from =0.52 to 1.25 (p = 0.01 to 0.005), with no safety issues reported. Five additional RCTs assessed suicidality as a safety measure, showing reductions in suicidal ideation with psilocybin (two studies) and MDMA-AT (three studies; p = 0.02 to 0.04). Among 24 non-randomized and cross-sectional studies, results were mixed. Psilocybin (three studies) reduced suicidal ideation, with odds ratios (OR) of 0.40–0.75. MDMA-AT (five studies in PTSD patients) had a pooled effect size of d = 0.61 (95% CI: 0.32–0.89). LSD (six studies) showed increased odds of suicidality, with odds ratios ranging from 1.15 to 2.08. Studies involving DMT (two studies) and multiple psychedelics (three studies) showed mixed results, with DMT studies not showing significant effects on suicidality and studies involving multiple psychedelics showing varying outcomes, some reporting reductions in suicidal ideation and others showing no significant change. **Conclusions**: The effect of psychedelic therapies on suicide-related outcomes remains inconclusive, highlighting the need for further trials to clarify safety and therapeutic mechanisms.

https://doi.org/10.3390/jcm14051416

Keywords: suicide; suicidal behavior; psychedelics; psilocybin; MDMA; psychiatric disorders; mood disorders; mental health

1. Introduction

Suicidal thoughts and behaviors, encompassing completed suicide, suicide attempts, and suicidal ideation, represent a major public health challenge and a significant contributor to global mortality [1]. Death by suicide accounts for approximately 1.4% of all deaths worldwide and ranks as the 10th leading cause of death in the United States [2]. Suicidal behavior arises from a complex interplay of factors, broadly categorized into predisposing elements and immediate stressors or triggers [3]. Mental disorders play a predominant role, with over 90% of individuals who die by suicide meeting the criteria for a psychiatric illness as outlined in the Diagnostic and Statistical Manual of Mental Disorders, Fourth Edition (DSM-IV) [4]. Among psychiatric conditions, mood disorders—primarily major depressive disorder (MDD) and bipolar disorder (BD)—are implicated in approximately 60% of completed suicides [5]. Notably, trauma burden and posttraumatic stress disorder (PTSD) significantly increase the risk of suicidal ideation and behaviors, further compounding the challenge of prevention and treatment [6]. Additional influences include the availability of lethal means, substance use (alcohol and drugs), access to mental health care, cultural and personal attitudes toward suicide, help-seeking behaviors, physical health conditions, marital status, age, and gender [3,7]. Current biological approaches to reduce suicidality remain limited in their effectiveness. Traditional treatments, such as antidepressants, cognitive behavioral therapy (CBT), and electroconvulsive therapy (ECT), have shown to reduce suicidal thoughts and behaviors in individuals with depression [8–10]. Additionally, pharmacotherapies such as clozapine and lithium, recognized for their anti-suicidal properties, also played a significant role in managing suicidality [11]. However, these interventions typically require several weeks to take effect, leaving many patients at significant risk of suicide during this period. Recent developments in rapid-acting antidepressants (RAADs), such as ketamine and its FDA-approved derivative esketamine (Spravato), represent promising advances in the treatment of acute suicidal ideation and behaviors, particularly in individuals with depression [12]. While these interventions can reduce symptoms within hours, their effects are limited to this population and do not address suicidality in a broader sense. Additionally, the short duration of effect following a single treatment and the unknown durability of their anti-suicidal properties with repeated administrations pose challenges to their clinical application [13]. Therefore, there is an urgent need for novel efficacious treatments to address this critical issue.

Serotonergic psychedelics, commonly known as "classic" psychedelics, include a range of substances such as psilocybin, dimethyltryptamine (DMT), ayahuasca, mescaline, and lysergic acid diethylamide (LSD) [14]. In contrast, 3,4-methylenedioxymethamphetamine (MDMA) is a distinct psychoactive compound considered an empathogen or entactogen that has also garnered attention for its therapeutic potential [14]. Classic psychedelics are naturally occurring, plant-derived or synthesized psychoactive substances that primarily function as serotonin 2A receptor agonists [15]. These compounds have the potential to induce profound experiences, which, in some cases, can enhance an individual's perceived quality of life [15]. Similarly, MDMA (3,4-methylenedioxymethamphetamine), though not a classic psychedelic, acts primarily as a serotonin-releasing agent and promotes prosocial effects, emotional openness, and enhanced therapeutic processing, which may also contribute to improvements in perceived quality of life [16,17]. Psychedelics, administered with psychological support, have been investigated in numerous randomized clinical trials

(RCTs) for a variety of psychiatric conditions, including MDD, BD, treatment-resistant depression (TRD), substance use disorders (SUDs), and PTSD [18–22]. Psychedelic therapies may also have potential benefits in reducing suicidality due to their ability to enhance emotional processing, facilitate personal insights, and promote a sense of interconnectedness, which can improve mental health and reduce self-destructive thoughts [23]. However, psychedelic use is also linked to adverse events, including heightened anxiety [24], and there have been reports suggesting an increase in suicidal ideations and behaviors in some individuals following LSD use [25].

Despite growing research on psychedelic therapies for psychiatric disorders such as depression, anxiety, substance use disorders, and PTSD, their effects on suicidality remain underexplored. Notably, many clinical trials on psychedelic therapies exclude participants with suicidal ideation, often assessed via the clinician-rated Columbia–Suicide Severity Rating Scale (C-SSRS), or those with borderline personality disorder (BPD)—a population at elevated risk for suicide and comprising a significant portion of psychiatric patients. Given the urgent need for treatments targeting individuals with acute and severe psychiatric symptoms, identifying therapies that can address suicidality in these high-risk groups is of profound importance. A systematic review is needed to evaluate the impact of psychedelic therapies on suicide risk, clarify their safety and therapeutic mechanisms, and guide future research and clinical practice. Such an assessment is crucial for understanding how psychedelic therapies can be safely integrated into treatment for individuals at high suicide risk. Therefore, in this systematic review, we aim to evaluate the effect of psychedelic therapies on suicidal-related outcomes.

2. Methods

This systematic review followed the Preferred Reporting Items for Systematic reviews and Meta-Analyses guidelines [26] and was registered on PROSPERO (registration ID: CRD42024611536).

2.1. Search Strategy

We conducted a comprehensive search in three databases (MEDLINE, Embase, and PsycINFO) via OVID, covering all records from inception through November 2024. We also searched Google Scholar and references of relevant studies. The following keywords were used: psilocybin or psilocibin or psilocybine or silocybin or psiloc* or shrooms or magic mushrooms or mushies or psilocybin-assisted therapy or PAP or psychedelics or MDMA or 3,4-methylenedioxymethamphetamine or ecstasy or molly or ayahuasca or LSD or lysergic acid diethylamide or DMT or dimethyltryptamine or mescaline or peyote or ibogaine or iboga or 5-MeO-DMT or salvinorin A or Salvia or bufotenin or 5-HO-DMT AND suicide or suicidal ideation or suicidality or suicidal thoughts or suicidal behavior or suicide attempt. No language or publication date restrictions were applied. Additionally, a search of registered clinical trials was conducted on ClinicalTrials.gov on 21 November 2024, using the same psychedelic agents paired with suicide-related terms.

2.2. Eligibility Criteria

Two reviewers (SM, TM) independently reviewed the title/abstract and full text of studies based on eligibility criteria. The screening process was conducted in Covidence (https://www.covidence.org/ (accessed on 1 November 2024). Conflicts between reviewers were resolved through discussion, and if disagreements persisted, a third reviewer was consulted to reach a consensus (VB). Studies were included if they met the following criteria: (1) original research of any study design; (2) evaluation of the effect or association of psychedelics or hallucinogens with suicide-related outcomes; (3) published in English. Secondary analyses were included only if their primary focus was on the effects of psychedelics on suicidal-related outcomes. Qualitative studies were also considered. Excluded studies were case reports, non-human studies, systematic reviews, narrative reviews, umbrella reviews, meta-analyses, letters, editorials, posters, conference abstracts, and studies not published in English. We chose to exclude systematic reviews and meta-analyses to ensure that our findings are based on primary data rather than synthesized evidence, thereby avoiding potential duplication of results. Regarding the exclusion of non-English studies, this decision was made to ensure consistency in data extraction and interpretation, as translations may introduce variability or misinterpretation of critical findings.

2.3. Data Extraction

Two reviewers (SM, TM) independently reviewed the full texts of eligible studies and extracted the following variables: author, year of publication, country, study design, participants, intervention, psychotherapy principle, outcome measure, results, and conclusion. Similar to the published studies, the following variables were extracted from the registered clinical trials: study characteristic, intervention, outcome measure, country, diagnosis, and estimated completion date. Additional extracted variables were the ClinicalTrials.gov identifier (i.e., an 11-digit alphanumeric identifier), trial status (i.e., not yet recruiting, recruiting, active, completed, etc.), estimated completion date, and projected sample size.

2.4. Quality Assessment

All studies included in this review were evaluated for quality by two independent assessors (SM, TM) using the JBI Critical Appraisal Tools Checklist for systematic reviews [27]. The specific checklists applied were tailored for RCTs and cohort studies. Lower-quality studies were not excluded; however, their methodological limitations were considered in the interpretation of findings. While a formal sensitivity analysis was not conducted, the influence of these studies was evaluated qualitatively, with particular attention to study limitations (Supplementary Materials Table S1).

3. Results

3.1. Search Results

An electronic OVID database search resulted in a total of 3074 records. We removed duplicate articles (n = 663) and screened the title/abstract of the remaining records (n = 2411). A total of 2346 articles were excluded based on title/abstract. We reviewed the full text of the remaining papers (n = 65) in detail based on our inclusion criteria. Out of 65 records, 26 records were excluded: 14 studies had the wrong study design, 4 did not include suicidal-related outcomes, 3 had insufficient results, 2 had the wrong intervention, 2 were not in English, and 1 had the wrong indication. Finally, 39 articles involving 1,671,773 participants (949 from intervention-based studies, 1,670,409 from population-based studies, and 415 from secondary analysis studies) met the inclusion criteria and were included in this systematic review. We also found one ongoing trial on ClinicalTrials.gov (accessed on 21 November 2024). The study selection details are indicated in Figure 1. The characteristics of the included studies are listed in Tables 1 and 2 and Figures 2–4.

Table 1. Characteristics of included intervention-based studies.

Author	Country	Study Design	Participants	Population	Relevant Exclusion Criteria	Intervention	Psychotherapy Principle	Outcome Measure	Results	Conclusion
						Psilocybin				
Carhartt-Harris, 2021 [28]	United Kingdom	RCT	Psilocybin group: $n = 30$, 11% female, mean age of 43.3 Placebo group: $n = 29$, 9% female, mean age of 39.1	MDD	Currently or previously diagnosed with psychotic disorder, family member with psychotic disorder, history of serious suicide attempts requiring hospitalization, or BPD	Psilocybin group: 2 doses of 25 mg Psilocybin3 weeks apart + 6 weeks of daily oral placebo Placebo group: 2 doses 1 mg of Psilocybin 3 weeks apart + 6 weeks of daily oral escitalopram. Both groups were given psychotherapy.	1 3-h preparation session, 2 4–6 h dosing sessions, 6 90 min integration sessions 3 integration sessions followed each dose. The first was in-person, and the second was over an online call. Length of these sessions was not specified.	SIDAS	Assessed as a secondary outcome. Change from baseline to 6 weeks. $n = 30$, Psilocybin group: −2.0 (95% CI; −4.3 to 0.0) $n = 29$, Placebo group: −0.8 (95% CI; −3.4 to 2.0) Between-group difference: −1.3 (95% CI = −6.5 to −0.3) Confidence intervals were not corrected for multiple comparisons.	Suggests that psilocybin has reduced suicide risk vs. escitalopram, but the intervals for the between group comparison were not corrected.
Davis, 2021 [29]	United States	RCT	$n = 27$, 67% women, mean age of 39.8 years	MDD	Personal or family history (first or second degree) of psychotic or bipolar disorders, medically significant suicide attempt, BP-I or II	Psilocybin at 20 mg/70 kg, followed by 30 mg/kg. Accompanied with psychotherapy. Session 1: 20 mg/70 kg Session 2: 30 mg/70 kg	8 h of preparation sessions, 2 day-long dosing sessions, no integration Immediate group received the intervention right after baseline screening, whereas the delayed group waited 8 weeks in between baseline and intervention.	Clinician-administered C-SSRS, ideation intensity subscales	Assessed as a secondary outcome. 24 completed the study. Remaining 3 opted out of study with no AE. Immediate group Baseline: 1.2 5 weeks post: 0.2 (p = ns) 8 weeks post: 0.2 (p = ns) Delayed group Baseline: 1.3 5 weeks post: 0.6 (p = ns) 8 weeks post: 0.5 (p = ns)	Psilocybin did not increase suicidal risk in MDD patients, regardless of delayed treatment.

Table 1. *Cont.*

Author	Country	Study Design	Participants	Population	Relevant Exclusion Criteria	Intervention	Psychotherapy Principle	Outcome Measure	Results	Conclusion
Goodwin, 2022 [19]	United States, Czech Republic, Denmark, Germany, Ireland, Netherlands, Portugal, Canada, Spain, United Kingdom	RCT	n = 233, 52% female, mean age of 39.8	TRD	Current or past history of schizophrenia, psychotic disorder (unless substance induced or due to a medical condition), bipolar disorder, delusional disorder, paranoid personality disorder, schizoaffective disorder, BPD, or any serious psychiatric comorbidity, clinically significant risk for suicide	Single dose of psilocybin at either 25 mg (n = 79), 10 mg (n = 75), or 1 mg (n = 79) All groups were given psychotherapy.	3 preparation sessions, 1 6–8 h dosing session, 2 integration sessions (time not specified)	Clinician-administered C-SSRS	Assessed as a safety measure. While individual scores were not, the number of participants exhibiting suicidal ideation and behavior per group was provided. Throughout all 12 weeks, Participants in the 25 mg and 10 mg groups exhibited higher suicidal ideation than in the 1 mg group. Baseline: 21 in the 25 mg group, 27 in the 10 mg group, 19 in the 1 mg group showed suicidal ideation (passive or no intent to plan) Baseline to week 3: 11 in the 25 mg group, 13 in the 10 mg group, and 7 in the 1 mg group showed increased suicidal risk. Here, 2 in the 25 mg and 2 in the 10 mg groups were noted for suicidal ideation with intent. Week 3 to week 12: 12 in the 25 mg, 12 in the 10 mg, and 12 in the 1 mg groups exhibited worsened suicidality. Here, 3 in the 25 mg group endorsed items on the behavior section of the C-SRSS, and 1 in the 10 mg group exhibited suicidal ideation with intent.	No clear evidence for reductions or increases in suicide risk due to psilocybin.

Table 1. *Cont.*

Author	Country	Study Design	Participants	Population	Relevant Exclusion Criteria	Intervention	Psychotherapy Principle	Outcome Measure	Results	Conclusion
Peck, 2022 [30]	United States	RCT	n = 10, 100% female, mean age of 28.3	Anorexia nervosa	Current or previously diagnosed psychotic disorder, substantial suicide risk, history of mania and borderline personality disorder	Single 25 mg dose of psilocybin with psychotherapy.	2 preparation sessions, 1 8 h dosing session, 2 90 min integration sessions	Clinician administered C-SSRS	Assessed as a safety measure. No increases in suicidal ideation throughout trial, and no suicidal behaviors present in follow-up visits	No evidence to suggest psilocybin increases suicidal risk.
Von Rotz, 2022 [31]	Switzerland	RCT	n = 52 Psilocybin n = 26, 61.5% female, mean age of 37.6 Placebo n = 26, 65.4% female, mean age of 35.9	MDD	Axis-II disorder symptoms associated with increased adverse emotional or behavioral reactions to intervention, psychosis spectrum disorders and/or mania symptoms in participants or first-degree relatives.	Single 0.215 mg/kg dose of psilocybin. Both groups were given psychotherapy.	2 1 h preparation sessions, 1 6 h dosing session, 3 1 h integration sessions	Clinician administered C-SSRS, intensity of ideation subscale	Assessed as a secondary outcome. Mean. Psilocybin Baseline: 0.50 14 days: 0.15 Change: −0.35 (p = 0.13, 95% CI: −0.10 to 0.71, d = 0.43) Placebo Baseline: 0.54 14 days: 0.46 Between-group difference not significant. (F[1, 50] = 1.40; p = 0.24)	No detectable impact of psilocybin on suicide risk.

Table 1. *Cont.*

Author	Country	Study Design	Participants	Population	Relevant Exclusion Criteria	Intervention	Psychotherapy Principle	Outcome Measure	Results	Conclusion
Raison, 2023 [32]	United States	RCT	n = 104, 50% female, mean age of 41.1 n = 51 given psilocybin, 47% female, mean age of 40.4	MDD	History of psychosis or mania, active suicidal ideation with intent.	Single 25 mg dose of psilocybin All groups were given psychotherapy.	6–8 h of preparatory sessions, 1 7–10 h dosing session, 4 h of integration sessions	Clinician administered C-SSRSor MADRS-SI	Assessed as a safety measure. No suicidal or self-injurious behavior occurred during the trial. All instances of ideation were passive. One participant receiving psilocybin and five receiving niacin had an increase in C-SSRS score from baseline to end of trial.	Little evidence of Psilocybin increasing suicide risk.
Ross et al., 2021 [33]	United States	RCT, secondary analysis	n = 11, 63.6% female, mean age of 60.3 n = 6 assigned to psilocybin first, 50% female, mean age of 57.5 n = 5 assigned to placebo first, 80% female, mean age of 63.6	Cancer patients with either adjustment with anxiety ± depression, acute stress disorder, generalized anxiety disorder (GAD), or anxiety disorder due to cancer.	Personal or immediate family history of schizophrenia, bipolar disorder, delusional disorder, paranoid disorder, and schizoaffective disorder.	Psilocybin at 0.3 mg/kg, crossed over with placebo. One group received psilocybin at the first dosing session and placebo at the second, whereas the other group received placebo first and psilocybin second. Both groups were given psychotherapy.	3 preparation sessions, 1st dosing session, cross over session (post dose integration + preparation for dose 2) over 7 weeks, 2nd dosing session, 3 integration sessions	Composite SI score using BDI-II and BSI	Composite score out of 100. Based on summed Z-scores of item 9 of BDI-II and item 9 of BSI, SI after dose 1 Psilocybin first Baseline: 70 8 h: 40 2 weeks: 40 7 weeks: 38 Placebo first Baseline: 66 8 h: 48 2 weeks: 52 7 weeks: 48 SI after dose 2 Both groups Baseline: 62 6.5 months post: 35	Authors note "acute and sustained reductions in SI… in patients with life threatening cancer". They report significant within-group improvements in SI.

Table 1. *Cont.*

Author	Country	Study Design	Participants	Population	Relevant Exclusion Criteria	Intervention	Psychotherapy Principle	Outcome Measure	Results	Conclusion
Carhart-Harris et al., 2018 [34]	United Kingdom	Open Label	$n = 20$, 30% female, mean age of 44.1	TRD	Current or previously diagnosed psychotic disorder or immediate family member with a diagnosed psychotic disorder	Two oral doses of psilocybin at 10 mg and 25 mg with psychotherapy.	1 preparation session, 2 dosing sessions	QIDS-SI, HAM-D-SI	Relevant items taken from primary outcome measures. Reported as mean change. QIDS-SI Change at 1 week post: −0.9 (95% CI = −0.4 to −1.4,; $p < 0.002$) Change at 2 weeks post: −0.85 (95% CI = −0.4 to −1.3; $p = 0.004$) Change at 3 weeks post: −0.8 (95% CI = −0.25 to −0.13; $p = 0.01$) Change at 5 weeks post: −0.7, 95% CI = −0.22 to −1.2; $p = 0.01$) HAM-D-SI Change at 1 week post: −0.95 (95% CI = −0.58 to −1.3; $p < 0.001$)	Authors note significant reductions at week 1 and 2 post treatment and nonsignificant changes 3 and 5 weeks out.

Table 1. *Cont.*

Author	Country	Study Design	Participants	Population	Relevant Exclusion Criteria	Intervention	Psychotherapy Principle	Outcome Measure	Results	Conclusion
Anderson et al., 2020 [35]	United States	Open Label	n = 18, 0% female, mean age of 59.2	OLTAS, Demoralization scale-II ≥ 8	Primary psychotic disorder, bipolar disorder I/II), severe major depressive episode, suicidal ideation with intent in the last three months or suicide attempt in last two years	A single 0.3–0.36 mg/kg dose of psilocybin with psychotherapy.	1 90 min preparation session, 1 8 h dosing session, 1 2 h individual psychotherapy session, 8–10 group psychotherapy sessions spread throughout 7-week trial period	Clinician-administered C-SSRS, ideation intensity subscale	Assessed as a safety measure. Mean. Baseline, week −3: 0.5 Week −1: 0.11 Day after drug, week 0: 0 Week 1 to 2: 0.11 End of treatment: 0.28 Reported no change in suicidal ideation over time, and no suicidal behavior detected during intervention.	No significant evidence to suggest increased suicide risk
Aaronson et al., 2024 [36]	United States	Open Label	n = 15, 60% female, mean age of 37.8	BP-II	History of BP-I disorder, schizophrenia, psychosis, delusions, paranoid, schizoaffective, or borderline personality disorder	A single 25 mg dose of psilocybin with psychotherapy.	3 preparation sessions, 1 8 h dosing session, 3 1 h integration sessions	Clinician-administered C-SSRS, ideation intensity subscale	Assessed as a safety measure. No patients attempted or committed suicide at any timepoints during the study.	No detectable impact on psilocybin-related suicide risk

Table 1. *Cont.*

Author	Country	Study Design	Participants	Population	Relevant Exclusion Criteria	Intervention	Psychotherapy Principle	Outcome Measure	Results	Conclusion
Ellis et al., 2024 [37]	United States	Open Label	*n* = 15, 13% female, mean of 43.2	Veterans with TRD	Current or past psychotic disorder, bipolar disorder, or personality disorder, current significant risk for suicide or engaged in suicidal behavior in the last three months	Single dose of 25 mg psilocybin with psychotherapy.	2 60 min and 1 90 min preparation sessions, 1 6–8 h dosing session, 3 90 min integration sessions	Clinician administered C-SSRS	Assessed as a safety measure. No observed increases in suicidal ideation from baseline, and no suicidal behavior present throughout the follow-up period.	No detectable impact on psilocybin-related suicide risk
MDMA-AT										
Mithoefer et al., 2018 [38]	United States	RCT	*n* = 26, 27% female, mean age of 37.2	PTSD	BP-I	Participants received MDMA-AT with 30 mg (*n* = 7), 75 mg (*n* = 7), or 125 mg (*n* = 12) All groups were given psychotherapy.	3 preparation sessions, 2 8 h dosing sessions, 3 integration sessions. Open-label crossover, 30 mg and 75 mg groups received 3 sessions of 100–125 mg	Clinician administered C-SSRS	Assessed as a safety measure. Numbers indicate participants with any positive ideation; C-SSRS ideation scale $\geq$ 1. Parenthesis indicate participants with serious ideation; C-SSRS ideation scale $\geq$ 4. 30 mg Baseline: 5(1) 1st session	Little evidence to suggest that MDMA may reduce suicidal risk in PTSD patients. There were no treatment emergent reports of suicidal ideation.

Table 1. *Cont.*

Author	Country	Study Design	Participants	Population	Relevant Exclusion Criteria	Intervention	Psychotherapy Principle	Outcome Measure	Results	Conclusion
									Pre-Drug: 1 Post-Drug: 1 Int. 1: 0 Int. 2: 1 Int. 3: 1 2nd session Pre-Drug: 0 During-Drug: 0 Int. 1: 0 Int. 2: 1 Int. 3: 2 3rd Session Pre-Drug: 1 During-Drug: 0 Int. 1: 0 Int. 2: 0 Int. 3: 0 75 mg Baseline: 6(2) 1st session Pre-Drug: 0 During-Drug: 0 Int. 1: 0 Int. 2: 0 Int. 3: 0 2nd session Pre-Drug: 0 During-Drug: 0 Int. 1: 0 Int. 2: 0 Int. 3: 0 3rd session Pre-Drug: 0	

Table 1. *Cont.*

Author	Country	Study Design	Participants	Population	Relevant Exclusion Criteria	Intervention	Psychotherapy Principle	Outcome Measure	Results	Conclusion
									During-Drug: 0 Int. 1: 0 Int. 2: 0 Int. 3: 0 125 mg Baseline: 11(5) 1st session Pre-Drug: 0 During-Drug: 0 Int. 1: 1 Int. 2: 2 Int. 3: 3 2nd session Pre-Drug: 1 During-Drug: 0 Int. 1: 0 Int. 2: 1 Int. 3: 2 Session 3 Pre-Drug: 0 During-Drug: 0 Int. 1: 1 Int. 2: 2 Int. 3: 2 Open label crossover. 30 mg and 75 mg groups received 100–125 mg MDMA for 3 more sessions 30 mg 4th session Pre-Drug: 0 During-Drug: 0 Int. 1: 1	

Table 1. *Cont.*

Author	Country	Study Design	Participants	Population	Relevant Exclusion Criteria	Intervention	Psychotherapy Principle	Outcome Measure	Results	Conclusion
									Int. 2: 0 Int. 3: 0 5th session Pre-Drug: 0 During-Drug: 0 Int. 1: 0 Int. 2: 0 Int. 3: 0 6th session Pre-Drug: 0 During-Drug: 0 Int. 1: 0 Int. 2: 0 Int. 3: 0 75 mg 4th session Pre-Drug: 0 During-Drug: 0 Int. 1: 0 Int, 2: 0 Int. 3: 0 5th session Pre-Drug: 1 During-Drug: 0 Int. 1: 0 Int. 2: 0 Int. 3: 0 6th session Pre-Drug: 0 During-Drug: 0 Int. 1: 0 Int. 2: 0 Int. 3: 0	

Table 1. *Cont.*

Author	Country	Study Design	Participants	Population	Relevant Exclusion Criteria	Intervention	Psychotherapy Principle	Outcome Measure	Results	Conclusion
Olatora et al., 2018 [39]	United States	RCT	Total $n = 28$, 67.9% female, mean age of 42 40 mg $n = 6$, 83.3% female, mean age of 40 100 mg $n = 9$, 66.7%, female mean age of 39.6 125 mg $n = 13$, 61.5% female, mean age of 44.6	PTSD	All personality disorders	2 separate doses of 40 mg, 100 mg, or 125 mg, followed by a supplemental half dose. All groups were given psychotherapy.	3 90 min preparatory sessions, 2 8 h dosing sessions, 3 integration sessions Open-label crossover, 100 mg and 125 mg groups received 1 session of 100–125 mg, accompanied by 3 integration sessions. 40 mg group received 3 sessions of 100–125 mg, accompanied by 1 preparatory session and 6 integration sessions.	Clinician-administered C-SSRS	Assessed as a safety measure. Numbers indicate participants with any positive ideation; C-SSRS ideation scale ≥ 1. Parenthesis indicate participants with serious ideation; C-SSRS ideation scale ≥ 4. RCT Phase 40 mg 1st session Baseline: 0 Pre-drug: 0 Post-drug: 0 Int. 1: 0 Int. 2: 1 Int. 3: 2 2nd session Baseline: 0 Pre-drug: 0 Post-drug: 0 Int. 1: 0 Int. 2: 0 Int. 3: 0 100 mg Baseline: 6 1st session Pre-drug: 5 Post-drug: 2	Authors observe greater suicide risk in active vs. comparator dose groups, but they did not exclude for past suicidal thinking in their patients.

Table 1. *Cont.*

Author	Country	Study Design	Participants	Population	Relevant Exclusion Criteria	Intervention	Psychotherapy Principle	Outcome Measure	Results	Conclusion
									Int. 1: 3 Int. 2: 3 Int. 3: 5 2nd session Pre-drug: 3 Post-drug: 3 Int. 1: 3 Int. 2: 3 Int. 3: 7 125 mg Baseline: 7 1st session Pre-drug: 3 Post-drug: 0 Int. 1: 0 Int. 2: 4 Int. 3: 5 2nd session Pre-drug: 3 Post-drug: 5 Int. 1: 0 Int. 2: 7 Int. 3: 9 Open-label crossover 100 mg 3rd session Pre-drug: 3 Post-drug: 2 Int. 1: 1 Int. 2: 3 Int. 3: 3 125 mg	

Table 1. *Cont.*

Author	Country	Study Design	Participants	Population	Relevant Exclusion Criteria	Intervention	Psychotherapy Principle	Outcome Measure	Results	Conclusion
									3rd session Pre-drug: 1 Post-drug: 3 Int. 1: 1 Int. 2: 1 Int. 3: 4 40 mg 4th session Pre-drug: 0 Post-drug: 1(1) Int. 1: 1(1) Int. 2: 0 Int. 3: 1 5th session Pre-drug: 0 Post-drug: 0 Int. 1: 0 Int. 2: 0 Int. 3: 0 6th session Pre-drug: 1 Post-drug: 0 Int. 1: 0 Int. 2: 1 Int. 3: 0	

Table 1. *Cont.*

Author	Country	Study Design	Participants	Population	Relevant Exclusion Criteria	Intervention	Psychotherapy Principle	Outcome Measure	Results	Conclusion
Mitchell et al., 2021 [40]	United States, Canada, Israel	RCT	Total $n = 90$, 65.5% female, mean age of 40.9 MDMA-AT group $n = 46$, 58.7% female, mean age of 43.5 Placebo group $n = 44$, 72.7% female, mean age of 38.2	PTSD	Primary psychotic disorder, BP-I, dissociative identity disorder, MDD with psychotic features, personality disorders	Session 1: Dose 1: 80 mg Dose 2: 40 mg (1.5–2.5 h after after dose 1) Session 2: Dose 1: 120 mg Dose 2: 60 mg (1.5–2.5 h after after dose 1) All groups were given psychotherapy.	3 preparatory sessions, 3 8 h dosing sessions, 9 integration sessions. Dosing sessions were spaced out 4 weeks apart, and 3 integration sessions occurred after each dosing session. The first integration session was the day after dosing, and the remaining two occurred in the following 3–4 weeks.	Clinician-administered C-SSRS	Assessed as a safety measure. Numbers indicate participants with any positive ideation; C-SSRS ideation scale ≥ 1. Parenthesis indicate participants with serious ideation; C-SSRS ideation scale ≥ 4. Placebo group Baseline: 14(1) 1st Session Pre-drug: 5(1) Post-drug: 6(1) Int. 1: 5(1) Int. 2: 11(1) Int. 3: 11(1) 2nd Session Pre-drug: 7(1) Post-drug: 3 Int. 1: 4(2) Int. 2: 8(2) Int. 3: 13(2) 3rd Session Pre-drug: 2 Post-drug: 1	Compared to placebo, MDMA did not increase suicide risk in patients with PTSD.

Table 1. *Cont.*

Author	Country	Study Design	Participants	Population	Relevant Exclusion Criteria	Intervention	Psychotherapy Principle	Outcome Measure	Results	Conclusion
									Int. 1: 4(1) Int. 2: 8(2) Int. 3: 9(2) MDMA-AT Baseline: 17 1st Session Post-drug: 9 Pre-drug: 2 Int. 1: 0 Int. 2: 9 Int. 3: 13 2nd Session Pre-drug: 7 Post-drug: 1 Int. 1: 3 Int.2: 5 Int.3: 11 3rd Session Pre-drug: 3 Post-drug: 0 Int. 1: 1 Int. 2: 6(1) Int. 3: 8	

Table 1. *Cont.*

Author	Country	Study Design	Participants	Population	Relevant Exclusion Criteria	Intervention	Psychotherapy Principle	Outcome Measure	Results	Conclusion
Mitchell et al. 2023 [22]	United States, Israel	RCT	$n = 104$, 71.2% female, mean age of 39.02 MDMA-AT group $n = 53$, 60.4% female, mean age of 38.2 Placebo $n = 51$, 82.4% female, mean age of 40	PTSD	Clinically significant suicide risk and comorbid personality disorders	Session 1: 80 mg dose + 40 mg half dose 2 h later Sessions 2 and 3: 120 mg dose + 60 mg half dose 2 h later All groups were given psychotherapy.	3 90 min preparation sessions 3 8 h dosing sessions, 9 90 min integration sessions Each dosing session was followed by 3 integration sessions.	Clinician-administered C-SSRS, ideation intensity and behavior subscales	Assessed as a safety measure. Numbers indicate participants with any positive ideation; C-SSRS ideation scale ≥ 0. Parenthesis indicate participants with serious ideation; C-SSRS ideation scale ≥ 4. Placebo Baseline: 12 1st Session Pre-drug: 4 Post-drug: 6 Int. 1: 2 Int. 2: 7 Int. 3: 10 2nd Session Pre-drug: 5 Post-drug: 5 Int. 1: 3 Int. 2: 4 Int. 3: 10 3rd Session Pre-drug: 4 Post-drug: 3(1) Int. 1: 2(1)	Suggests that MDMA-AT does not increase suicide risk in PTSD patients.

Table 1. *Cont.*

Author	Country	Study Design	Participants	Population	Relevant Exclusion Criteria	Intervention	Psychotherapy Principle	Outcome Measure	Results	Conclusion
									Int. 2: 3 Int. 3: 8 MDMA-AT Baseline: 13 1st Session Pre-drug: 3 Post-drug: 2 Int. 1: 2 Int. 2: 3 Int. 3: 4 2nd Session Pre-drug: 2 Post-drug: 3 Int. 1: 2 Int. 2: 4 Int. 3: 4 3rd Session Pre-drug: 4 Post-drug: 3 Int. 1: 2 Int. 2: 5 Int. 3: 11(1)	

Table 1. *Cont.*

Author	Country	Study Design	Participants	Population	Relevant Exclusion Criteria	Intervention	Psychotherapy Principle	Outcome Measure	Results	Conclusion
						DMT				
Davis et al., 2023 [41]	Mexico	Longitudinal, prospective	n = 86, 0% female, mean age of 42.88	Trauma-exposed military veterans	Current or past psychotic spectrum disorders or BD-I, or symptoms of impaired reality testing	10 mg/kg Ibogaine + 3 doses of 5-MeO-DMT (5 mg, 10 mg, 15 mg). Fourth (30 mg) and fifth doses (45 mg) if needed. Given with psychotherapy.	Day 1: Preparation session, ibogaine dosing Day 2: Ibogaine integration Day 3: Preparation, 5MeO-DMT dosing Following days: Integration in groups and individually	DSI-SS	Baseline (n = 86): 1.03 1 month (n = 71): 0.60 3 month (n = 62): 0.70 6 month (n = 52): 0.67 Change from baseline to 1 month: −0.53 (p = <0.01)	Ibogaine and 5-MeO-DMT assisted psychotherapy moderately reduced suicidal ideation in trauma exposed veterans.
Davis et al., 2020 [42]	Mexico	Longitudinal study, retrospective	51 participants, 4% female, mean age of 40.4	Military veterans with cognitive and physical trauma	Current or past psychotic spectrum disorders or bipolar I disorder, or symptoms of impaired reality testing	10 mg/kg Ibogaine + 3 doses of 5-MeO-DMT (5 mg, 10 mg, 15 mg). Fourth (30 mg) and fifth doses (45 mg) if needed. Given with psychotherapy.	Day 1: Preparation session, ibogaine dosing Day 2: Ibogaine integration Day 3: Preparation, 5MeO-DMT dosing Following days: Integration in groups and individually	DSI-SS	n = 41 completed the study; 10 refused to respond. 1 month pre-treatment: 2.7 1 month post-treatment: 0.4 Change: −2.3 (p = <0.001)	Ibogaine and 5-MeO-DMT decrease suicidal ideation in traumatized military veterans.

Table 1. *Cont.*

Author	Country	Study Design	Participants	Population	Relevant Exclusion Criteria	Intervention	Psychotherapy Principle	Outcome Measure	Results	Conclusion
Ragnhildstveit et al., 2023 [43]	United States	Longitudinal, prospective	$n = 1$, female, 23 years old	PTSD	NA	10–15 mg of 5-MeO-DMT via vaporized bufotoxin from *Incilius alvarius* with psychotherapy.	1 dosing session, followed by weekly follow-ups	BHS	Baseline: 17 24 h: 8 1 month: 4 3 month: 9 6 month: 3 12 month: 8	5-MeO-DMT decreases feelings of hopelessness and suicidality in the case of a 23-year-old woman with PTSD.
Zeifman et al., 2019 [44]	Brazil	Secondary analysis, RCT	Total $n = 29$, 72% female, mean age of 42.04 Drug group $n = 14$, 72% female, mean age of 39.71	Treatment resistant unipolar MDD	Imminent suicidal risk, personal or family history of schizophrenia, bipolar affective disorder, mania, or hypomania.	1 mL/kg dose of ayahuasca containing 0.36 mg/mL DMT, with no psychotherapy	1 8 h dosing session	MADRS-SI	Between-group effects 1 day: d = 0.58 (95% CI = −1.32 to 0.17) 2 days: d = 0.56 (95% CI = −1.30 to 0.18) 7 days: d = 0.67 (95% CI = −1.42 to 0.08) Ayahuasca within-group effects 1 day: d = 1.33 (95% CI = 1.25 to 3.18, $n = 14$) 2 days: d = 1.42 (95% CI = 1.50 to 3.74, $n = 13$) 7 days: d = 1.19 (95% CI = 1.21 to 3.50, $n = 14$)	Relative to placebo, ayahuasca did not significantly reduce suicidality in patients with unipolar MDD

Table 1. *Cont.*

Author	Country	Study Design	Participants	Population	Relevant Exclusion Criteria	Intervention	Psychotherapy Principle	Outcome Measure	Results	Conclusion
Zeifman et al., 2021 [45]	Brazil	Secondary analysis, open label	$n = 17$, 82% female, mean age of 42.71	MDD	Presence of active psychotic symptoms, a diagnosis of bipolar or psychotic disorder, or a history of antidepressant or substance-induced mania or hypomania	2.2 mL/kg dose of ayahuasca containing 0.8 mg/mL DMT, with no psychotherapy.	1 4 h dosing session	MADRS-SI	$n = 15$; 2 participants showed 0 suicidality at baseline and were excluded from analysis Baseline: 2.40 1 day: 0.53 7 days: 0.53 14 days: 0.53 21 days: 0.33	Ayahuasca is associated with reduced suicidality among MDD patients within a day of administration, and effects last for at least 21 days post dosing.
LSD										
Gasser et al., 2015 [46]	United States	RCT	$n = 10$, 60% female, mean age of 51.1	Anxiety associated with life-threatening disease	Not mentioned	2 doses of 200 μg LSD with psychotherapy	6–8 therapy sessions in 3 months of which 2 included LSD experience	Semi-structured interview at 12-month follow-up	33% of participants reported "... no more suicidal thoughts, less depressed feelings"	No evidence to suggest that LSD alters suicidal thinking

Abbreviations: AE: adverse event. RCT: randomized controlled trial. MDD: major depressive disorder. TRD: treatment-resistant depression. PTSD: post-traumatic stress disorder. BP-I: bipolar I disorder. BP-II: bipolar II disorder. BPD: borderline personality disorder. OLTAS: older long-term acquired immunodeficiency syndrome survivor. MADRS-SI: Montgomery–Åsberg Depression Rating Scale-Suicidality Item. C-SSRS: Columbia–Suicide Severity Rating Scale. C-SSRS-IIS: C-SSRS intensity of ideation subscale. DSI-SS: Depressive Symptom Index-Suicidality Subscale. Composite SI: Composite Suicidality Item. BHS: Beck Hopelessness Scale. BDI-II: Beck Depression Inventory II. BSI: Brief Symptom Inventory. QIDS-SI: Quick Inventory of Depressive Symptomatology-Suicidality item. HAM-D-SI: Hamilton Depression Rating Scale-Suicidality item. SIDAS: Suicidal Ideation Attributes Scale. MDMA-AT: 3,4-methylenedioxymethamphetamine-assisted therapy. Int.: integration.

Table 2. Characteristics of included population studies.

Author	Country	Study Design	Participants	Population	Intervention	Psychotherapy Principle	Outcome Measure	Results	Conclusion
Psilocybin									
Carbonaro et al., 2016 [47]	United States	Cross-sectional	$n = 1993$, 22% female, mean age of 30	Healthy, taken psilocybin before and experienced distress during their trip	NA	NA	Qualitative responses made by researchers	5 participants reported increased suicidality, whereas 6 reported decreased suicidality	Unmonitored psilocybin use can result in distressing experiences that increase suicidality. However, a similar amount of participants report decreased suicidality after drug use.
MDMA									
Celine et al., 2019 [48]	France	Cross-sectional	$n = 26,351$ participants, age 17	Healthy	NA	NA	ESCAPAD (no year provided)	Suicidal ideation in ecstacy/amphetamine users vs. non users OR: 2.42 aOR: 2.74 (no *p*-value reported)	Ecstacy/amphetamine use, relative to no use, was associated with increased suicide ideation even when adjusted for covariates.
Kim et al., 2011 [49]	United States	Cross-sectional	$n = 19,301$, aged 12–17	Healthy	NA	NA	NSDUH (2000)	OR of ecstasy use and suicidal behaviors (adjusted for family and individual factors): Suicidal ideation: 1.5 ($p \leq 0.05$) Suicide attempt: 5.5 ($p \leq 0.001$)	Ecstacy use among adolescents was associated with increased odds of suicidal ideation and even greater odds of suicidal attempt.

Table 2. *Cont.*

Author	Country	Study Design	Participants	Population	Intervention	Psychotherapy Principle	Outcome Measure	Results	Conclusion
					LSD				
Han et al., 2022 [50]	United States	Cross-sectional	n = 69,916, aged 12–17	Healthy	NA	NA	NSDUH (2015–2019)	OR of past year LSD use vs. never used LSD on suicidal ideation OR: 2.4 aOR: 1.2 OR of lifetime but no past year use vs. never used LSD on suicidal ideation OR: 2.0 aOR: 1.1 (no p-values reported)	LSD users had a slightly higher risk of suicidal ideation than non LSD users.
Yockey et al., 2019 [51]	United States	Cross-sectional	n = 13,840, 51.6% female, aged 12–17	Healthy	NA	NA	NSDUH (2017)	OR of Lifetime LSD use vs. no use on thoughts about suicide OR: 2.46 ($p < 0.001$) aOR: 1.381 ($p < 0.001$)	LSD use was associated with increased thoughts of suicide

Table 2. *Cont.*

Author	Country	Study Design	Participants	Population	Intervention	Psychotherapy Principle	Outcome Measure	Results	Conclusion
Not Specified/Multiple Psychedelic Studies									
Wong et al., 2013 [52]	United States	Cross-sectional	$n = 73{,}183$, 49.3% female, mean age of 16.0, school-going adolescents	Healthy	NA	NA	YRBSS (2001–2009)	OR of hallucinogen use vs. no use on: (* = $p < 0.0001$) Suicide ideation OR: 3.3 * aOR: 1.8 * Suicide plan: OR: 4.0 * aOR: 1.9 * Suicide attempt OR: 4.9 * aOR: 2.1 * Severe suicide attempt OR: 10.4 * aOR: 3.4 * OR of ecstasy use vs. no use compared to non users: (* = $p < 0.0001$) Suicide ideation OR: 3.1 * aOR: 1.6 * Suicide plan OR: 4.3 * aOR: 1.5 * Suicide attempt OR: 5.0 * aOR: 1.9 * Severe suicide attempt OR: 10.7 * aOR: 2.9 *	Hallucinogen and ecstacy use are associated with increased suicidal ideation and planning, suicide attempt, and severe suicide attempt. Notably, ecstasy has a weaker association with these parameters than hallucinogen use.

Table 2. *Cont.*

Author	Country	Study Design	Participants	Population	Intervention	Psychotherapy Principle	Outcome Measure	Results	Conclusion
Hendricks et al., 2015 [53]	United States	Cross-sectional	n = 27,235 psychedelic users, 37.2% female, aged 12–17	Healthy	NA	NA	NSDUH (2008–2012)	Classic psychedelics defined as DMT, mescaline, LSD, psilocybin, peyote, OR of lifetime classic psychedelic use vs. no use on: Past year suicidal thinking: 0.86 Past year suicidal planning: 0.71 Past year suicidal attempt: 0.64 (no p-values reported)	Lifetime classic psychedelic use is associated with reduced suicidal thinking, planning, and attempt
Argento, 2017 [54]	Canada	Longitudinal, prospective	290 participants, 100% women	Healthy, marginalized sex workers	NA	NA	AESHA (2010–2014)	OR of lifetime psychedelic use vs. no use on suicidality: OR: 1.00 (p = 0.995) aOR: 0.40 (p = 0.036)	Psychedelic use is independently associated with reduced suicidality in a population of sex workers.

Table 2. *Cont.*

Author	Country	Study Design	Participants	Population	Intervention	Psychotherapy Principle	Outcome Measure	Results	Conclusion
Argento, 2018 [55]	Canada	Longitudinal, prospective	340 participants, 100% women	Healthy, marginalized sex workers	NA	NA	AESHA (2010–2017)	Psychedelics defined: LSD, MDMA, psilocybin OR of psychedelic vs. no use on suicidal behavior: Prescription opioid users (psychedelic use vs. no use): 0.69 vs. 2.91 ($p = 0.016$) Cocaine users: 0.39 vs. 4.69 ($p = 0.001$) Crack users: 1.31 vs. 4.08 ($p = 0.326$) Crystal Meth users: 1.98 vs. 4.51 ($p = 0.206$) Heroin users: 0.88 vs. 2.15 ($p = 0.170$)	Psychedelic use moderated suicidality among prescription opioid, cocaine, crack, crystal meth, and heroin using sex workers.

Table 2. *Cont.*

Author	Country	Study Design	Participants	Population	Intervention	Psychotherapy Principle	Outcome Measure	Results	Conclusion
Sexton, 2019 [56]	United States	Cross-sectional	n = 273,720, 21% female, aged 12–17	Healthy	NA	NA	NSDUH (2008–2016)	Classic psychedelics defined as LSD, mescaline, DMT, psilocybin). Novel psychedelics defined as $5HT_{2AR}$ agonists with similar PK and PD to psychedelics. OR of lifetime novel psychedelic use vs. lifetime classic but not novel psychedelic use: Suicidal thinking: 1.4 (p = 0.0180) Suicidal planning: 1.6 (p = 0.0285) Past year suicide attempt: 1.2 (p = 0.6310) OR of lifetime novel psychedelic use vs. no novel or classic psychedelic use: Suicidal thinking: 1.3 (p = 0.0749) Suicidal planning: 1.4 (p = 0.1196) Past year suicide attempt: 0.9 (p = 0.8813)	Novel psychedelic use was associated with increased suicidal thinking and planning, relative to both classic and no psychedelic use.

Table 2. *Cont.*

Author	Country	Study Design	Participants	Population	Intervention	Psychotherapy Principle	Outcome Measure	Results	Conclusion
Sexton, 2020 [57]	United States	Cross-sectional	n = 356,046, 51.5% female, aged 12–17	Healthy	NA	NA	NSDUH (2008–2017)	Lifetime classic tryptamine use vs. no use on past-year suicidal thinking: aOR = 0.79 Lifetime novel phenethylamine use vs. no use on past year suicidal thinking: aOR = 1.60 (No p-values reported)	While lifetime tryptamine use may decrease suicidal thinking, novel phenethylamine use is associated with increased suicidal thinking.
Zeifman, 2020 [58]	United States	Secondary analysis, two longitudinal studies	n = 104, 29.8% female, mean age of 29.28	Non-clinical, but not healthy	NA	Participants planned to use a psychedelic and responded to surveys before/after use.	Composite SI (QIDS-SI + SIDAS)	Psychedelics defined: psilocybin, LSD, ayahuasca, 5-MeO-DMT, Salvia divinorum, mescaline, ibogaine Composite score ranging from 1 to −1. Baseline: 0.48 2 weeks: −0.19 ($p < 0.001$; baseline to 2 weeks) 4 weeks: −0.47 ($p < 0.003$; 2 weeks to 4 weeks)	Intentional psychedelic use is associated with reductions in suicidality.

Table 2. *Cont.*

Author	Country	Study Design	Participants	Population	Intervention	Psychotherapy Principle	Outcome Measure	Results	Conclusion
Zeifman, 2020 [58]	United States	Secondary analysis, two longitudinal studies $n = 254$, 45.3% female, mean age of 43.61	Non-clinical	NA	Participants planning to use psychedelics in the presence of a facilitator.	Composite SI (QIDS-SI + SIDAS)	Psychedelics defined: psilocybin, LSD, ayahuasca, 5-MeO-DMT, Salvia divinorum, mescaline, ibogaine, Composite score ranging from 1 to −1. Baseline: 0.16 4 weeks: −0.28 ($p < 0.001$ from baseline to 4 weeks)	Intentional psychedelic use in the presence of a facilitator is associated with reductions in suicidality.	
Desai, 2022 [59]	United States	Cross-sectional	$n = 10{,}504$, 37.6% female, school-going adolescents	Healthy	NA	NA	YRBSS (2001–2019)	Psychedelics defined: LSD, PCP, mescaline, mushrooms OR for hallucinogen users vs. non users: Considered suicide 1.31 ($p = 0.03$) Made a suicide plan 1.44 ($p = 0.03$) Attempted suicide: 1.15 ($p = 0.395$) Injurious suicide attempt: 1.39 ($p = 0.118$)	Hallucinogen use is associated with increased suicidal ideation and attempt in school-going adolescents.

Table 2. *Cont.*

Author	Country	Study Design	Participants	Population	Intervention	Psychotherapy Principle	Outcome Measure	Results	Conclusion
Jones, 2022 [60]	United States	Cross-sectional	$n = 5983$ psychedelic users, 41% female, mean of 16.08, aged 12–17	Healthy	NA	NA	NSDUH (2004–2019)	Psychedelics defined: LSD, psilocybin, peyote, mescaline aOR of Psychedelic use vs. no use on: (* = $p \leq 0.05$) Lifetime suicidal thinking: MDMA: 0.96 Psilocybin: 0.84 * LSD: 1.19 * Peyote: 0.99 Mescaline: 0.80 Lifetime suicidal planning: MDMA: 1.12 Psilocybin: 0.78 * LSD: 1.36 * Peyote: 1.29 Mescaline: 0.72 Lifetime suicidal attempt: MDMA: 1.15 Psilocybin: 0.77 * LSD: 1.23 * Peyote: 1.24 Mescaline: 0.71	While psilocybin use was associated with reduced suicidal thoughts and behaviors, LSD use is associated with increased suicidal thoughts and behaviors. MDMA was not associated with suicidal thoughts and behaviors, and results for peyote and mescaline are nonsignificant as well.

Table 2. *Cont.*

Author	Country	Study Design	Participants	Population	Intervention	Psychotherapy Principle	Outcome Measure	Results	Conclusion
Jones, 2022 [25]	United States	Cross-sectional	Total $n = 484,732$, aged 12–17 MDMA users $n = 34,416$, 42.2% female Psilocybin users $n = 45,565$, 33.5% female	Healthy	NA	NA	NSDUH (2008–2019)	OR of MDMA vs. no use on: Suicidal thinking: 0.9 ($p = 0.01$) Suicidal planning: 0.88 ($p = 0.05$) Suicide attempt: 1.00 (no *p*-value reported) OR of psilocybin vs. no use on: Suicidal thinking: 0.9 ($p = 0.01$) Suicidal planning: 0.88 ($p = 0.08$) Suicide attempt: 0.85 ($p = 0.07$) OR of LSD use vs. no use on suicidal thinking: 1.07 ($p = 0.05$)	MDMA and psilocybin are associated with decreased suicidal thinking and planning. Psilocybin is also associated with reduced suicide attempts. Unlike MDMA and psilocybin, LSD is associated with increased suicidal thinking.

Table 2. *Cont.*

Author	Country	Study Design	Participants	Population	Intervention	Psychotherapy Principle	Outcome Measure	Results	Conclusion
Yang, 2022 [61]	United States	Cross-sectional	n = 241,675, aged 12–17	Healthy	NA	NA	NSDUH (2015–2020)	Tryptamines defined as DMT, AMT, Foxy aOR of LSD use vs. no use on Suicidal thinking: 1.21 ($p < 0.001$) Suicidal planning: 1.14 (p = ns) Suicidal attempt: 1.27 (p = ns) aOR of tryptamine (DMT/AMT/Foxy) use vs. no use on Suicidal thinking: 1.14 (p = ns) Suicidal planning: 1.81 ($p < 0.01$) Suicidal attempt: 1.16 (p = ns) aOR of Salvia divinorum vs. no use on Suicidal thinking: 1.41 ($p < 0.05$) Suicidal planning: 1.74 (p = ns) Suicidal attempt: 2.05 (p = ns) aOR of ecstasy use vs. no use on Suicidal thinking: 0.86 ($p < 0.05$) Suicidal planning: 0.80 (p = ns) Suicidal attempt: 0.83 (p = ns)	LSD use is associated with increased suicidal thinking, planning, and attempt. Salvia divinorum has an even greater association with such parameters than LSD, while ecstasy has a weaker association. Tryptamine effects on suicidal planning, thinking, and attempt are comparable to LSD, except that suicidal planning has a stronger association with tryptamine use.

Table 2. *Cont.*

Author	Country	Study Design	Participants	Population	Intervention	Psychotherapy Principle	Outcome Measure	Results	Conclusion
Giugovaz, 2024 [62]	United States	Cross-sectional	n = from 25,800 to 42,800 per year, on average 53.6% female, aged 12–17	Healthy	NA	NA	NSDUH (2008–2020)	Psychedelics defined: LSD, MDMA, psilocybin OR for hallucinogen psilocybin users vs. non users: Suicidal ideation: 0.46 Suicidal planning: 0.56 Suicidal attempt: 1.01	LSD, MDMA, and psilocybin use is associated with reduced suicidal ideation and planning among adolescents.
Soboka, 2024 [63]	Canada	Cross-sectional	n = 22,500, 39% female, mean age of 37.09	Healthy	NA	NA	MHA intake (2020–2021)	aOR of psychedelic use vs. no use on Mild suicide risk: 2.04 ($p < 0.001$) Moderate/high suicide risk: 3.54 ($p < 0.001$)	Psychedelic use was moderately associated with mild suicide risk, and has an even stronger association with moderate/high suicide risk.

Relevant Items on Outcome Measures

NSDUH: The NSDUH annually collects data via online and in-person interviews and includes questions on the following suicidal outcomes: ideation (i.e., at any time in the past 12 months, did you seriously think about trying to kill yourself?), planning (during the past 12 months, did you make any plans to kill yourself?), and attempt (i.e., in the past 12 months, did you try to kill yourself?). Answers to these questions are "yes", "no", "I don't know", and "I don't want to answer".

YRBSS: Four dichotomized questions on the survey asked about the following suicide-related outcomes: considered suicide (during the past 12 months, did you ever seriously consider attempting suicide?), made a suicide plan (during the past 12 months, did you make a plan about how you would attempt suicide?), attempted suicide (during the past 12 months, how many times did you actually attempt suicide?), had an injurious suicide attempt (if you attempted suicide during the past 12 months, did any attempt result in an injury, poisoning, or overdose that had to be treated by a doctor or nurse?).

MHA Intake: The following dichotomous suicide-related questions were asked: "Have you had thoughts about suicide or wanting to be dead in the past two weeks?" "Have you tried to kill yourself or attempt suicide in the past?" "Do you have thoughts of suicide now?" If participants had answered yes to any one of these questions, they were further interviewed and classified into a risk group by a clinician using their judgement and Nova Scotia's suicide risk assessment and intervention tool (SRAI).

Abbreviations: AE: adverse event. OR: odds ratio. aOR: odds ratio adjusted for covariates. PD: pharmacodynamics. PK: pharmacokinetics. Composite SI: Composite Suicidality Item. QIDS-SI: Quick Inventory of Depressive Symptomatology-Suicidality item. SIDAS: Suicidal Ideation Attributes Scale. NSDUH: National Survey on Drug Use and Health. YRBSS: Youth Risk Behavior Surveillance System. ESCAPAD: The Survey on Health and Drug Use on National Defence and Citizenship Day. MHA Intake: Mental Health and Addictions intake program of Nova Scotia. AESHA: An Evaluation of Sex Workers Health Access.

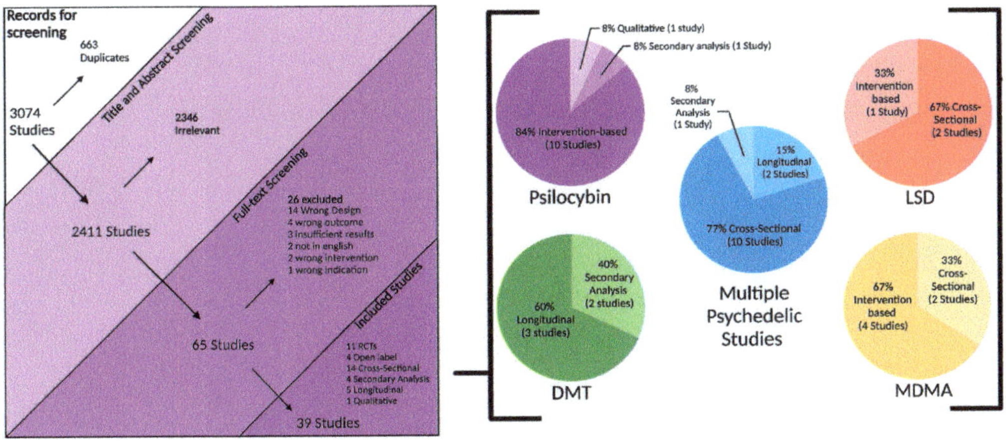

Figure 1. Study flow diagram.

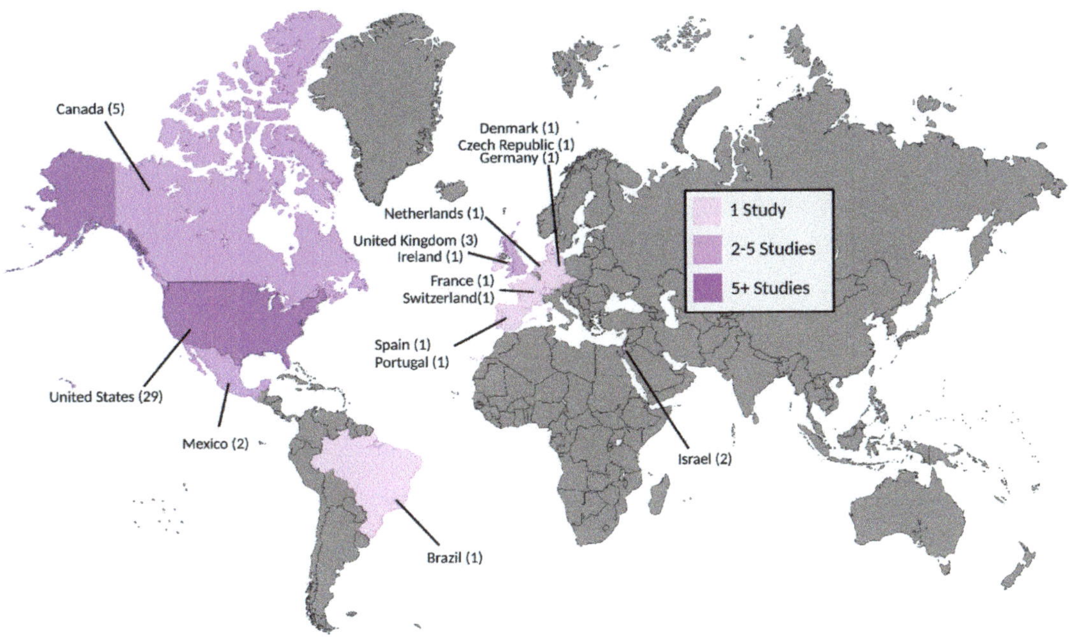

Figure 2. Countries of included studies. Number of studies for a given country are included in parentheses.

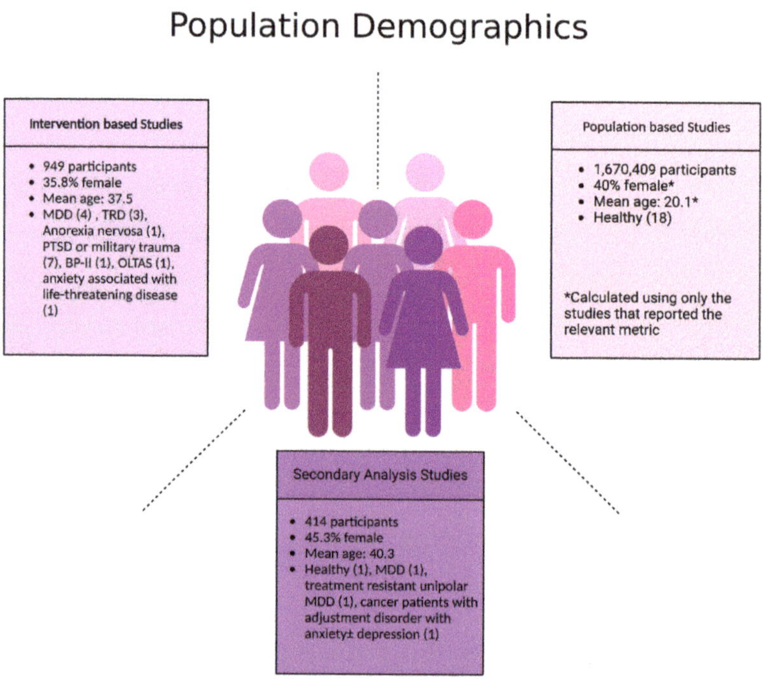

Figure 3. Population demographics of participants in included studies. Abbreviations: MDD: major depressive disorder; TRD: treatment-resistant depression; PTSD: post-traumatic stress disorder; BP-II: Bipolar II disorder; OLTAS: older long-term acquired immunodeficiency syndrome survivors.

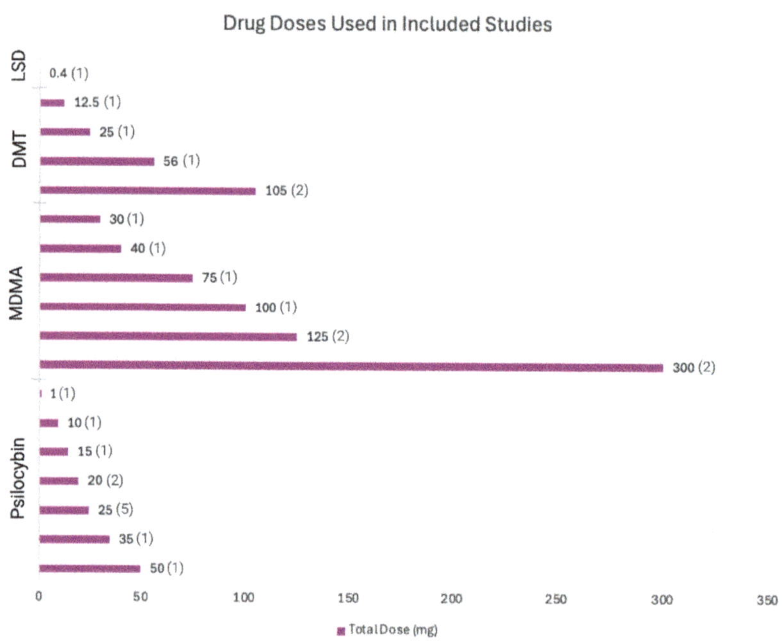

Figure 4. Drug doses used in included studies.

3.2. Registered Clinical Trial

We found one trial that had the identifier NCT05220410, which is currently recruiting participants. The estimated completion date for the study is April 2024, and it is being conducted in the United States. This is an interventional phase 2 trial with a single-group assignment and no masking. The projected sample size is 20 participants. The intervention involves administering 25 mg of psilocybin, and the primary outcome measure is the Columbia–Suicide Severity Rating Scale (C-SSRS). The trial focuses on individuals with TRD with chronic suicidal ideation.

3.3. Psilocybin

Six RCTs, four open-label trials, one qualitative cross-sectional study, and one secondary analysis investigated the effects of psilocybin on suicidal ideation and attempt.

3.3.1. RCTs with Suicide as Safety or Secondary Outcome

MDD

Carhartt-Harris et al. (2021) examined the effects of psilocybin on suicidal thoughts through the Suicidal Ideation Attributes Scale (SIDAS; out of 50, 5 items out of 10) in MDD patients [28]. Their psilocybin group received two doses of 25 mg psilocybin 3 weeks apart (and daily placebo capsules), whereas their comparator group received two doses of 1 mg psilocybin with 6 weeks of oral escitalopram. All participants also received psychological support. The investigators reported a −2.0 change in the psilocybin group (95% CI = −4.3 to 0.0), a −0.8 change in the placebo group (95% CI = −3.4 to 2.0), and a between-group difference of −1.3 (95% CI = −6.5 to −0.3) from baseline to 6 weeks post dosing, but these were not corrected for multiple comparisons [28]. Davis et al. (2021) administered two doses of psilocybin (20 mg/kg, followed by 30 mg/kg) with psychotherapy to patients with MDD [29]. Patients either received treatment directly after baseline screening (immediate group) or after 8 weeks (delayed group). As a secondary outcome, Davis et al. assessed patients at baseline and clinical endpoints (i.e., time of follow-up) with the clinician-administered C-SSRS intensity of ideation subscale (C-SSRS-ISS; 0 out of 5), and found non-significant reductions in suicidal ideation from baseline (immediate: 1.2, delayed: 1.3; p = ns) to 5 (immediate: 0.2, delayed: 0.6; p = ns) and 8 (immediate: 0.2, delayed: 0.4; p = ns) weeks out [29]. They state that in general, suicidal ideation was low at baseline and trended lower after treatment [29]. Importantly, as participants with medically significant attempts for suicide were excluded from this study, observed C-SSRS-IIS scores may be lower among this population than otherwise. Raison et al. (2023) also investigated MDD patients and conducted an RCT using a single 25 mg dose of psilocybin with psychotherapy [32]. In their safety assessment, they report that no patients showed signs of suicidal behavior at any timepoint during the trial, as measured through the clinician-administered C-SSRS-IIS or the Montgomery–Åsberg Depression Rating Scale-Suicidality Item (MADRS-SI; out of 6) [32]. However, one participant receiving psilocybin and five receiving placebo niacin had an increase in C-SSRS suicidal ideation score from baseline to the end of the trial [32]. von Rotz et al. (2022) gave MDD patients a single 0.215 mg/kg dose of psilocybin with therapy. Although they reported a mean within-group change of −0.35 in patient suicidal ideation as measured via the clinician-administered C-SSRS-ISS (95% CI = −0.10 to 0.71; d = 0.43; p = 0.13), they also report nonsignificant differences between experimental and placebo groups ($F_{(1,50)} = 1.40$; p = 0.24) [31].

TRD

Goodwin et al. (2022) conducted an RCT to observe the effects of a single, randomized dose of psilocybin at 1 mg ($n = 79$), 10 mg ($n = 75$), or 25 mg ($n = 79$) with psychological support in TRD patients. They used the clinician-administered C-SSRS and considered suicidal ideation with intent or endorsement of the suicidal behavior section of the scale as a serious adverse event (AE) [19]. Throughout all 12 weeks, participants exhibiting suicidal ideation or behavior were higher in the 25 mg and 10 mg groups, relative to the 1 mg group [19]. Twenty-one (27%) patients in the 25 mg group, twenty-seven (36%) in the 10 mg group, and nineteen (24%) in the 1 mg group showed suicidal ideation (passive or active with no intent to plan) at baseline [19]. From baseline to week 3, 11 (13.9%) in the 25 mg group, 13 (17.3%) in the 10 mg group, and 7 (8.9%) in the 1 mg group exhibited increased suicidal risk [19]. Of these patients, some reported serious, suicide-related AEs: two (4.5%) in the 25 mg group (suicidal ideation with intent), two in the 10 mg (7%) group (suicidal ideation with intent), and no patients in the 1 mg group [19]. From week 3 to week 12, 12 (15.2%) in the 25 mg, 12 (16.0%) in the 10 mg, and 12 (15.2%) in the 1 mg dose groups exhibited worsened suicidality. Here, serious suicide-related AEs were reported by three patients in the 25 mg group (three endorsement of suicidal behavior section of C-SSRS) and one in the 10 mg group (one suicidal ideation with intent). As participants at clinically significant risk for suicide were excluded from this study, the adverse events reported here are not part of longstanding behavioral trends [19].

Anorexia Nervosa

Peck et al. (2022) examined the safety of a single 25 mg dose with psychotherapy in 10 women with anorexia nervosa and reported no increases in suicidal risk as per the C-SSRS [30].

3.3.2. Open-Label Trials with Suicide as a Safety or Secondary Outcome

TRD

Carhart-Harris et al. (2018) conducted their own open-label trial with TRD patients, giving them two oral doses of psilocybin at 10 mg and 25 mg. Using the Quick Inventory of Depressive Symptomatology-Suicidality item (QIDS-SI; out of three) and the Hamilton Depression Rating Scale-Suicidality item (HAM-D-SI; out of four), they report significant reductions in QIDS-SI scores for suicide risk from baseline to 1 week (−0.9, 95% CI = −0.4 to −1.4; $p < 0.002$) and 2 weeks (−0.85, 95% CI = −0.4 to −1.3; $p = 0.004$) post dosing [34]. Scores at 3 weeks (−0.8, 95% CI = −0.25 to −1.3, $p = 0.01$) and 5 weeks (−0.7, 95% CI = −0.22 to −1.2, $p = 0.01$) show trend reductions but were non-significant [34]. Ellis et al. (2024) also conducted an open-label trial using a 25 mg dose with psychotherapy among 15 military veterans with TRD, most (73%, $n = 11$) of whom had PTSD [37]. Using the clinician-administered C-SSRS as part of their safety assessment, they reported no increases in suicidal ideation from baseline and that no suicidal behavior was present throughout the follow-up period [37].

BD-II

Aaronson et al. (2024) conducted an open-label trial for the use of 25 mg of psilocybin with psychotherapy for major depressive episodes in patients with bipolar type-II disorder (BD-II) [36]. Study clinicians assessed suicidal risk using the C-SSRS-IIS as part of their safety measures and found that the main effect on timepoint was non-significant. They also reported that no patients attempted or completed suicide at any timepoints during the study [36].

OLTAS

Anderson et al. (2020) worked with older long-term acquired immunodeficiency syndrome survivors (OLTAS) with moderate to severe demoralization, as quantified by a score of ≥9 on the Demoralization Scale-II [35]. Patients were given 0.3–0.36 mg/kg doses of psilocybin with group psychotherapy. While the investigators reported no changes in C-SSRS-IIS scores over time nor any suicidal behavior during the intervention period, one patient (out of eighteen) attempted suicide at their 3-month follow-up [35].

3.3.3. Secondary Analyses in Cancer Patients with Adjustment Disorder

Ross et al. (2021) conducted a secondary analysis assessing patient suicidal ideation in their 2016 trial where they administered a single 0.3 mg/kg dose of psilocybin with psychotherapy in cancer patients who were diagnosed with adjustment disorder with anxiety ± depression, acute stress disorder, generalized anxiety disorder (GAD), or anxiety disorder due to cancer [33]. Patients received psilocybin and placebo niacin (250 mg) in a crossover design. They used their own composite SI (suicidal ideation) measure, comprised of item nine of the Beck Depression Inventory-II (BDI-II) and item nine of the Brief Symptom Inventory (BSI) [33]. Ross et al. reported a significant within-group reduction of SI at 6.5 months from baseline ($p < 0.001$) but did not observe significant between-group effects [33].

3.3.4. Qualitative Studies in Previous Healthy Psilocybin Users

Carbonaro et al. (2016) conducted a cross-sectional study asking previous healthy psilocybin users to rate their most distressing experience while on the drug [47]. Participants responded qualitatively to questions made by the investigators, some of which asked about suicidality. Out of 1993 respondents, six reported complete remission of suicidal thoughts after taking psilocybin (timeline not specified), whereas five reported increased suicidal thinking and behaviors during their experience [47]. Increased suicidality outcomes were reported as attempt to overdose and waking up in an intensive care unit (one participant), attempting to shoot themselves in the head (one participant), pre-existing depression exacerbated by psilocybin and leading to suicide attempt (one participant), and increased salience of suicidal thoughts during the experience (three participants) [47]. The context of psilocybin use (i.e., alone, one other person, small group, large group) was not reported in relation to suicidality outcomes.

3.4. *MDMA-Assisted Therapy*

Four RCTs and two cross-sectional studies examined the effects of MDMA-assisted therapy (MDMA-AT) on suicide risk as well as different suicide-related outcomes (i.e., ideation intensity, behavior).

3.4.1. RCTs Assessing Suicidality as a Safety Measure in PTSD Patients

Mithoefer et al. (2018) conducted a double-blinded RCT in PTSD patients who received MDMA at a dose of 30 mg, 75 mg, or 125 mg with psychotherapy, followed by a supplemental half dose [38]. After the final RCT endpoint, the 30 mg and 75 mg groups were invited to participate in a 125 mg open-label crossover for three more sessions. The investigators stated in their safety assessment that by all post-treatment endpoints, the percentage of participants reporting suicidal ideation and behavior was reduced compared with baseline lifetime and pretreatment reports, as measured by the clinician-administered C-SSRS [38]. They also reported that there were no treatment-emergent reports of suicidal ideation [38]. Olatora et al. (2018) also ran their own double-blinded RCT with an open-label phase, where they administered to PTSD patients 40 mg, 100 mg, or 125 mg of MDMA with psychotherapy and with a supplemental half dose [39]. After the RCT endpoint, patients received either one (100 mg and 125 mg groups) or three (40 mg group) doses of 100–125 mg MDMA in an open-label crossover. While the investigators reported higher clinician-administered C-SSRS scores in the 100 mg and 125 mg groups, they did not exclude for past suicidal thinking during patient recruitment [39]. Therefore, unlike most similar studies, 28.6% of treatment-receiving participants were already impacted by symptoms of suicidal behavior before participating, and it is unclear to what extent MDMA or their medical history attributed to trends in C-SSRS scores [39]. Mitchell et al.'s (2021) RCT administered two doses of MDMA to PTSD patients through two sessions (first session: 80 + 40 mg half dose; second session: 120 + 60 mg half dose) with psychotherapy [40]. MDMA, when compared to a placebo, did not increase suicidal risk in patients with PTSD at all follow-up timepoints, as measured by a study clinician using the C-SSRS intensity of ideation subscale in their safety assessment [40]. Mitchell et al. ran another RCT in 2023 administering MDMA to PTSD patients using the same dosing regimen and found that from baseline to end of intervention, MDMA-AT did not increase suicidal risk relative to placebo in patients as scored by the clinician-administered C-SSRS [22].

3.4.2. Cross-Sectional Studies: Survey Data in Non-Clinical Populations

Celine et al. (2019) looked at France's national survey on health and drug use, ESCAPAD, and found that among French adolescents, ecstasy use is associated with increased suicide risk relative to non-users ([odds ratio] OR = 2.42, [adjusted OR] aOR = 2.74; [no p-values reported]) [48]. Here, adjusting the OR is accounting for covariates that influence the outcome variable, i.e., suicide risk, and is therefore controlling for confounding effects. Kim et al. (2011) conducted their own cross-sectional study using multinomial logistic regression analysis on data from the United States National Survey on Drug Use and Health (NSDUH), where, while not adjusted for confounders, they found that ecstasy use among American adolescents was associated with higher suicidal ideation and attempt compared to non-use (ideation OR: 1.5 [$p \leq 0.05$], attempt OR: 5.5 [$p < 0.001$]) [49].

3.5. *DMT and Ibogaine*

In total, two prospective longitudinal (one cohort and one single-case), one retrospective longitudinal, and two secondary analyses (one of a RCT and one of an open-label trial) provided reports on the effect of DMT and ibogaine on suicidal behavior.

3.5.1. Observational Studies in Persons with Military Trauma or PTSD

Davis et al. (2023) collected prospective data from a clinical treatment program about an open-label trial treating trauma-exposed military veterans. Patients were treated with 10 mg/kg ibogaine, followed by three doses of 5-Meo-DMT, at 5 mg, 10 mg, and 15 mg, accompanied by psychotherapy [41]. Fourth (30 mg) and fifth doses (45 mg) were administered if the patient did not reach an altered state of consciousness. The investigators reported a −0.53 ($p < 0.01$) decrease in the DSI-SS (Depressive Symptom Inventory-Suicide Subscale; out of 0 to 12) between baseline and one month post treatment [41]. Davis et al. (2020) also conducted a longitudinal, retrospective study using the same treatment regimen and found a −2.3 ($p < 0.0001$) decrease in DSI-SS scores from one month pretreatment to one month post treatment in military veterans with cognitive and physical trauma [42]. Ragnhildstveit et al. (2023) followed a 23-year-old woman with PTSD, administering to her a bufotoxin extract containing 10–15 mg of DMT. Immediately, within 24 h and for 12 months following treatment, the patient's Beck Hopelessness Scale (BHS; out of 20) scores dropped below the cut-off for suicidal ideation and behavior (> 9) [43]. The investigators considered this drop a significant and large reduction in the patient's suicide risk.

3.5.2. Secondary Analyses in MDD Patients

Zeifman et al. (2019) conducted a secondary analysis of an RCT for treatment-resistant patients with unipolar MDD [44]. They assessed baseline patient characteristics using the MADRS-SI for a population that either received a placebo or a single 1 mL/kg dosing of ayahuasca (containing 0.36 mg/mL of DMT) with no psychotherapy. They report moderate between-group effects for decreases in MADRS-SI scores at one day (d = 0.58, 95% CI = −1.32 to 0.17), two days (d = 0.56, 95% CI = −1.30 to 0.18), and seven days (d = 0.67, 95% CI = −1.42 to 0.08) after intervention [44]. Within the ayahuasca group, there were large effect sizes for decreases in MADRS-SI at one day (d = 1.33; 95% CI 1.25 to 3.18; $n = 14$), two days (d = 1.42; 95% CI 1.50 to 3.74; $n = 13$), and seven days (d = 1.19; 95% CI 1.21 to 3.50; $n = 14$) [44]. Zeifman et al. (2021) conducted another secondary analysis on an open-label trial for MDD patients receiving 2.2 mL/kg dose of ayahuasca (itself containing 0.8 mg/mL of DMT) with no psychotherapy and found rapid reductions in suicidality, as measured through MADRS-SI scores, that remained 21 days after intervention [45].

3.6. *LSD*

One RCT and two cross-sectional studies examined LSD effects in patient and non-clinical populations, respectively.

3.6.1. RCT for Patients with Anxiety Associated with Life-Threatening Disease

Gasser et al. (2015) ran an RCT for patients with anxiety associated with life-threatening disease, giving them two doses of 200 μg LSD with psychotherapy in 4-to-6-week intervals. At their 12-month follow up, 33% of patients reported "no more suicidal thoughts" and "less depressed feelings" [46].

3.6.2. Cross-Sectional Studies: Retrospective Survey Data in Non-Clinical Populations

Han et al. (2022) conducted multivariable analyses using NSDUH data from 2015 to 2019 and found that past-year LSD use, relative to non-use, was associated with mildly elevated suicidal ideation among adolescents (OR = 2.4 [no p-values reported]). They controlled for confounding variables and reported an adjusted OR of 1.2 (no p-value reported) [50]. Yockey et al. (2019) examined the 2017 NSDUH results and also used multi-variable analyses to conclude that lifetime LSD use among adolescents was significantly associated with more frequent thoughts about suicide (OR = 2.46 [$p < 0.001$], aOR = 1.381 [$p < 0.001$]) [51].

3.7. *Not Specified/Multiple Psychedelic Studies*

From our search, ten cross-sectional, two longitudinal, and one secondary analysis (of two longitudinal studies) examined the effects of psychedelics but either used multiple psychedelics or did not specify which psychedelics they assessed.

3.7.1. Longitudinal Studies

Argento et al. conducted two overlapping longitudinal studies using a cohort of women belonging to Vancouver, Canada's An Evaluation for Sex Workers Health Access (AESHA) cohort [54,55]. At baseline, they excluded any participants who reported previous suicidal thoughts or attempts in this analysis. They then followed participants annually for several years and later tested for associations between changes in suicidality and psychedelic use (e.g., LSD, MDMA, and psilocybin) [54,55]. Argento et al. (2017) used AESHA data from January 2010 to August 2014 and found that lifetime psychedelic use was independently associated with reduced suicidality in a population of sex workers after adjusting for covariates (OR = 1.00 [$p = 0.995$], aOR = 0.40 [$p = 0.036$]) [54]. In their follow-up study, Argento et al. (2018), using data from January 2010 to February 2017, looked at associations between psychedelic use and suicidal behaviors in users of different drugs [55]. They observed that psychedelic use moderated suicidal ideation in prescription opioid users ([OR = psychedelic use vs. no psychedelic use]; OR = 0.69 vs. 2.91 [$p = 0.016$]; aOR = 0.36 vs. 2.59 [$p = 0.036$]) and cocaine users (OR = 0.39 vs. 4.69 [$p = 0.001$] [55]. While not significant, they also tested for the effect of psychedelic use in crack users (OR = 1.31 vs. 4.08 [$p = 0.326$]), crystal meth users (OR = 1.98 vs. 4.51 [$p = 0.206$]), and heroin users (OR = 0.99 vs. 2.15 [$p = 0.170$]) [55].

3.7.2. Cross-Sectional Studies: Retrospective Survey Data in Non-Clinical Populations

Guigovaz et al. (2024) used regression analyses on NSDUH data from 2008 to 2020 and found that hallucinogen use, (e.g., MDMA, LSD, psilocybin) among adolescents is not significantly associated with increased suicidal ideation, planning, or attempt (OR = 0.46, 0.56, and 1.14 respectively; [no p-values reported]) [62]. Sexton et al. also conducted analyses using the NSDUH [56,57]. In 2019, Sexton et al. looked at the NSDUH from 2008 to 2016 and found that lifetime novel psychedelic use (e.g., 2-[4-Bromo-2,5-dimethoxyphenyl]-ethanamine; 2C-B, 2,5-dimethoxy-4-iodophenethylamine; 2CI) compared to lifetime classic psychedelic use (e.g., LSD, mescaline, DMT, psilocybin) was associated with increased odds of suicide ideation (OR = 1.4 [$p = 0.0180$]), planning (OR = 1.6 [$p = 0.0285$]), and attempt (OR = 1.2 [$p = 0.6310$]) [56]. They also found that lifetime novel psychedelic use, compared to no lifetime psychedelic use, was associated with increased odds of suicide ideation (OR = 1.3 [$p = 0.0749$]) and planning (OR = 1.4 [$p = 0.1196$]) but not attempt (OR = 0.9 [$p = 0.8813$]) [56]. Novel psychedelics were defined as serotonin 2A receptor (5HT2AR) agonists with similar pharmacokinetics and pharmacodynamics to classic psychedelics [56]. In 2020, Sexton et al. analyzed the NSDUH from 2008 to 2017 [57]. They focused on associations between suicide and either lifetime classic tryptamine or novel phenylethylamine use. When adjusting for covariates, while they found that increased past-year suicidal thinking was not associated with lifetime classic tryptamine use (aOR = 0.79 [no p-value reported]), they did observe an association with novel phenylethylamine use (aOR = 1.60 [no p-value reported]) [57]. Hendricks et al. (2015) also looked at the NSDUH and found that in 2008–2012, lifetime classic psychedelic use, relative to no use, was associated with reduced past-year suicidal thinking (OR = 0.86 [no p-value reported]), planning (OR = 0.71 [no p-value reported]), and attempt (OR = 0.64 [no p-value reported]) [53]. Here, odds ratios are not adjusted for confounders. Jones et al. (2022) looked at the NSDUH from 2008 to 2019 and reported that neither MDMA or psilocybin are associated with increased suicidal planning (OR = 0.9 [$p = 0.01$]), thinking (MDMA: OR = 0.88 [$p = 0.05$]; psilocybin: OR = 0.88 [$p = 0.08$]), or attempt (MDMA: OR = 1.00 [p = non-significant; ns]; psilocybin: OR = 0.85 [$p = 0.07$]) [25]. However, unlike MDMA and psilocybin, LSD was associated with increased odds of suicidal thinking (OR = 1.07 [$p = 0.05$]) [25]. Again, odds ratios were not adjusted for confounders. Another article published by Jones et al. in 2022 looked at NSDUH data from 2004 to 2019 [60]. They report that while psilocybin use is associated with reduced suicidal thoughts (aOR = 0.84 [$p \leq 0.05$]) and behaviors (suicidal planning: aOR = 0.78 [$p \leq 0.05$]; suicidal attempt: aOR = 0.77 [$p \leq 0.05$]), LSD use is associated with increased suicidal thinking (aOR = 1.19 [$p \leq 0.05$]) and behaviors (suicidal planning: aOR = 1.36 [$p \leq 0.05$]; suicidal attempt: aOR = 1.23 [$p \leq 0.05$]) [60]. MDMA, peyote, and mescaline were examined as well but were nonsignificant and not distinctly associated with suicidal ideation or behavior [60]. Yang et al. (2022) looked at associations of LSD, tryptamine (DMT/AMT [a-methyltryptamine]/Foxy [5-methoxy-diisopropyltryptamine]), Salvia divinorum, and MDMA use with suicidal thinking, planning, and attempt from NSDUH data (2015 to 2020) [61]. Compared to non-users, LSD was associated with greater suicidal ideation (OR = 1.21 [$p < 0.001$]), planning (OR = 1.14 [p = ns]), and attempt (OR = 1.27 [p = ns]) [61]. Where Salvia divinorum use was associated with even greater ideation (OR = 1.41 [$p < 0.05$]), planning (OR = 1.74 [p = ns]), and attempt (OR = 2.05 [p = ns]) than LSD, ecstasy was associated with lesser ideation (OR = 0.86 [$p < 0.05$]), planning (OR = 0.80 [p = ns]), and attempt (OR = 0.83 [p = ns]) [61]. Tryptamine effects on suicidal ideation (OR = 1.14 [p = ns]) and attempt (OR = 1.16 [p = ns]) were comparable to LSD, but tryptamines were associated with increased suicidal planning (OR = 1.81 [$p < 0.01$]) [61]. Desai et al. (2022) used data from the Youth Risk Behavior Surveillance System (YRBSS) by the United States Centers for Disease Control and Prevention, which targets school-going adolescents [59]. The investigators found that relative to non-users, hallucinogen-(e.g., LSD, PCP [phencyclidine], mescaline, or mushrooms)-using high schoolers more often considered suicide (OR = 1.31 [$p = 0.03$]), made a suicide plan (OR = 1.44 [$p = 0.03$]), attempted suicide (OR = 1.15 [$p = 0.395$]), or had an injurious suicide attempt (OR = 1.39 [$p = 0.118$]) [59]. Importantly, these associations were not adjusted for confounders. Wong et al. used the YRBSS from 2001 to 2009 to examine if hallucinogen and ecstasy use were associated with suicidal behaviors [52]. They found that hallucinogen-using high schoolers, compared to non-users, exhibited higher suicide ideation (OR = 3.3, aOR = 1.8; [both $p \leq 0.0001$]), planning (OR = 4.0, aOR = 1.0; [both $p \leq 0.0001$]), suicide attempt (OR = 4.9, aOR = 2.1; [both $p \leq 0.0001$]), or severe suicide attempt (OR = 10.4, aOR = 3.4; [both $p \leq 0.0001$]) [52]. Interestingly, ecstasy use was also positively associated with such parameters, but to a reduced extent (ideation: OR = 3.1, aOR = 1.6 [both $p > 0.0001$]; planning: OR = 4.3, aOR = 1.5 [both $p > 0.0001$]; attempt: OR = 5.0, aOR = 1.9 [both $p > 0.0001$]; severe attempt: OR = 10.7, aOR = 2.9 [both $p > 0.0001$]) [52]. Soboka et al. (2024) examined Nova Scotia's Mental Health and Addiction (MHA) intake program data from 2020 to 2021 and tested participant data for associations with suicide risk [63]. They considered past suicide attempts, suicidal thoughts two weeks before the interview, and suicidal ideation during the interview in defining suicide risk. They report that psychedelic use, when adjusted for covariates, was positively associated with mild (aOR = 2.04 [$p < 0.001$]) and even moderate/high (aOR = 3.54 [$p < 0.001$]) suicide risk [63].

3.7.3. Secondary Analyses

Zeifman et al. (2020) performed a secondary analysis on two longitudinal, observational studies [58]. They used a composite suicidal ideation score (composite SI) made of the single-item QIDS-SI and the five-item Suicidal Ideation Attributes Scale (SIDAS; out of 50), ranging from 1 to −1. In their first study, Zeifman et al. used a convenience sample of participants planning to use a psychedelic of choice (e.g., psilocybin, LSD, ayahuasca, 5-Meo-DMT, Salvia divinorum, mescaline, or ibogaine) and reported that relative to baseline, psychedelic use was associated with significant reductions in suicidal ideation at 2 weeks (0.48 to −0.19 [$p < 0.001$]) and 4 weeks (0.48 to −0.47 [$p < 0.001$]) [58]. In the second study, participants planned to use psychedelics in the presence of a facilitator: an individual who would guide them through the process. Once again, psychedelic use was associated with a significant reduction in suicidal ideation from baseline to 4 weeks post psychedelic use (0.16 to −0.28 [$p < 0.001$]) [58].

4. Discussion

In this systematic review, we evaluated the effects of psychedelics on suicidal-related outcomes using 39 studies. Psilocybin was studied in multiple trials focusing on its effects on suicidal ideation and behavior, primarily in patients with depression and other psychiatric conditions. In summary, while clinical trials have supported the potential of psychedelics, especially psilocybin, in reducing suicidality in patients with psychiatric conditions, findings from observational and cross-sectional studies on general or adolescent populations suggested mixed or negative associations. However, these studies are limited by unknown confounding variables, such as the potential for increased substance use among individuals with mental health conditions or the reverse association, where those with suicidality may engage in greater substance use. Additionally, the lack of baseline data or detailed population characteristics severely limits the interpretability of these findings regarding the effects of psychedelics on suicidality, underscoring the need for further rigorous investigation.

Suicidality is a multifaceted and complex phenomenon that can manifest across a range of psychiatric disorders, including mood disorders, anxiety, PTSD, substance use disorders, and chronic pain [64]. While most pharmacological treatments are designed to target the primary disorder with the assumption that improving the underlying condition will also alleviate suicidality, this approach may be overly reductive. Suicidality may persist even in the absence of other symptoms, suggesting that treating the primary disorder may not always be sufficient to address the risk of suicide [65]. Consequently, it is critical to reconsider the assumption that treating the underlying condition inherently resolves suicidality. A more nuanced approach that evaluates suicidality as a distinct clinical target, independent of the underlying disorder, may offer more effective and tailored therapeutic interventions. This is analogous to the use of hypnotic medications to address sleep disturbances, irrespective of the underlying psychiatric condition, and could lead to more focused strategies for managing suicidality in clinical practice.

Several RCTs have reported positive effects of psychedelic administration on suicide risk, with most trials finding moderate between-group effect sizes for reductions in suicidality. Some studies reported rapid effects of psychedelics on suicidal ideations, potentially similar to ketamine [66], which is an important advantage given the limitations of current treatments due to their delayed onset of action. However, the limited reporting on the timing of suicide outcome assessments prevents definitive conclusions. Antidepressants and ECT typically take up to two weeks to show therapeutic effects [67,68], making psychedelics a critical alternative for patients with suicidal ideations without intent or plan, offering a potentially life-saving intervention when time is of the essence. The mechanisms by which psychedelics may reduce suicidality are complex and multifaceted, with one primary mechanism being the promotion of neuroplasticity, enhancing the brain's ability to process and reframe negative beliefs and emotional experiences associated with suicidality [69,70]; however, these effects are closely influenced by factors such as set (mindset), setting (environment), and therapeutic integration [69,70]. Importantly, combining psychedelics with evidence-based therapies such as CBT may offer additional benefits [71]. Meta-analytic evidence suggests that CBT reduces suicide attempts by half in those who attempted suicide in the previous six months, making it a valuable adjunctive or follow-up intervention [72]. Moreover, psychedelics could be leveraged to address potentially modifiable factors associated with higher suicide risk, such as hopelessness, anxiety, impulsivity, psychotic symptoms, and the impact of stressful life events (e.g., financial stress, victimization) [73]. By promoting a shift in perspective on life stresses and alleviating emotional burdens, psychedelics, when combined with therapies like CBT, may more effectively target these underlying factors, further supporting reductions in suicidality [74]. Future studies should investigate the efficacy of integrated psychedelic-assisted therapy approaches to maximize therapeutic outcomes in this high-risk population.

Psychedelics also increase connectivity in brain regions involved in emotional regulation and self-reflection, facilitating emotional processing and alleviating feelings of hopelessness and despair [75]. Additionally, reductions in experiential avoidance—identified as an indirect effect in a clinical trial and as a correlate in two naturalistic studies—may contribute to decreases in suicidality by enabling individuals to confront and process difficult thoughts and emotions rather than suppressing them [58,76]. Psychedelics enable profound emotional experiences that allow individuals to confront unresolved trauma and suppressed emotions, potentially leading to emotional catharsis [77]. This is thought to be mediated by serotonin system interactions, particularly through the 5-HT2A receptor, which plays a crucial role in mood regulation [78]. The therapeutic context, which typically involves supportive, guided environments, also contributes to the reduction in suicidality by fostering trust, safety, and emotional processing, potentially leading to shifts in perspective and enhanced meaning or connectedness. The combination of psychedelics' unique mechanisms of action, along with their rapid therapeutic effects, presents a promising option for individuals at high risk of suicide [79]. However, it is important to note that individuals at high suicide risk, including those with a history of attempts reported during screening, have been systematically excluded from included studies, limiting the generalizability of current findings to this population. Additionally, BPD has also been underrepresented in these trials, despite the elevated suicide risk associated with this group [79]. Further, while psychedelics offer rapid reductions in symptoms, the inconsistent reporting of safety outcomes across trials represents a significant limitation, particularly in studies addressing suicide outcomes. Specifically, many trials rely on scales designed to measure broader psychiatric disorders rather than directly assessing suicidality. When suicidality is evaluated, it is often through single-item measures or scales with only 2–3 questions, which fail to capture the complexity of suicidality, including its chronicity, acuity, risk level, and predisposing factors [72]. Additionally, the timing of these measurements is not always consistent, leaving uncertainty about when suicidal outcomes were assessed in relation to the psychedelic intervention. Another concern is the ambiguous categorization of suicidal outcomes—whether they are treated as adverse effects or primary outcomes [72]. If considered adverse effects, suicidality may not be systematically monitored or directly inquired about, risking underreporting when left to participant-initiated disclosures. This lack of standardization in assessing and reporting suicidal outcomes undermines a comprehensive evaluation of the risk-benefit profile of psychedelics. For comparison, ketamine and esketamine demonstrate significant short-term benefits, but their effects are often transient, requiring repeated dosing, and come with their own safety considerations [13]. Therefore, further research is essential to identify which individuals are most likely to benefit from psychedelics, to evaluate their safety in high-risk populations, and to address the caveats associated with their clinical application. Our search of clinicaltrials.gov yielded only one trial with a primary outcome focused on suicide prevention, underscoring the need for additional studies in this area.

Suicidal ideation and attempts are assessed in clinical trials as a safety measure due to concerns about the potential for increased suicidal thoughts following psychedelic administration. The C-SSRS is the most commonly used tool to evaluate suicidal ideation in these studies. While the majority of trials report no increase in suicidal risk during the study period, some severe adverse events, including suicidal ideation following psychedelic use, have been documented [79]. Additionally, one study has reported death by suicide following psilocybin administration [80]. Prior to their death by suicide, the participant exhibited no signs of behavioral impairment and showed no adverse effects during follow-up later that day or in the subsequent days [80]. However, the authors noted that this was not attributed to the intervention. In clinical trials, the controlled environment and support from trained professionals are intended to mitigate these risks, yet the unpredictable nature of psychedelic experiences means that some individuals may react in ways that are difficult to anticipate. As such, ongoing monitoring and individualized care are crucial components of ensuring participant safety, particularly for those with a history of mental health issues. Increased suicidal ideations, planning, and attempts have also been reported in population-based studies, though these findings have been inconsistent. Some studies suggest that psychedelics were associated with increased odds of suicidal behaviors in certain individuals, while others reported no significant association, and some demonstrated reduced suicidal behaviors following psychedelic use. These mixed results may be due to several factors, such as differences in study design, participant characteristics, and the specific contexts in which psychedelics are used. The intensity of the psychedelic experience itself—often involving profound emotional and psychological shifts—can vary widely among individuals, which may influence the risk of adverse outcomes. These mixed findings highlight the complexity of the relationship between psychedelics and suicidality, suggesting that further research is needed to clarify the potential risks and identify factors that may increase vulnerability to adverse outcomes. Factors such as prior mental health conditions, personal history of trauma, and the setting in which psychedelics are administered may all play a role in determining the effects on suicidality. As a result, personalized treatment approaches and careful risk assessment are essential for ensuring participant safety, particularly for those with pre-existing mental health concerns.

This systematic review added to the literature by synthesizing existing research on the effects of psychedelic therapies—specifically psilocybin and other serotonergic psychedelics—on suicidality in individuals with psychiatric disorders. By focusing on RCTs, observational studies, and other relevant data, this review evaluated the potential of psychedelics as a treatment for suicide risk. It highlighted the methodological gaps in current research, such as the exclusion of high-risk populations, inconsistent definitions of suicidality, and limited longitudinal data. Additionally, this review discussed the implications for clinical practice and future research directions, providing an evidence-based foundation for the safe integration of psychedelic therapies into psychiatric care, particularly for individuals at high risk for suicide. Given these findings, it is clear that psychedelic therapies hold promise for addressing suicidality in psychiatric patients, particularly when combined with psychotherapy. However, due to methodological limitations and a lack of data from high-risk populations, it is premature to implement these therapies as standard practice. Further research is required to better understand their long-term efficacy, safety, and optimal treatment protocols. Only through rigorous clinical trials that include high-risk individuals and consistent outcome measures can we determine the potential role of psychedelics in clinical settings.

Limitations

The limitations of this review include several factors that may affect the validity and generalizability of the results. First, the sample size is insufficient to detect significant effects, limiting the ability to generalize findings to broader populations. Selection bias is another concern, as participants may not be randomly selected or fully representative of the target population. Additionally, higher-risk patients are often excluded, which limits the study's external validity and generalizability. Confounding variables, such as unmeasured factors influencing the outcomes, could also distort the findings. Moreover, the short duration of the study limits the ability to assess long-term effects or trends, which may be important in understanding sustained outcomes. If a study is cross-sectional, it can only establish associations, not causality, which is a significant limitation. Furthermore, the absence of subgroup analyses for specific psychedelics and populations limited the ability to assess the nuanced effects across different types of psychedelics and varied populations. The lack of data suitable for a meta-analysis prevented a more comprehensive synthesis of results across studies. Additionally, publication bias may lead to an overrepresentation of positive findings, as studies with negative or null results are less likely to be published, which may influence the conclusions drawn. These limitations should be carefully considered when interpreting the findings. Ethical considerations, accessibility, and scalability of psychedelic therapies are critical issues that must be addressed in future research. The potential for these therapies to be widely implemented in clinical settings depends on overcoming significant barriers related to their cost, regulatory approval, and the need for trained professionals to administer them safely. Additionally, the mechanisms by which psychedelics exert their therapeutic effects remain not fully understood, highlighting a need for further research into their pharmacodynamics and neurobiological mechanisms. Furthermore, although certain adverse effects have been identified, there is a clear gap in the systematic evaluation of potential long-term risks associated with psychedelic use, such as exacerbation of mental health symptoms or emergence of new psychological issues. These concerns must be addressed to ensure the safe and effective use of psychedelics in treating psychiatric disorders.

5. Future Directions

Future research should focus on well-designed longitudinal studies that consistently define and assess suicide-related outcomes, account for confounding factors, and evaluate long-term safety and efficacy. Expanding inclusion criteria to encompass high-risk populations will be critical in determining whether psychedelics can be safely and effectively used for suicide risk reduction. Standardizing adverse event reporting, including suicidality, is essential to clarify potential risks. Addressing these gaps will provide a clearer understanding of whether psychedelics have a meaningful role in managing suicidality in clinical and real-world settings.

6. Conclusions

While clinical trials suggest that psychedelics, particularly psilocybin, may reduce suicide-related outcomes in individuals with psychiatric disorders, the evidence remains inconclusive. Reductions in suicidality appear closely linked to improvements in comorbid symptoms such as depression, PTSD, and anxiety, rather than a direct effect on suicidality itself. Methodological limitations, including inconsistent definitions of suicide-related outcomes, reliance on single-item measures, and variability in outcome assessment timing, weaken the strength of current findings. Additionally, observational and cross-sectional studies indicate more variable results, with some evidence suggesting increased suicidality in certain populations. The exclusion of high-risk individuals from clinical trials further limits the generalizability of these findings. At present, there is insufficient evidence to support the clinical use of psychedelics for suicide prevention, and further research is needed to determine their safety and efficacy in this context. Given these factors, it remains premature to conclude that psychedelics have a definitive role in mitigating suicidality.

Supplementary Materials: The following supporting information can be downloaded at https://www.mdpi.com/article/10.3390/jcm14051416/s1.

Author Contributions: Conceptualization: S.M. and V.B.; methodology: S.M. and V.B.; formal analysis: S.M. and T.M.; investigation: S.M., T.M. and V.B.; writing—original draft preparation: S.M. and T.M.; writing—review and editing, all authors; supervision: V.B. All authors have read and agreed to the published version of the manuscript.

Funding: This research did not receive any specific grant from funding agencies in the public, commercial, or not-for-profit sectors.

Institutional Review Board Statement: Not applicable.

Informed Consent Statement: Not applicable.

Data Availability Statement: Not applicable.

Conflicts of Interest: Richard Zeifman received funding from the NYU Langone Psychedelic Medicine Research Training program (funded by MindMed) and the Canadian Institutes of Health Research (Grant Number: 202110MFE-472921-HTB-272687). Jennifer Swainson, Lisa Burback, Olga Winkler, and Yanbo Zhang are supported by the Academic Medicine and Health Services Program (AMHSP), a joint program funded by the University of Alberta and Alberta Health Services to ensure physicians affiliated with Alberta's faculties of medicine are compensated for providing patient care along with their work related to research, innovation, education, administration, and leadership. Jennifer Swainson has received honoraria for speaking or advisory roles from Abbvie, Bausch Health, Biron, Eisai, Idorsia, Janssen, Lundbeck, Novo Nordisk, and Otsuka. Rakesh Jetly is the CMO of Mydecine Innovation Group. Muhammad I. Husain is supported by the Cameron Wilson Chair in Depression Studies from the University of Toronto. He is leading contracted research for Compass Pathways Ltd and has served as an advisor to Mindset Pharma, Psyched Therapeutics, and Wake Network. Venkat Bhat is supported by an Academic Scholar Award from the University of Toronto Department of Psychiatry and has received research funding from the Canadian Institutes of Health Research, Brain & Behavior Foundation, Ontario Ministry of Health Innovation Funds, Royal College of Physicians and Surgeons of Canada, Department of National Defence (Government of Canada), New Frontiers in Research Fund, Associated Medical Services Inc. Healthcare, American Foundation for Suicide Prevention, Roche Canada, Novartis, and Eisai. David Erritzoe is acting as a paid scientific advisor for Aya Biosciences, Lophora Aps, Clerkenwell Health, Mindstate Design Lab. Manish Jha has received contract research grants from Acadia Pharmaceuticals, Neurocrine Bioscience, Navitor/Supernus and Janssen Research and Development; has received honorarium to serve as Section Editor of the Psychiatry and Behavioral Health Learning Network and as Guest Editor for Psychiatric Clinics of North America from Elsevier; has received consultant fees from Eleusis Therapeutics US, Janssen Global Services, Janssen Scientific Affairs, Boehringer Ingelheim and Guidepoint Global; has received fees to serve on Data Safety and Monitoring Board for Worldwide Clinical Trials (Eliem and Inversargo), Vicore Pharma and IQVIA (Click); and honoraria for educational presentations from North American Center for Continuing Medical Education, Medscape/WebMD, Clinical Care Options, H.C. Wainwright and Company and Global Medical Education.

References

1. Masango, S.M.; Rataemane, S.T.; Motojesi, A.A. Suicide and suicide risk factors: A literature review. *S. Afr. Fam. Pract.* **2008**, *50*, 25–29. [CrossRef]
2. Centers for Disease Control and Prevention: WISQARS: Fatal Injury Reports, National, and Regional, 1999–2018. Available online: https://webappa.cdc.gov/sasweb/ncipc/mortrate.html (accessed on 20 February 2020).
3. Mann, J.J. A current perspective of suicide and attempted suicide. *Ann. Intern. Med.* **2002**, *136*, 302–311. [CrossRef] [PubMed]
4. Mann, J.J.; Apter, A.; Bertolote, J.; Beautrais, A.; Currier, D.; Haas, A.; Hegerl, U.; Lonnqvist, J.; Malone, K.; Marusic, A.; et al. Suicide prevention strategies: A systematic review. *JAMA* **2005**, *294*, 2064–2074. [CrossRef] [PubMed]
5. Baldessarini, R.J.; Tondo, L. Suicidal risks in 12 DSM-5 psychiatric disorders. *J. Affect. Disord.* **2020**, *271*, 66–73. [CrossRef] [PubMed]
6. Panagioti, M.; Gooding, P.A.; Triantafyllou, K.; Tarrier, N. Suicidality and posttraumatic stress disorder (PTSD) in adolescents: A systematic review and meta-analysis. *Soc. Psychiatry Psychiatr. Epidemiol.* **2015**, *50*, 525–537. [CrossRef] [PubMed]
7. Stack, S. Contributing factors to suicide: Political, social, cultural and economic. *Prev. Med.* **2021**, *152*, 106498. [CrossRef] [PubMed]
8. Kaminski, J.A.; Bschor, T. Antidepressants and suicidality: A re-analysis of the re-analysis. *J. Affect. Disord.* **2020**, *266*, 95–99. [CrossRef] [PubMed]
9. Wu, H.; Lu, L.; Qian, Y.; Jin, X.H.; Yu, H.R.; Du, L.; Fu, X.L.; Zhu, B.; Chen, H.L. The significance of cognitive-behavioral therapy on suicide: An umbrella review. *J. Affect. Disord.* **2022**, *317*, 142–148. [CrossRef] [PubMed]
10. Peltzman, T.; Shiner, B.; Watts, B.V. Effects of electroconvulsive therapy on short-term suicide mortality in a risk-matched patient population. *J. ECT* **2020**, *36*, 187–192. [CrossRef] [PubMed]
11. Müller-Oerlinghausen, B.; Lewitzka, U. The contributions of lithium and clozapine for the prophylaxis and treatment of suicidal behavior. In *Biological Aspects of Suicidal Behavior*; Karger Publishers: Basel, Switzerland, 2016; Volume 30, pp. 145–160.
12. Chen, C.C.; Zhou, N.; Hu, N.; Feng, J.G.; Wang, X.B. Acute Effects of Intravenous Sub-Anesthetic Doses of Ketamine and Intranasal Inhaled Esketamine on Suicidal Ideation: A Systematic Review and Meta-Analysis. *Neuropsychiatr. Dis. Treat.* **2023**, *19*, 587–599. [CrossRef] [PubMed] [PubMed Central]

13. Siegel, A.N.; Di Vincenzo, J.D.; Brietzke, E.; Gill, H.; Rodrigues, N.B.; Lui, L.M.W.; Teopiz, K.M.; Ng, J.; Ho, R.; McIntyre, R.S.; et al. Antisuicidal and antidepressant effects of ketamine and esketamine in patients with baseline suicidality: A systematic review. *J. Psychiatr. Res.* **2021**, *137*, 426–436. [CrossRef] [PubMed]
14. Mendes, F.R.; dos Santos Costa, C.; Wiltenburg, V.D.; Morales-Lima, G.; Fernandes, J.A.; Filev, R. Classic and non-classic psychedelics for substance use disorder: A review of their historic, past and current research. *Addict. Neurosci.* **2022**, *3*, 100025. [CrossRef]
15. Griffiths, R.R.; Richards, W.A.; McCann, U.; Jesse, R. Psilocybin can occasion mystical-type experiences having substantial and sustained personal meaning and spiritual significance. *Psychopharmacology* **2006**, *187*, 268–283. [CrossRef]
16. Heifets, B.D.; Olson, D.E. Therapeutic mechanisms of psychedelics and entactogens. *Neuropsychopharmacology* **2024**, *49*, 104–118. [CrossRef]
17. Wardle, M.C.; de Wit, H. MDMA alters emotional processing and facilitates positive social interaction. *Psychopharmacology* **2014**, *231*, 4219–4229. [CrossRef] [PubMed]
18. Rosenblat, J.D.; Meshkat, S.; Doyle, Z.; Kaczmarek, E.; Brudner, R.M.; Kratiuk, K.; Mansur, R.B.; Schulz-Quach, C.; Sethi, R.; Abate, A.; et al. Psilocybin-assisted psychotherapy for treatment resistant depression: A randomized clinical trial evaluating repeated doses of psilocybin. *Med* **2024**, *5*, 190–200. [CrossRef]
19. Goodwin, G.M.; Aaronson, S.T.; Alvarez, O.; Arden, P.C.; Baker, A.; Bennett, J.C.; Bird, C.; Blom, R.E.; Brennan, C.; Brusch, D.; et al. Single-dose psilocybin for a treatment-resistant episode of major depression. *N. Engl. J. Med.* **2022**, *387*, 1637–1648. [CrossRef]
20. Bogenschutz, M.P.; Ross, S.; Bhatt, S.; Baron, T.; Forcehimes, A.A.; Laska, E.; Mennenga, S.E.; O'Donnell, K.; Owens, L.T.; Podrebarac, S.; et al. Percentage of heavy drinking days following psilocybin-assisted psychotherapy vs placebo in the treatment of adult patients with alcohol use disorder: A randomized clinical trial. *JAMA Psychiatry* **2022**, *79*, 953–962. [CrossRef]
21. Meshkat, S.; Kaczmarek, E.; Doyle, Z.; Brudner, R.M.; Gomes, F.A.; Blainey, M.G.; Weiglein, G.; McIntyre, R.S.; Mansur, R.B.; Rosenblat, J.D. Psilocybin-Assisted Psychotherapy for Treatment-Resistant Depression in Bipolar II Disorder. *Psychedelic Med.* **2024**, *5*, 190–200.e5. [CrossRef]
22. Mitchell, J.M.; Ot'alora, G.M.; van der Kolk, B.; Shannon, S.; Bogenschutz, M.; Gelfand, Y.; Paleos, C.; Nicholas, C.R.; Quevedo, S.; Balliett, B.; et al. MDMA-assisted therapy for moderate to severe PTSD: A randomized, placebo-controlled phase 3 trial. *Nat. Med.* **2023**, *29*, 2473–2480. [CrossRef]
23. Thiessen, M.S.; Walsh, Z.; Bird, B.M.; Lafrance, A. Psychedelic use and intimate partner violence: The role of emotion regulation. *J. Psychopharmacol.* **2018**, *32*, 749–755. [CrossRef]
24. Hinkle, J.T.; Graziosi, M.; Nayak, S.M.; Yaden, D.B. Adverse events in studies of classic psychedelics: A systematic review and meta-analysis. *JAMA Psychiatry* **2024**, *81*, 1225–1235. [CrossRef]
25. Jones, G.M.; Nock, M.K. MDMA/ecstasy use and psilocybin use are associated with lowered odds of psychological distress and suicidal thoughts in a sample of US adults. *J. Psychopharmacol.* **2022**, *36*, 46–56. [CrossRef]
26. Page, M.J.; McKenzie, J.E.; Bossuyt, P.M.; Boutron, I.; Hoffmann, T.C.; Mulrow, C.D.; Shamseer, L.; Tetzlaff, J.M.; Akl, E.A.; Brennan, S.E.; et al. The PRISMA 2020 statement: An updated guideline for reporting systematic reviews. *bmj* **2021**, *372*, n71. [CrossRef]
27. Porritt, K.; Gomersall, J.; Lockwood, C. JBI's systematic reviews: Study selection and critical appraisal. *Am. J. Nurs.* **2014**, *114*, 47–52. [CrossRef] [PubMed]
28. Carhart-Harris, R.; Giribaldi, B.; Watts, R.; Baker-Jones, M.; Murphy-Beiner, A.; Murphy, R.; Martell, J.; Blemings, A.; Erritzoe, D.; Nutt, D.J. Trial of Psilocybin versus Escitalopram for Depression. *N. Engl. J. Med.* **2021**, *384*, 1402–1411. [CrossRef]
29. Davis, A.K.; Barrett, F.S.; May, D.G.; Cosimano, M.P.; Sepeda, N.D.; Johnson, M.W.; Finan, P.H.; Griffiths, R.R. Effects of Psilocybin-Assisted Therapy on Major Depressive Disorder: A Randomized Clinical Trial. *JAMA Psychiatry* **2021**, *78*, 481–489. [CrossRef]
30. Peck, S.K.; Shao, S.; Gruen, T.; Yang, K.; Babakanian, A.; Trim, J.; Finn, D.M.; Kaye, W.H. Psilocybin therapy for females with anorexia nervosa: A phase 1, open-label feasibility study. *Nat. Med.* **2023**, *29*, 1947–1953. [CrossRef]
31. von Rotz, R.; Schindowski, E.M.; Jungwirth, J.; Schuldt, A.; Rieser, N.M.; Zahoranszky, K.; Seifritz, E.; Nowak, A.; Nowak, P.; Jäncke, L.; et al. Single-dose psilocybin-assisted therapy in major depressive disorder: A placebo-controlled, double-blind, randomised clinical trial. *EClinicalMedicine* **2022**, *56*, 101809. [CrossRef]
32. Raison, C.L.; Sanacora, G.; Woolley, J.; Heinzerling, K.; Dunlop, B.W.; Brown, R.T.; Kakar, R.; Hassman, M.; Trivedi, R.P.; Robison, R.; et al. Single-Dose Psilocybin Treatment for Major Depressive Disorder: A Randomized Clinical Trial. *JAMA* **2023**, *330*, 843–853. [CrossRef]
33. Ross, S.; Agin-Liebes, G.; Lo, S.; Zeifman, R.J.; Ghazal, L.; Benville, J.; Franco Corso, S.; Bjerre Real, C.; Guss, J.; Bossis, A.; et al. Acute and Sustained Reductions in Loss of Meaning and Suicidal Ideation Following Psilocybin-Assisted Psychotherapy for Psychiatric and Existential Distress in Life-Threatening Cancer. *ACS Pharmacol. Transl. Sci.* **2021**, *4*, 553–562. [CrossRef]

34. Carhart-Harris, R.L.; Bolstridge, M.; Day, C.M.J.; Rucker, J.; Watts, R.; Erritzoe, D.E.; Kaelen, M.; Giribaldi, B.; Bloomfield, M.; Pilling, S.; et al. Psilocybin with psychological support for treatment-resistant depression: Six-month follow-up. *Psychopharmacology* **2018**, *235*, 399–408. [CrossRef] [PubMed]
35. Anderson, B.T.; Danforth, A.; Daroff, P.R.; Stauffer, C.; Ekman, E.; Agin-Liebes, G.; Trope, A.; Boden, M.T.; Dilley, P.J.; Mitchell, J.; et al. Psilocybin-assisted group therapy for demoralized older long-term AIDS survivor men: An open-label safety and feasibility pilot study. *EClinicalMedicine* **2020**, *27*, 100538. [CrossRef] [PubMed]
36. Aaronson, S.T.; van der Vaart, A.; Miller, T.; LaPratt, J.; Swartz, K.; Shoultz, A.; Lauterbach, M.; Sackeim, H.A.; Suppes, T. Single-Dose Synthetic Psilocybin With Psychotherapy for Treatment-Resistant Bipolar Type II Major Depressive Episodes: A Nonrandomized Open-Label Trial. *JAMA Psychiatry* **2024**, *81*, 555–562. [CrossRef]
37. Ellis, S.; Bostian, C.; Feng, W.; Fischer, E.; Schwartz, G.; Eisen, K.; Lean, M.; Conlan, E.; Ostacher, M.; Aaronson, S.; et al. Single-dose psilocybin for U.S. military Veterans with severe treatment-resistant depression—A first-in-kind open-label pilot study. *J. Affect. Disord.* **2025**, *369*, 381–389. [CrossRef] [PubMed]
38. Mithoefer, M.C.; Mithoefer, A.T.; Feduccia, A.A.; Jerome, L.; Wagner, M.; Wymer, J.; Holland, J.; Hamilton, S.; Yazar-Klosinski, B.; Emerson, A.; et al. 3,4-methylenedioxymethamphetamine (MDMA)-assisted psychotherapy for post-traumatic stress disorder in military veterans, firefighters, and police officers: A randomised, double-blind, dose-response, phase 2 clinical trial. *Lancet Psychiatry* **2018**, *5*, 486–497. [CrossRef] [PubMed]
39. Ot'alora, G.M.; Grigsby, J.; Poulter, B.; Van Derveer, J.W., 3rd; Giron, S.G.; Jerome, L.; Feduccia, A.A.; Hamilton, S.; Yazar-Klosinski, B.; Emerson, A.; et al. 3,4-Methylenedioxymethamphetamine-assisted psychotherapy for treatment of chronic posttraumatic stress disorder: A randomized phase 2 controlled trial. *J. Psychopharmacol.* **2018**, *32*, 1295–1307. [CrossRef] [PubMed]
40. Mitchell, J.M.; Bogenschutz, M.; Lilienstein, A.; Harrison, C.; Kleiman, S.; Parker-Guilbert, K.; Ot'alora, G.M.; Garas, W.; Paleos, C.; Gorman, I.; et al. MDMA-assisted therapy for severe PTSD: A randomized, double-blind, placebo-controlled phase 3 study. *Nat. Med.* **2021**, *27*, 1025–1033. [CrossRef] [PubMed]
41. Davis, A.K.; Xin, Y.; Sepeda, N.; Averill, L.A. Open-label study of consecutive ibogaine and 5-MeO-DMT assisted-therapy for trauma-exposed male Special Operations Forces Veterans: Prospective data from a clinical program in Mexico. *Am. J. Drug Alcohol. Abuse.* **2023**, *49*, 587–596. [CrossRef]
42. Davis, A.K.; Averill, L.A.; Sepeda, N.D.; Barsuglia, J.P.; Amoroso, T. Psychedelic Treatment for Trauma-Related Psychological and Cognitive Impairment Among US Special Operations Forces Veterans. *Chronic Stress* **2020**, *4*, 2470547020939564. [CrossRef]
43. Ragnhildstveit, A.; Khan, R.; Seli, P.; Bass, L.C.; August, R.J.; Kaiyo, M.; Barr, N.; Jackson, L.K.; Gaffrey, M.S.; Barsuglia, J.P.; et al. 5-MeO-DMT for post-traumatic stress disorder: A real-world longitudinal case study. *Front. Psychiatry.* **2023**, *14*, 1271152. [CrossRef]
44. Zeifman, R.J.; Palhano-Fontes, F.; Hallak, J.; Arcoverde, E.; Maia-Oliveira, J.P.; Araujo, D.B. The Impact of Ayahuasca on Suicidality: Results From a Randomized Controlled Trial. *Front. Pharmacol.* **2019**, *10*, 1325. [CrossRef] [PubMed]
45. Zeifman, R.J.; Singhal, N.; Dos Santos, R.G.; Sanches, R.F.; de Lima Osório, F.; Hallak, J.E.C.; Weissman, C.R. Rapid and sustained decreases in suicidality following a single dose of ayahuasca among individuals with recurrent major depressive disorder: Results from an open-label trial. *Psychopharmacology* **2021**, *238*, 453–459. [CrossRef]
46. Gasser, P.; Kirchner, K.; Passie, T. LSD-assisted psychotherapy for anxiety associated with a life-threatening disease: A qualitative study of acute and sustained subjective effects. *J. Psychopharmacol.* **2015**, *29*, 57–68. [CrossRef] [PubMed]
47. Carbonaro, T.M.; Bradstreet, M.P.; Barrett, F.S.; MacLean, K.A.; Jesse, R.; Johnson, M.W.; Griffiths, R.R. Survey study of challenging experiences after ingesting psilocybin mushrooms: Acute and enduring positive and negative consequences. *J. Psychopharmacol.* **2016**, *30*, 1268–1278. [CrossRef]
48. Céline, B.; François, B.; Stanislas, S. Physical and psychosocial factors associated with psychostimulant use in a nationally representative sample of French adolescents: Specificities of cocaine, amphetamine, and ecstasy use. *Addict. Behav.* **2019**, *92*, 208–224. [CrossRef]
49. Kim, J.; Fan, B.; Liu, X.; Kerner, N.; Wu, P. Ecstasy use and suicidal behavior among adolescents: Findings from a national survey. *Suicide Life Threat. Behav.* **2011**, *41*, 435–444. [CrossRef]
50. Han, B.; Blanco, C.; Einstein, E.B.; Compton, W.M. Mental health conditions and receipt of mental health care by illicit lysergic acid diethylamide (LSD) use status among young adults in the United States. *Addiction* **2022**, *117*, 1794–1800. [CrossRef] [PubMed]
51. Yockey, R.A.; King, K.A.; Vidourek, R.A. "Go ask Alice, when she's 10-feet tall": Psychosocial correlates to lifetime LSD use among a national sample of US adults. *J. Psychedelic Stud.* **2019**, *3*, 308–314. [CrossRef]
52. Wong, S.S.; Zhou, B.; Goebert, D.; Hishinuma, E.S. The risk of adolescent suicide across patterns of drug use: A nationally representative study of high school students in the United States from 1999 to 2009. *Soc. Psychiatry Psychiatr. Epidemiol.* **2013**, *48*, 1611–1620. [CrossRef] [PubMed]
53. Hendricks, P.S.; Thorne, C.B.; Clark, C.B.; Coombs, D.W.; Johnson, M.W. Classic psychedelic use is associated with reduced psychological distress and suicidality in the United States adult population. *J. Psychopharmacol.* **2015**, *29*, 280–288. [CrossRef]

54. Argento, E.; Strathdee, S.A.; Tupper, K.; Braschel, M.; Wood, E.; Shannon, K. Does psychedelic drug use reduce risk of suicidality? Evidence from a longitudinal community-based cohort of marginalised women in a Canadian setting. *BMJ Open* **2017**, *7*, e016025. [CrossRef]
55. Argento, E.; Braschel, M.; Walsh, Z.; Socias, M.E.; Shannon, K. The moderating effect of psychedelics on the prospective relationship between prescription opioid use and suicide risk among marginalized women. *J. Psychopharmacol.* **2018**, *32*, 1385–1391. [CrossRef] [PubMed]
56. Sexton, J.D.; Crawford, M.S.; Sweat, N.W.; Varley, A.; Green, E.E.; Hendricks, P.S. Prevalence and epidemiological associates of novel psychedelic use in the United States adult population. *J. Psychopharmacol.* **2019**, *33*, 1058–1067. [CrossRef] [PubMed]
57. Sexton, J.D.; Nichols, C.D.; Hendricks, P.S. Population Survey Data Informing the Therapeutic Potential of Classic and Novel Phenethylamine, Tryptamine, and Lysergamide Psychedelics. *Front. Psychiatry* **2020**, *10*, 896. [CrossRef] [PubMed]
58. Zeifman, R.J.; Wagner, A.C.; Watts, R.; Kettner, H.; Mertens, L.J.; Carhart-Harris, R.L. Post-Psychedelic Reductions in Experiential Avoidance Are Associated With Decreases in Depression Severity and Suicidal Ideation. *Front. Psychiatry* **2020**, *11*, 782. [CrossRef]
59. Desai, S.; Jain, V.; Xavier, S.; Du, W. Hopelessness, Suicidality, and Co-Occurring Substance Use among Adolescent Hallucinogen Users-A National Survey Study. *Children* **2022**, *9*, 1906. [CrossRef]
60. Jones, G.; Arias, D.; Nock, M. Associations between MDMA/ecstasy, classic psychedelics, and suicidal thoughts and behaviors in a sample of U.S. adolescents. *Sci. Rep.* **2022**, *12*, 21927. [CrossRef]
61. Yang, K.H.; Han, B.H.; Palamar, J.J. Past-year hallucinogen use in relation to psychological distress, depression, and suicidality among US adults. *Addict. Behav.* **2022**, *132*, 107343. [CrossRef] [PubMed]
62. Giugovaz, A.; Grassi, M.; Marchetti, I. Substance addictions and suicidal thoughts and behaviors: Evidence from a multi-wave epidemiological study. *Psychiatry Res.* **2024**, *334*, 115821. [CrossRef] [PubMed]
63. Soboka, M.; Stewart, S.H.; Tibbo, P.; Wang, J. Substance use and risk of suicide among adults who sought mental health and addiction specialty services through a centralised intake process in Nova Scotia: A cross-sectional study. *BMJ Open* **2024**, *14*, e086487. [CrossRef] [PubMed]
64. Xu, Y.E.; Barron, D.A.; Sudol, K.; Zisook, S.; Oquendo, M.A. Suicidal behavior across a broad range of psychiatric disorders. *Mol. Psychiatry* **2023**, *28*, 2764–2810. [CrossRef]
65. Dunlop, B.W.; Polychroniou, P.E.; Rakofsky, J.J.; Nemeroff, C.B.; Craighead, W.E.; Mayberg, H.S. Suicidal ideation and other persisting symptoms after CBT or antidepressant medication treatment for major depressive disorder. *Psychol. Med.* **2019**, *49*, 1869–1878. [CrossRef]
66. Hochschild, A.; Grunebaum, M.F.; Mann, J.J. The rapid anti-suicidal ideation effect of ketamine: A systematic review. *Prev. Med.* **2021**, *152*, 106524. [CrossRef] [PubMed]
67. Kellner, C.H.; Fink, M.; Knapp, R.; Petrides, G.; Husain, M.; Rummans, T.; Mueller, M.; Bernstein, H.; Rasmussen, K.; O'Connor, K.; et al. Relief of expressed suicidal intent by ECT: A consortium for research in ECT study. *Am. J. Psychiatry* **2005**, *162*, 977–982. [CrossRef] [PubMed]
68. Simon, G.E.; Savarino, J.; Operskalski, B.; Wang, P.S. Suicide risk during antidepressant treatment. *Am. J. Psychiatry* **2006**, *163*, 41–47. [CrossRef]
69. De Vos, C.M.; Mason, N.L.; Kuypers, K.P. Psychedelics and neuroplasticity: A systematic review unraveling the biological underpinnings of psychedelics. *Front. Psychiatry* **2021**, *12*, 724606. [CrossRef] [PubMed]
70. Underwood, M.D.; Arango, V. Evidence for neurodegeneration and neuroplasticity as part of the neurobiology of suicide. *Biol. Psychiatry* **2011**, *70*, 306–307. [CrossRef]
71. Lam, R.W.; Kennedy, S.H.; Adams, C.; Bahji, A.; Beaulieu, S.; Bhat, V.; Blier, P.; Blumberger, D.M.; Brietzke, E.; Chakrabarty, T.; et al. Canadian Network for Mood and Anxiety Treatments (CANMAT) 2023 Update on Clinical Guidelines for Management of Major Depressive Disorder in Adults: Réseau canadien pour les traitements de l'humeur et de l'anxiété (CANMAT) 2023: Mise à jour des lignes directrices cliniques pour la prise en charge du trouble dépressif majeur chez les adultes. *Can. J. Psychiatry* **2024**, *69*, 07067437241245384.
72. Büscher, R.; Torok, M.; Terhorst, Y.; Sander, L. Internet-based cognitive behavioral therapy to reduce suicidal ideation: A systematic review and meta-analysis. *JAMA Netw. Open* **2020**, *3*, e203933. [CrossRef]
73. Schimmers, N.; Breeksema, J.J.; Smith-Apeldoorn, S.Y.; Veraart, J.; van den Brink, W.; Schoevers, R.A. Psychedelics for the treatment of depression, anxiety, and existential distress in patients with a terminal illness: A systematic review. *Psychopharmacology* **2022**, *239*, 15–33. [CrossRef]
74. Fauvel, B.; Strika-Bruneau, L.; Piolino, P. Changes in self-rumination and self-compassion mediate the effect of psychedelic experiences on decreases in depression, anxiety, and stress. *Psychol. Conscious. Theory Res. Pract.* **2023**, *10*, 88. [CrossRef]
75. Smigielski, L.; Scheidegger, M.; Kometer, M.; Vollenweider, F.X. Psilocybin-assisted mindfulness training modulates self-consciousness and brain default mode network connectivity with lasting effects. *NeuroImage* **2019**, *196*, 207–215. [CrossRef] [PubMed]

76. Zeifman, R.J.; Wagner, A.C.; Monson, C.M.; Carhart-Harris, R.L. How does psilocybin therapy work? An exploration of experiential avoidance as a putative mechanism of change. *J. Affect. Disord.* **2023**, *334*, 100–112. [CrossRef]
77. Lindegaard, T. Do psychedelics facilitate emergence of unconscious psychological processes? *Psychodyn. Psychiatry* **2023**, *51*, 270–286. [CrossRef]
78. Szigeti, B.; Heifets, B. Expectancy effects in psychedelic trials. *Biol. Psychiatry Cogn. Neurosci. Neuroimaging* **2024**, *9*, 512–521. [CrossRef] [PubMed]
79. Zhang, G.; Stackman, R.W., Jr. The role of serotonin 5-HT2A receptors in memory and cognition. *Front. Pharmacol.* **2015**, *6*, 225. [CrossRef] [PubMed]
80. Griffiths, R.R.; Johnson, M.W.; Carducci, M.A.; Umbricht, A.; Richards, W.A.; Richards, B.D.; Cosimano, M.P.; Klinedinst, M.A. Psilocybin produces substantial and sustained decreases in depression and anxiety in patients with life-threatening cancer: A randomized double-blind trial. *J. Psychopharmacol.* **2016**, *30*, 1181–1197. [CrossRef]

Journal of
Clinical Medicine

MDPI

Article

Validation of the Colombian–Spanish Suicidality Scale for Screening Suicide Risk in Clinical and Community Settings

Ana María Arenas Dávila [1,*], Katherine Pastrana Arias [1], Óscar Mauricio Castaño Ramírez [1], Pamela Van den Enden [1], Juan Carlos Castro Navarro [1], Santiago González Giraldo [1], Doris Mileck Vera Higuera [1] and Keith M. Harris [2]

[1] Department of Mental Health, Universidad de Caldas, Manizales 170004, Colombia; k-tpa@hotmail.com (K.P.A.); oscar.castano@ucaldas.edu.co (Ó.M.C.R.); pamelavandenenden@gmail.com (P.V.d.E.); jcnmdpsi@gmail.com (J.C.C.N.); santiago.gonzalez@ucaldas.edu.co (S.G.G.); doris.vera@ucaldas.edu.co (D.M.V.H.)

[2] Independent Researcher, Brisbane 4073, Australia; esensei@yahoo.com

[*] Correspondence: ana.7720138416@ucaldas.edu.co

Abstract: Background/Objective: This study aimed to validate the eight-item Suicidality Scale (SS) in Spanish in a Colombian sample to aid in suicide risk assessment, given the pressing need for accurate, accessible tools in resource-strained settings. **Methods**: A sample of 313 participants, drawn from both clinical and community settings, was used to evaluate the psychometric properties of the SS through tests of internal consistency, item response theory (IRT), and comparisons with clinical risk evaluations. **Results**: The SS demonstrated strong psychometric properties, with high internal consistency ($\omega = 0.96$) and a significant correlation with clinical risk assessments ($r = 0.84$). Model fit indices confirmed a unidimensional eight-item structure with low error rates, while item response analysis revealed strong item discrimination. No differential item functioning was observed by gender or psychiatric diagnosis, supporting its consistency across demographics. Items on past suicide attempts and desire to live were excluded as they did not improve scale performance. Variability within risk levels suggests that individual differences may require clinical judgment. **Conclusions**: The findings validate the Colombian–Spanish SS as a valuable tool for suicide risk assessment, usable in both self-report and clinician-administered formats. Its brief, culturally adapted structure supports its utility in resource-limited environments, providing an accessible option for rapid screening. While the SS effectively categorizes general risk, further longitudinal studies are recommended to enhance its applicability in guiding clinical decisions and long-term risk management.

Keywords: validation studies; suicide prevention; suicide; clinical decision making; Colombia; translations

1. Introduction

Suicide stands as one of the most critical global public health challenges, demanding urgent efforts to develop reliable tools for early detection and timely intervention [1]. Each year, suicide accounts for 1.5% of all deaths worldwide [2], disproportionately affecting vulnerable populations and developing regions where mental health resources are often limited [3].

In Colombia, where suicide rates are 7.5 per 100,000 for women and 13.7 per 100,000 for men [4,5], prevention efforts are significantly hindered by limited access to mental healthcare, particularly in rural areas [6]. Additionally, the pervasive influence of socioeconomic stressors on mental health, including intramarital conflicts and financial difficulties, is exacerbated by the country's ongoing issues with violence and economic instability [7–10]. Addressing these challenges requires culturally adapted, accessible, and psychometrically sound tools that align with the UN Sustainable Development Goals, advancing equitable healthcare and reducing global mental health inequalities [11].

Several instruments are used in Colombia to assess suicide risk, including the Scale for Suicide Ideation (SSI) [12], the Self-Rated Scale for Suicide Ideation (Sr-SSI) [13], the Modified Scale for Suicide Ideation (MSSI) [14], the SAD PERSONS Scale [15], and the Plutchik Suicide Risk Scale [16]. Among these, only the Plutchik Suicide Risk Scale has been validated within the Colombian context [17]. However, existing tools often present challenges, including excessive length, the need for specialized training, or potential inaccuracies in risk estimation, making them impractical in clinical settings.

Accurately assessing suicidal intent is crucial for evaluating both immediate and long-term risk of suicide. To date, the accuracy of suicide prediction models is inadequate [7]. To improve this situation, it is helpful to be guided by well-validated psychological theories, such as attitude formation. The tripartite model of attitudes (e.g., toward suicide or death) comprises three correlated but distinct components: affect, behavior, and cognition [18,19]. Evidence has shown that these are useful factors to measure the risk of current and future suicidal behaviors. The affective component encompasses hopelessness the wish to live (WTL) and the wish to die (WTD), which are considered part of a "motivational dimension" in suicidality [20–23]. The relationship between suicidality and affect is supported by mixed evidence. Cognitive aspects, such as death-related ideation and suicidal thoughts, are also predictors of suicide risk [23–28].

Behavioral components, such as past suicide attempts, are considered predictors of suicidality, though there is mixed evidence regarding their predictive strength. While some studies present past attempts as very strong predictors, others do not find an association that is as robust. Additionally, non-suicidal self-harm (NSSH) has not been shown to provide additional predictive value when included in models that already account for suicidal cognition and behaviors [27,29–38]. Suicidality, viewed as a latent trait, reflects the interplay of these dimensions.

The Suicidal Affect–Behaviors–Cognition Scale (SABCS) is grounded in the tripartite model. Developed using item response theory (IRT), the SABCS assesses suicidality as a unidimensional construct encompassing affective, behavioral, and cognitive dimensions. It has demonstrated high internal consistency and strong construct validity, and has been validated across diverse populations [39].

Based on its strong psychometrics, we aimed to validate the SABCS to assess suicide risk in Hispanic populations. However, the six-item SABCS was recently part of a large psychometric project, which resulted in the development of the eight-item Suicidality Scale (SS) [39], including items on past suicide attempts and WTL. The SS studies showed that the behavioral items did not function well across broad and diverse samples. Only a behavioral intention item—on the possibility of future suicide attempts—demonstrated strong validity for inclusion in a clinically useful risk assessment. The final eight-item SS demonstrated strong psychometric properties across ages 13–80, genders, and other demographic variables, with no evidence of differential item functioning (DIF).

The present study aimed to test the validity of the SS in Hispanic communities and psychiatric samples in Colombia. After a critical evaluation of the ensemble of items and their relevance for the local population, the decision was made to develop and validate a culturally and Spanish language-adapted suicide risk assessment (SRA) based on the SS. As a distinct construct, the resulting eight-item Spanish Suicidality Scale (S-SS) struck a balance between being a brief, easy-to-administer tool and being sufficiently precise to capture key elements of suicide risk without overwhelming the evaluator with additional questions. The S-SS will be made freely available through Creative Commons BY (free culture) licensing.

2. Materials and Methods

2.1. Ethics and Open Science

This study complied with the ethical standards outlined by national and institutional human experimentation committees and the Helsinki Declaration of 1975, revised in 2008. Ethical approval was granted by the Ethics Committee of Universidad de Caldas

(ACTA No 003 de 2021, consecutive number CBCS-007). The research further adhered to Colombian guidelines for human research [40] and the World Medical Association's Declaration of Helsinki [41].

Aligned with open science principles and the United Nations Sustainable Development Goals [11], this study aims to promote equitable access to scientific findings. The data and analysis code are openly accessible at https://osf.io/fze6j/ (accessed on 22 July 2023).

Funding was provided by the Territorial de Salud de Caldas, which did not influence the study's design, implementation, or reporting, thereby ensuring no conflicts of interest.

2.2. Recruitment and Administration

Participants were recruited in person between March and June 2021. After providing informed consent, they completed the SS-S and demographic questions. The self-report questionnaire required less than five minutes, and no incentives were provided for participation.

All participants underwent semi-structured psychiatric evaluations conducted by licensed psychiatrists or psychiatric residents. They were classified as "diagnosed" if they met the criteria for at least one mental health disorder according to the DSM-5 criteria, while those who did not were categorized as "non-diagnosed." If, during the assessment, any participant was identified as being at risk of suicide, regardless of their psychiatric diagnosis, they were referred for further evaluation by the team to determine the necessary interventions.

Privacy was protected through the assignment of unique identifiers.

2.3. Design and Procedure

This study used a cross-sectional descriptive design to validate the SRA tailored to the Colombian population. As outlined in Figure 1, the methodological framework encompassed scale selection, translation, cultural adaptation, and validation through community and clinical testing. Data collection included the administration of the SRA and a comprehensive evaluation of psychometric properties.

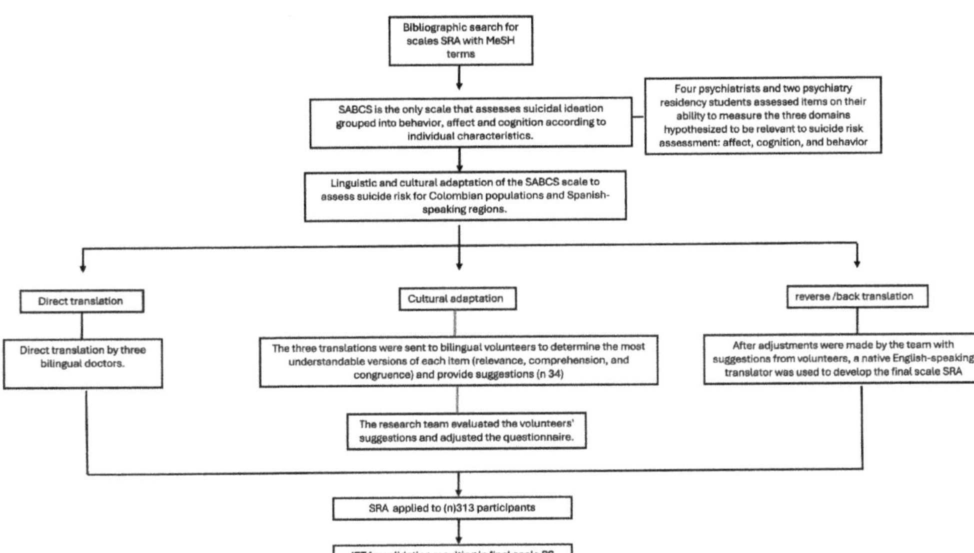

Figure 1. Study design and procedure flowchart. The methodological framework for validating the SS (Suicidality Scale) [39].

2.4. Translation and Adaptation

The SRA included the eight-item SS and two supplementary items. It was translated and culturally adapted to ensure relevance for Spanish-speaking communities.

A committee of six mental health experts (four psychiatrists and two psychiatry residents) evaluated the SRA, composed of the eight-item SS and two supplementary items (history of suicide attempts and wish to live), for their ability to measure affect, cognition, and behavior.

Direct translations were performed by three bilingual clinicians and refined based on feedback from 34 volunteers, who rated item clarity and validity. Suggestions were incorporated, and the final questionnaire underwent back-translation by a native-English-speaking translator. We similarly verified the linguistic equivalence to Colombian–Spanish. A sample of over 300 participants was selected for initial validation, following [42].

Development of the SS found that suicidal behaviors were not of sufficient value for assessing current risk at the population level. Nevertheless, the authors recommended including behavior items for supplementary information. The SS demonstrated strong psychometric properties and validity across individuals with English as a first or second language, gender, and those ages 13–80. The SS can be applied by clinicians, people without clinical training, or can be self-administered and includes descriptions of suicidality levels based on IRT analyses. For this study, we included the eight cognitive and affective SS items, plus two supplementary items: past suicide attempts (Attempt), ranging from none to "at least once really wanted to die"; and wish to live (WTL), a reverse-scored polar opposite to the wish to die (WTD) item included in the SS. We aimed to critically examine the validity of all items, including supplementary items, for inclusion in a final Spanish SS. See Appendix A for total items and responses.

2.5. Clinical Ratings

Evaluations for clinical participants were conducted by licensed psychiatrists and psychiatry residents who classified participants into predefined suicide risk categories based on gatekeeper training protocols and professional expertise. Among the 313 participants, 1.6% were categorized as ultra-high risk, 14.1% as high risk, 13.1% as moderate risk, 19.5% as low risk, and 55.3% as having no identifiable risk.

2.6. Analyses

We used the R psych package to conduct a multimodel approach to evaluate the SRA items and scale critically. Analyses included minimum residual factor analysis (FA, direct oblimin rotation), which produces an unweighted least squares solution that is robust for skewed data [43]. This included common variance, item communalities (h2), factor loadings, and model fit (Tucker–Lewis Index, TLI; root mean square error of approximation, RMSEA). Hierarchical cluster analysis and bifactor analysis also included model fit, error, and item loadings. We calculated McDonald's omega (ω), bootstrapped 1000 iterations, as a robust estimate of internal consistency for congeneric scales [44]. For IRT analyses, we used the graded response model [45–47]. Analyses were conducted with the open-source R statistical environment, v.4.2.0 [48] including the following packages: ltm [49], lordif [50], and coefficient alpha [51].

We also tested item monotonicity and linearity through rest-score plots [52]. Graded response model (GRM) analyses also led to creating individual person scores derived from empirical Bayesian estimates [49]. These IRT-derived theta values are based on unique item characteristics and response patterns. In contrast, traditional sum scores assume all items are equally weighted and all item steps are equivalent. We examined invariance by demographics (e.g., age, sex, residence) and clinical factors (psychiatric diagnosis) through differential item functioning (DIF). DIF is recommended over confirmatory factor analysis (CFA) and other invariance tests [53]. The lordif package uses GRM modeling to detect evidence of DIF through R^2 change ($\geq$0.02).

3. Results

The SRA, including the SS along with the clinical evaluation, was administered to all 313 participants. Demographic characteristics of the participants included an age range of 18–65 years (M = 35.29), with 42% female and 58% male. The sample was composed of single people, followed by smaller proportions who were married, cohabitating, separated, divorced, or widowed. The majority of participants identified as Mestizo (nearly 95%), with smaller groups identifying as White, Mulatto, Indigenous, or Afro-Colombian. About four out of five participants lived in urban areas, while the remainder resided in rural settings. Socioeconomic status was predominantly concentrated in the middle–lower range, with nearly three-quarters falling within social strata 2 and 3 on Colombia's six-tier classification system.

3.1. Psychometric Properties and Scale Reliability

The SS included eight core items assessing suicidality and two supplementary items—Attempt and wish to live. Table 1 shows that core items demonstrated consistent variability and near-normal distributions, supporting their reliability. In contrast, WTL and Attempt showed greater variability and deviation from normality, with WTL displaying moderate skewness and kurtosis and Attempt contributing less to scale reliability. SS person scores demonstrated lower skewness and kurtosis. Individual standard residuals ranged from −0.87 to 2.87 and can be found in the data file with the other data at https://osf.io/fze6j/ (accessed on day 22 July 2023).

Table 1. Suicidality Scale and item characteristics (N = 313).

Item/Scale	Range	*M*	*SD*	Skew	Kurtosis
DKS	1–6	1.59	1.25	2.16	6.63
WTD	1–6	1.89	1.57	1.58	4.09
Dead	1–6	2.16	1.76	1.26	3.03
Debate	1–6	2.72	1.79	1.11	2.73
Ideation	1–6	1.95	1.61	1.55	4.05
Predict	1–6	1.63	1.26	2.14	6.69
Meaning	1–6	2.33	1.84	1.06	2.57
RFD	1–6	1.59	1.23	2.19	6.89
SS sum	8–48	15.41	10.91	1.49	1.08
SS person	−0.80–3.08	0.10	1.04	0.94	−0.17
WTLr	1–6	1.88	1.55	1.57	4.06
Attempt	1–4	1.75	1.19	1.17	2.58

Note: SE skew (SES) = 0.14; SE kurtosis = 0.28. DKS = desire to kill self; WTD = wish to die; RFD = reason for dying; sum = sum score; person = graded response model-derived person score; SS = Suicidality Scale; WTLr = wish to live, reverse-scored.

We examined the psychometric properties of all ten SRA items. Table 2 contains the final SS item diagnostics of our four-step analyses. First, we tested the general unidimensionality and suitability of the items through these four different psychometric models, with a critical view of each item's specific properties. The analyses can be considered to be in order of sophistication, with cluster analyses providing general item and cluster properties and GRM providing the most advanced information. However, each test contributes unique and meaningful results that are useful for testing and confirming scale validity. Hierarchical cluster analysis showed high loadings across the eight final items and provided support for a unidimensional item set. Next, factor analysis (minimum residual) confirmed strong common factor loadings, a unidimensional item set, and strong commonalities, with one exception. RFD showed a somewhat low communality (<0.60) but was still moderately strong. Bifactor analyses further supported a unidimensional model, with high loadings and communalities and no evidence of meaningful subgroup factors.

Table 2. Colombian–Spanish Suicidality Scale item characteristics.

Item	Clus	FA		BA		GRM		
		L	h^2	g	h^2	LL	UL	a
Dead	0.91	0.91	0.83	0.87	0.90	0.29	1.69	3.68
Ideation	0.85	0.86	0.73	0.87	0.92	0.52	1.83	3.49
Debate	0.86	0.86	0.73	0.83	0.77	0.17	1.64	3.22
Predict	0.88	0.87	0.75	0.84	0.90	0.77	2.47	2.48
DKS	0.88	0.87	0.76	0.83	0.85	0.93	2.49	3.55
Meaning	0.85	0.85	0.72	0.81	0.81	0.07	1.47	3.13
WTD	0.91	0.92	0.84	0.87	0.83	0.60	2.05	3.57
RFD	0.77	0.77	0.59	0.72	0.63	1.00	2.91	2.80

Note: Clus = hierarchical cluster analysis; FA = minimum residual factor analysis; BA = bifactor analysis (Schmid–Leiman); L = common factor loading; g = general factor; h^2 = communalities; DKS = desire to kill self; WTD = wish to die; RFD = reason for dying.

GRM results showed that all items had high discrimination, other than Attempt. For WTL, discrimination was moderately high but below 2.0. These results indicate that the Attempt item does not make a sufficient contribution to measuring suicidality and that WTL is somewhat weaker than other items. We next conducted rest-score plots and found a lack of linearity between WTLr and other items, demonstrating that this item is related to the latent trait but inconsistent with others. Figure 2 shows the GRM item characteristic curves, illustrating the b values, with the area under each line representing the item's information function (the amount of information on the latent trait that that item provides).

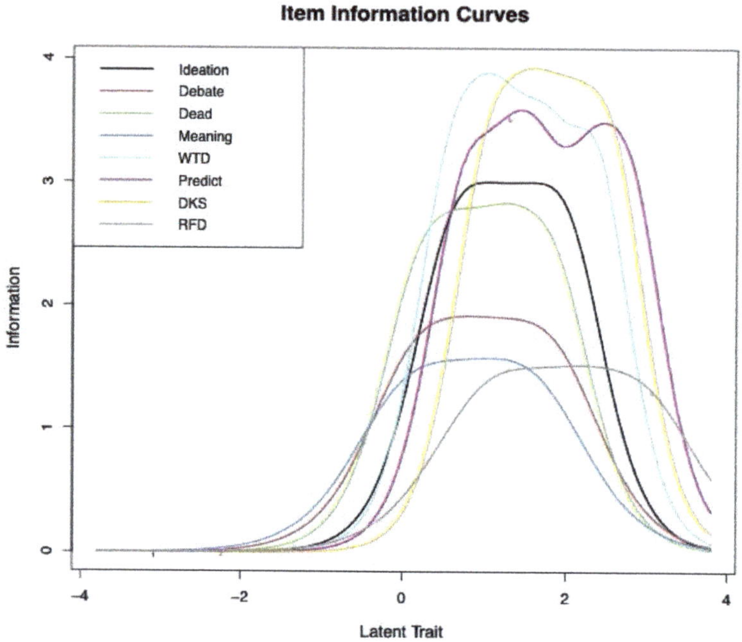

Figure 2. Suicidality Scale item characteristic curves.

3.2. Construct Validity

Exploratory factor analysis confirmed the unidimensionality of the SS. A single-factor solution accounted for 68.5% of the variance in suicidality, with most items achieving acceptable factor loadings (≥0.71). The Attempt item fell below acceptable thresholds, supporting its limited utility. High communalities further supported the scale's ability to encapsulate suicidality as a unified latent construct.

We further tested for group invariance to determine whether the SS exhibited any bias across groups. The results showed no differential item functioning (DIF) for gender or psychiatric diagnosis ($\Delta R^2 < 0.02$). Due to sample size and distribution limitations, DIF analyses for other variables were not conducted. Instead, we examined the SS across the full sample and by age groups. As shown in Table 3, diagnostics were nearly identical; all fit indices were very high, and error was reasonably low. All conditions similarly exhibited strong internal consistency.

Table 3. Colombian–Spanish Suicidality Scale diagnosis across ages.

Scale	Cluster			FA		BA			ω	95% CI
	Fit	RMSR	V	TLI	RMSEA	ω^h	ECV	RMSEA		
SS	0.98	0.05	0.74	0.88	0.19	0.89	0.84	0.08	0.96	[0.95, 0.96]
Age1	0.98	0.05	0.76	0.85	0.22	0.92	0.84	0.20	0.96	[0.95, 0.97]
Age2	0.98	0.06	0.75	0.83	0.23	0.87	0.80	0.03	0.96	[0.95, 0.96]
Age3	0.96	0.09	0.67	0.62	0.32	0.76	0.65	0.26	0.94	[0.56, 0.98]

Note: FA = minimum residual factor analysis; BA = bifactor analysis; RMSR = root mean square of residuals; TLI = Tucker–Lewis Index of factoring reliability; RMSEA = root mean square error of approximation; V = variance; ω^h = general factor variance; ECV = explained common variance; ω = internal consistency, bootstrapped 1000 iterations. SS = Suicidality Scale; Age1 = 18–25 (n = 93); Age2 = 26–49 (n = 158); Age3 = 50–84 (n = 64).

The SS performed well for younger age groups but showed lower factorability and higher error for participants over 50 years. This is likely due to the small subsample size but warrants further review.

3.3. Clinical and Test Evaluations

We then compared SS person scores and sum scores with clinical decisions for these participants. First, we tested for demographic confounds, finding small but statistically significant associations between SS scores with sex and age, with males and younger participants reporting higher suicidality (*ps* < 0.05). Bootstrapped partial correlations (controlling for sex and age) showed strong correlations between clinical assessments, made on a five-point ordered categorical scale, with SS sum scores with r = 0.82, 95% CI [0.78, 0.87] and SS person scores with r = 0.84, 95% CI [0.79, 0.88]. However, Figure 3 shows some important variance; clinical ratings matched sum scores and person scores at the non-risk and highest risk levels. However, clinical ratings appear to better match the person scores than the sum scores at the low to moderate risk levels.

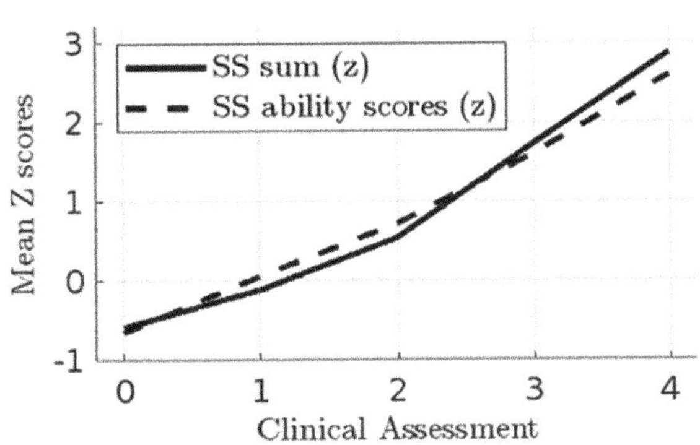

Figure 3. Correlations between clinical and Suicidality Scale assessments.

4. Discussion

Following the adaptation and field testing of Colombian–Spanish suicide risk assessment questions, we developed a concise, evidence-based Spanish Suicidality Scale (S-SS) designed for use in Hispanic communities. The SS has been validated across diverse populations, demonstrating strong psychometric properties in both clinical and community settings, as well as across different demographic groups and psychiatric diagnoses. Clinical evaluations showed strong correlations with S-SS scores while also identifying some important distinctions. These results highlight the S-SS's potential to guide clinical decision making by focusing on the most prevalent symptoms of suicidality, supported by this and additional evidence.

The S-SS offers several benefits. It can be used as a self-report and it does not require prior specialized training for application and interpretation, allowing it to be used in a variety of settings. However, an improved understanding of interpreting latent trait measures would be helpful across the mental health field. The S-SS is briefer, at eight items, compared to other tests. For example, the Self-Rated Scale For Suicide Ideation—SRSSI—includes 19 items [13]; the Modified Scale For Suicide Ideation—MSSI—has 18 items [14]; and the Plutchik scale, which is the only SRA previously validated in Colombia, has 26 items. This parsimony makes it more favorable for assessing risk in an emergency or primary care service where there is little time per consultation [17]. The SS and S-SS present as a unique construct, evaluating three dimensions of suicide: affect (e.g., Wish to die), behavioral intentions (Predict), and cognition (e.g., Debate). In addition, other scales (e.g., SADPERSONS) apparently overestimate suicide risk, leading to the hospitalization of patients who do not require it [15,54].

To make the best use of our data, we utilized IRT and bifactor analysis, and conducted DIF. These analytical approaches provide deeper insights into the latent trait under investigation [55]. IRT-derived person (ability) scores enable precise identification of an individual's position on the underlying suicidality continuum. Additionally, these methods help determine which questions yield the most informative responses, allowing for greater emphasis on those items when assessing suicide risk.

We tested ten items, but after reviewing multimodel analyses, we found that items related to previous suicide attempts and WTL provided less information on the latent trait of suicide. These items were not invalid, but they did not perform well across a broad sample. There are likely two different issues here. First, suicidal behaviors are rare and, therefore, most people respond "no" to such items, while those who respond "yes" may have attempted or planned suicide years ago but are now mentally healthy and not suicidal. That reduces the benefit of such an item other than for important biographical information. Secondly, reverse-scored items sometimes fail to function well. The WTL item showed weakness across our psychometric analyses, similar to that of the larger SS study [39]. It could be that WTL is capturing information on a trait that is related but distinct to suicidality.

However, the suicide attempts item, in particular and along with a suicide plans item, can provide valuable additional biographic data. While that data can aid the understanding and treatment of patients, those items did not demonstrate sufficient validity for inclusion in scale scores. Once removed, the fit indices for the 8-item version were higher than for the 10-item version, showing that their removal contributes to a better fit of the model data, consistent with the English and Chinese studies [39].

It was notable that the clinician ratings corresponded better to the IRT-derived person scores than to sum scores. There was strong agreement at the lowest and highest risk levels, but it seems clinicians are picking up on additional information to make their decisions at low to moderate risk levels. That appears to offer some validation for the accuracy of person scores over the simple summing of all items.

Limitations

There are important limitations to this study, such as sample size and the need for testing mid- and long-term suicidal outcomes through longitudinal study. However, the greatest limitation may be in deciding how patients should be placed into outcome categories, ranging from immediate discharge to emergency care. SS cutoff scores (e.g., low risk, moderate risk, or high risk) are very appealing, and many scales include them. However, this study and all known studies on suicide measurement have demonstrated that such cutoff values are built on false assumptions, as scale items demonstrate varying weights, discrimination levels, etc. There are, fortunately, highly useful means for making the most of these instruments.

Scores should serve as a guide rather than dictate clinical decisions. The S-SS is most effective in a comprehensive evaluation, with scores interpreted along a spectrum. Low scores generally suggest low or no suicidality, high scores indicate severe risk necessitating immediate intervention, and intermediate scores call for careful clinical judgment. This approach avoids rigid reliance on arbitrary cutoffs while leveraging the scale's strengths. Furthermore, the self-report S-SS is designed to be accessible, eliminating the need for literacy or specialized training in interviewer-administered protocols, making it suitable for use in developing regions. Importantly, the clinician-administered SS has proven effective, with no reported issues.

5. Conclusions

The S-SS showed strong psychometrics and represents a step forward in accurate risk assessment for adults and diverse populations. Importantly, the S-SS was developed through community involvement as a localized instrument. It is not enough to create a high-quality tool; local knowledge and skills are required for sustainable use and future development. The S-SS is free culture licensed, allowing for free use and modification. This can aid communities and individuals who require high-quality risk assessments but who have limited resources.

The S-SS is a valuable tool for monitoring therapeutic progress. Administering the scale at multiple intervals allows clinicians to track changes in risk levels following psychotherapeutic or pharmacological interventions. This functionality supports tailored adjustments to care and provides insights into treatment effectiveness. While more longitudinal studies are needed to assess the scale's utility in shaping treatment directions, its dual role in initial risk assessment and ongoing evaluation can enhance clinical outcomes and promote sustained mental health recovery.

Our study suggests that the SS-S should be evaluated in additional demographic subgroups and compared with other suicide instruments validated in Central and South America. It is also important to study suicide risk assessment in younger age groups. Despite the fact that suicide risk is a very difficult health factor to assess, with the validation of this scale, we come a little closer to understanding this mental health problem.

Author Contributions: Conceptualization, J.C.C.N. and D.M.V.H.; methodology, A.M.A.D., K.P.A. and Ó.M.C.R.; software, K.M.H.; validation, A.M.A.D. and K.P.A.; formal analysis, K.M.H., A.M.A.D. and K.P.A.; investigation, A.M.A.D., K.P.A., P.V.d.E. and S.G.G.; resources, A.M.A.D. and K.P.A.; data curation, A.M.A.D., K.P.A., P.V.d.E. and S.G.G.; writing—original draft preparation, A.M.A.D. and K.P.A.; writing—review and editing, K.M.H. and Ó.M.C.R.; visualization, A.M.A.D., K.P.A. and Ó.M.C.R.; supervision, Ó.M.C.R. and D.M.V.H.; project administration, A.M.A.D. and K.P.A.; funding acquisition, Ó.M.C.R. All authors have read and agreed to the published version of the manuscript.

Funding: This research was partly funded by Dirección Territorial de Salud de Caldas, Caldas, Colombia (150.25.4.0327 de 2021). The funding agency played no role in the research methods or analyses.

Institutional Review Board Statement: The study was conducted in accordance with the Declaration of Helsinki and approved by the Ethics Committee of Facultad de Ciencias para la Salud, Universidad de Caldas (Consecutive CBCS-007, 3 March 2021).

Informed Consent Statement: Consent was obtained from all subjects involved in the study.

Data Availability Statement: The original contributions presented in the study are included in the article, further inquiries can be directed to the corresponding author/s.

Acknowledgments: We would like to acknowledge the contributions of Dirección Territorial de Salud de Caldas, Clínica San Juan de Dios de Manizales, and Universidad de Caldas for their assistance on earlier parts of the project.

Conflicts of Interest: The authors declare that there are no conflicts of interest.

Appendix A

ESCALA COLOMBIANA DE RIESGO DE SUICIDIO

Nos gustaría hacerte algunas preguntas personales relacionadas con el suicidio. Por favor respóndelas de la manera más precisa posible.

PREGUNTA 1: ¿Con qué frecuencia has pensado en suicidarte durante el último año?

- Nunca (1) (2) (3) (4) (5) (6) Muy frecuentemente.

PREGUNTA 2: Recientemente, ¿has tenido una discusión interna (en tu cabeza) acerca de vivir o morir?

- Nunca (1) (2) (3) (4) (5) (6) Muy Frecuentemente.

PREGUNTA 3: Últimamente, ¿has tenido pensamientos acerca de que estarías mejor muerto(a)?

- Nunca. (1) (2) (3) (4) (5) (6) Muy Frecuentemente.

PREGUNTA 4: ¿Recientemente, has tenido el sentimiento de que tu vida no tiene sentido?

- Nunca (1) (2) (3) (4) (5) (6) Muy Frecuentemente.

PREGUNTA 5: Recientemente, ¿qué tanto has deseado morir?

- No deseo para nada morir (1) (2) (3) (4) (5) (6) Mucho.

PREGUNTA 6: ¿Qué tan probable es que en el futuro cercano intentes suicidarte?

- No hay ninguna probabilidad (1) (2) (3) (4) (5) (6) Es muy probable.

PREGUNTA 7: En una escala del 1 al 6 siendo 1 la ausencia de deseos de suicidarte, y 6 un deseo intenso de hacerlo ¿dónde te ubicas?

- No tengo deseos de suicidarme (1) (2) (3) (4) (5) (6) Tengo un deseo intenso de suicidarme.

PREGUNTA 8: En una escala del 1 al 6 evalúa, ¿qué tantas razones tienes para VIVIR o MORIR?

- Tengo más razones para VIVIR que para morir (1) (2) (3) (4) (5) (6) Tengo más para MORIR que para vivir.

References

1. World Health Organization. Global Health Estimates 2016: Deaths by Cause, Age, Sex, by Country and by Region, 2000–2016. Geneva. 2018. Available online: https://www.who.int/data/gho/data/themes/mortality-and-global-health-estimates (accessed on 22 July 2023).
2. Naghavi, M. Global, regional, and national burden of suicide mortality 1990 to 2016: Systematic analysis for the Global Burden of Disease Study 2016. *BMJ* **2019**, *364*, 194. [CrossRef] [PubMed]
3. World Health Organization. Suicide. 2024. Available online: https://www.who.int/news-room/fact-sheets/detail/suicide (accessed on 22 July 2023).
4. Chaparro-Narváez, P.; Díaz-Jiménez, D.; Castañeda-Orjuela, C. Tendencia de la mortalidad por suicidio en las áreas urbanas y rurales de Colombia, 1979–2014. *Biomédica* **2019**, *39*, 339–353. [CrossRef] [PubMed]
5. Instituto Nacional de Medicina Legal y Ciencias Forenses. Sistema de Información Clínica y Odontología Forense-SICLICO Forenses-Grupo Centro de Referencia Nacional Sobre Violencia. 2019. Available online: https://www.medicinalegal.gov.co/ (accessed on 22 July 2023).
6. Ayala García, J.; La salud en Colombia: Más cobertura, pero menos acceso [Internet]. Bogotá, Colombia: Banco de la República. 2014. Available online: https://www.banrep.gov.co/sites/default/files/publicaciones/archivos/dtser_204.pdf (accessed on 22 July 2023).

7. Castro Moreno, L.S.; Fuertes Valencia, L.F.; Pacheco García, O.E.; Muñoz Lozada, C.M. Risk factors associated with suicide attempt as predictors of suicide, Colombia, 2016–2017. *Rev. Colomb. Psiquiatr.* **2023**, *52*, 176–184. [CrossRef]
8. González Zapata, C. Factores de Riesgo para la Incidencia de Suicidio en la Región Cafetera de Colombia. 2022. Available online: https://repositorio.ucaldas.edu.co/handle/ucaldas/17604 (accessed on 15 June 2023).
9. Cañon-Ayala, M.J.; Perdomo-Jurado, Y.E.; Caro-Delgado, A.G. Spatiotemporal analysis of suicide attempts in Colombia from 2018 to 2020. *Cad. Saúde Pública* **2024**, *40*, e00119323. [CrossRef]
10. Arenas, Á.; Gómez-Restrepo, C.; Rondón, M. Factores asociados a la conducta suicida en Colombia. Resultados de la Encuesta Nacional de Salud Mental 2015. *Rev. Colomb. Psiquiatr.* **2016**, *45*, 68–75. [CrossRef]
11. United Nations General Assembly. Resolution adopted by the General Assembly on 25 September 2015. Transforming Our World: The 2030 Agenda for Sustainable Development (Resolution 70/1). New York. 2015. Available online: https://sdgs.un.org/2030agenda (accessed on 22 July 2023).
12. Beck, A.T.; Kovacs, M.; Weissman, A. Assessment of suicidal intention: The Scale for Suicide Ideation. *J. Consult. Clin. Psychol.* **1979**, *47*, 343–352. [CrossRef]
13. Beck, A.T.; Steer, R.A.; Ranieri, W.F. Scale for Suicide Ideation: Psychometric properties of a self-report version. *J. Clin. Psychol.* **1988**, *44*, 499–505. [CrossRef] [PubMed]
14. Miller, I.W.; Norman, W.H.; Bishop, S.B.; Dow, M.G. The Modified Scale for Suicidal Ideation: Reliability and validity. *J. Consult. Clin. Psychol.* **1986**, *54*, 724–725. [CrossRef]
15. Patterson, W.M.; Dohn, H.H.; Bird, J.; Patterson, G.A. Evaluation of suicidal patients: The SAD PERSONS scale. *Psychosomatics* **1983**, *24*, 343–349. [CrossRef]
16. Koslowsky, M.; Bleich, A.; Greenspoon, A.; Wagner, B.; Apter, A.; Solomon, Z. Assessing the validity of the Plutchik Suicide Risk Scale. *J. Psychiatr. Res.* **1991**, *25*, 155–158. [CrossRef]
17. Rangel-Garzón, C.X.; Suárez-Beltrán, M.F.; Escobar-Córdoba, F. Escalas de evaluación de riesgo suicida en atención primaria. *Rev. La Fac. Med. Univ. Nac.* **2015**, *63*, 707–716. [CrossRef]
18. Eagly, A.H.; Chaiken, S. *The Psychology of Attitudes*; Harcourt Brace Jovanovich College: Fort Worth, TX, USA, 1993.
19. Harris, K.M.; Syu, J.-J.; Lello, O.D.; Chew, Y.L.E.; Willcox, C.H.; Ho, R.H.M. The ABC's of suicide risk assesment: Applying a tripartite approach to individial evaluations. *PLoS ONE* **2015**, *10*, e0127442. [CrossRef] [PubMed]
20. Beck, A.T.; Brown, G.; Berchick, R.J.; Stewart, B.L.; Steer, R.A. Relationship between hopelessness and ultimate suicide: A replication with psychiatric outpatients. *Am. J. Psychiatry* **1990**, *147*, 190–195. [CrossRef]
21. Beck, A.T.; Kovacs, M.; Weissman, A. Hopelessness and suicidal behavior. An overview. *JAMA* **1975**, *234*, 1146–1149. [CrossRef]
22. Kovacs, M.; Beck, A.T. Maladaptive cognitive structures in depression. *Am. J. Psychiatry* **1978**, *35*, 525–533. [CrossRef]
23. Baca-Garcia, E.; Perez-Rodriguez, M.M.; Oquendo, M.A.; Keyes, K.M.; Hasin, D.S.; Grant, B.F.; Blanco, C. Estimating risk for suicide attempt: Are we asking the right questions? Passive suicidal ideation as a marker for suicidal behavior. *J. Affect. Disord.* **2011**, *134*, 327–332. [CrossRef]
24. Michel, K.; Maltsberger, J.T.; Jobes, D.A.; Leenaars, A.A.; Orbach, I.; Stadler, K.; Dey, P.; Young, R.A.; Valach, L. Discovering the truth in attempted suicide. *Am. J. Psychother.* **2002**, *56*, 424–437. [CrossRef]
25. Winters, N.C.; Myers, K.; Proud, L. Ten-year review of rating scales. III: Scales assessing suicidality, cognitive style, and self-esteem. *J. Am. Acad. Child Adolesc. Psychiatry* **2002**, *41*, 1150–1181. [CrossRef]
26. Shneidman, E.S. The suicidal mind. In *Review of Suicidology*; Maris, R.W., Silverman, M.M., Canetto, S.S., Eds.; Guilford Press: New York, NY, USA, 1997; pp. 22–41.
27. Horwitz, A.G.; Czyz, E.K.; King, C.A. Predicting Future Suicide Attempts Among Adolescent and Emerging Adult Psychiatric Emergency Patients. *J. Clin. Child Adolesc. Psychol.* **2014**, *44*, 751–761. [CrossRef]
28. Brown, G.K.; Beck, A.T.; Steer, R.A.; Grisham, J.R. Risk factors for suicide in psychiatric outpatients: A 20-year prospective study. *J. Consult. Clin. Psychol.* **2000**, *68*, 371–377. [CrossRef]
29. Tran, T.; Luo, W.; Phung, D.; Harvey, R.; Berk, M.; Kennedy, R.L.; Venkatesh, S. Risk stratification using data from electronic medical records better predicts suicide risks than clinician assessments. *BMC Psychiatry* **2014**, *14*, 76. [CrossRef] [PubMed]
30. Bilén, K.; Ottosson, C.; Castrén, M.; Ponzer, S.; Ursing, C.; Ranta, P.; Ekdahl, K.; Pettersson, H. Deliberate self-harm patients in the emergency department: Factors associated with repeated self-harm among 1524 patients. *Emerg. Med. J. EMJ* **2011**, *28*, 1019–1025. [CrossRef] [PubMed]
31. Harriss, L.; Hawton, K.; Zahl, D. Value of measuring suicidal intent in the assessment of people attending hospital following self-poisoning or self-injury. *Br. J. Psychiatry J. Ment. Sci.* **2005**, *186*, 60–66. [CrossRef] [PubMed]
32. Suokas, J.; Suominen, K.; Isometsä, E.; Ostamo, A.; Lönnqvist, J. Long-term risk factors for suicide mortality after attempted suicide--findings of a 14-year follow-up study. *Acta Psychiatr. Scand.* **2001**, *104*, 117–121. [CrossRef]
33. Osman, A.; Bagge, C.L.; Gutierrez, P.M.; Konick, L.C.; Kopper, B.A.; Barrios, F.X. The Suicidal Behaviors Questionnaire-Revised (SBQ-R): Validation with clinical and nonclinical samples. *Assessment* **2001**, *8*, 443–454. [CrossRef]
34. Beck, R.W.; Morris, J.B.; Beck, A.T. Cross-validation of the Suicidal Intent Scale. *Psychol. Rep.* **1974**, *34*, 445–446. [CrossRef]
35. Kovacs, M.; Beck, A.T.; Weissman, A. The communication of suicidal intent. A reexamination. *Arch. Gen. Psychiatry* **1976**, *33*, 198–201. [CrossRef]

36. Misson, H.; Mathieu, F.; Jollant, F.; Yon, L.; Guillaume, S.; Parmentier, C.; Raust, A.; Jaussent, I.; Slama, F.; Leboyer, M.; et al. Factor analyses of the Suicidal Intent Scale (SIS) and the Risk-Rescue Rating Scale (RRRS): Toward the identification of homogeneous subgroups of suicidal behaviors. *J. Affect. Disord.* **2010**, *121*, 80–87. [CrossRef]
37. Hubers, A.A.M.; Moaddine, S.; Peersmann, S.H.M.; Stijnen, T.; van Duijn, E.; van der Mast, R.C.; Dekkers, O.M.; Giltay, E.J. Suicidal ideation and subsequent completed suicide in both psychiatric and non-psychiatric populations: A meta-analysis. Epidemiol. *Psychiatr. Sci.* **2018**, *27*, 186–198. [CrossRef]
38. Demesmaeker, A.; Chazard, E.; Hoang, A.; Vaiva, G.; Amad, A. Suicide mortality after a nonfatal suicide attempt: A systematic review and meta-analysis. *Aust. N. Z. J. Psychiatry* **2022**, *56*, 603–616. [CrossRef]
39. Harris, K.M.; Wang, L.; Mu, G.M.; Lu, Y.; So, C.; Zhang, W.; Ma, J.; Liu, K.; Wang, W.; Zhang, M.W.-b.; et al. Measuring the suicidal mind: The 'open source' Suicidality Scale, for adolescents and adults. *PLoS ONE* **2023**, *18*, e0282009. [CrossRef] [PubMed]
40. Ministerio de Salud. Resolución 8430 de 1993. Ministerio de Salud y Protección Social, República de Colombia. 1993; pp. 1–19. Available online: https://www.minsalud.gov.co/sites/rid/Lists/BibliotecaDigital/RIDE/DE/DIJ/RESOLUCION-8430-DE-1993.PDF (accessed on 22 July 2023).
41. World Medical Association. World Medical Association Declaration of Helsinki: Ethical principles for medical research involving human subjects. *JAMA* **2013**, *310*, 2191–2194. [CrossRef] [PubMed]
42. Clark, L.A.; Watson, D. Constructing validity: Basic issues in objective scale development. *Psychol. Assess.* **1995**, *7*, 309–319. [CrossRef]
43. Flora, D.B.; LaBrish, C.; Chalmers, R.P. Old and new ideas for data screening and assumption testing for exploratory and confirmatory factor analysis. *Front. Psychol.* **2012**, *3*, 55. [CrossRef] [PubMed]
44. Revelle, W.; Zinbarg, R.E. Coefficients alpha, beta, omega, and the glb: Comments on Sijtsma. *Psychometrika* **2009**, *74*, 145–154. [CrossRef]
45. Samejima, F. Graded response model. In *Encyclopedia of Social Measurement*; Kempf-Leonard, K., Ed.; Academic Press: Cambridge, MA, USA, 2004; pp. 77–82.
46. de Ayala, R.J. *The Theory and Practice of Item Response Theory*; Guilford Press: New York, NY, USA, 2009.
47. Embretson, S.E.; Reise, S.P. *Item Response Theory for Psychologists*; Lawrence Erlbaum Associates, Inc.: Mahwah, NJ, USA, 2000.
48. R Core Team. *R: A Language and Environment for Statistical Computing*; Version 4.1.1; R Foundation for Statistical Computing: Vienna, Austria, 2021. Available online: https://www.R-project.org (accessed on 22 July 2023).
49. Rizopoulos, D. ltm: An R Package for Latent Variable Modeling and Item Response Analysis. *J. Stat. Softw.* **2006**, *17*, 1–25. [CrossRef]
50. Choi, S.W.; Gibbons, L.E.; Crane, P.K. lordif: An R Package for Detecting Differential Item Functioning Using Iterative Hybrid Ordinal Logistic Regression/Item Response Theory and Monte Carlo Simulations. *J. Stat. Softw.* **2011**, *39*, 1–30. [CrossRef]
51. Zhang, Z.; Yuan, K.-H. Robust coefficients alpha and omega and confidence intervals with outlying observations and missing data: Methods and software. *Educ. Psychol. Meas.* **2016**, *76*, 387–411. [CrossRef]
52. Meijer, R.R.; Egberink, I.J.L. Investigating invariant item ordering in personality and clinical scales: Some empirical findings and a discussion. *Educ. Psychol. Meas.* **2012**, *72*, 589–607. [CrossRef]
53. Meade, A.W.; Lautenschlager, G.J. A Comparison of Item Response Theory and Confirmatory Factor Analytic Methodologies for Establishing Measurement Equivalence/Invariance. *Organ. Res. Methods* **2004**, *7*, 361–388. [CrossRef]
54. Bullard, M.J. Problems of suicide risk management in the emergency department without fixed, full-time emergency physician. Chang. *Yi Xue Za Zhi* **1993**, *16*, 30–38.
55. Hays, R.D.; Morales, L.S.; Reise, S.P. Item response theory and health outcomes measurement in the 21st century. *Med. Care* **2000**, *38* (Suppl. 9), II28–II42. [CrossRef] [PubMed]

Journal of
Clinical Medicine

MDPI

Article

Suicidal Thoughts and Behaviors Among Health Care Trainees, Staff and Faculty at an Academic Medical Center

Sijia Zhang [1,*], Sidney Zisook [2], Judy Davidson [3], Desiree Shapiro [2] and Neal Doran [2,4]

1 School of Medicine, University of California, San Diego, CA 92093, USA
2 Department of Psychiatry, University of California, San Diego, CA 92093, USA; szisook@health.ucsd.edu (S.Z.); dlshapiro@health.ucsd.edu (D.S.); nmdoran@health.ucsd.edu (N.D.)
3 Health Sciences, University of California, San Diego, CA 92121, USA; jdavidson@health.ucsd.edu
4 Mental Health Care Line, VA San Diego Healthcare System, San Diego, CA 92161, USA
* Correspondence: siz004@health.ucsd.edu

Abstract: Background/Objectives: Health care workers are at greater risk for death by suicide compared to the general population and are less likely to seek assistance. More information about correlates of suicidality and treatment-seeking behavior are needed to reduce risk. **Methods**: The American Foundation for Suicide Prevention developed an Interactive Screening Program to identify and engage at-risk staff and trainees in health care settings. The study reports on the prevalence and demographic and clinical predictors of current suicidal thoughts, behaviors and mental health treatment at a single site (n = 5898) from 2009 to 2024. **Results**: The study found that 18.2% of respondents reported current suicidal thoughts and behaviors. These were more common among respondents who were younger, male, and who identified as a race/ethnicity other than non-Hispanic White. Suicidal thoughts and behaviors were more likely among those with higher PHQ-8 scores ($OR = 1.23$, $p < 0.01$) and those who endorsed maladaptive coping behaviors, hopelessness, loneliness, stress and nervousness (*OR*s 1.36–3.04, *p*s < 0.01). Current mental health treatment was more likely among women, non-Hispanic White respondents compared with Asian or Pacific Islander respondents, and nurses relative to physicians. Mental health treatment was also associated with higher PHQ-8 scores, lifetime suicide attempts, difficulty controlling eating and alcohol consumption, and recent feelings of anxiety, stress and nervousness. **Conclusions**: Findings suggest a continued need to identify and engage health care trainees and staff who are at risk for suicide and to establish new approaches to linking these individuals to resources or interventions aimed at reducing risk. The study identified male and/or Asian/Pacific Islander-identifying health care workers who reported intense loneliness and/or hopelessness, use of non-prescription drugs and recent suicidal thoughts and/or behaviors as high-risk individuals who may require enhanced methods of outreach, identification, acceptance and accessibility of treatment.

Keywords: suicide; suicide risk; depression; intense affective states; health care workforce; mental health care; workplace wellness

1. Introduction

Most people who experience suicidal ideation (SI) do not die by suicide and many individuals who die by suicide have never reported SI [1]. However, failure to identify SI may be a missed opportunity for prevention, especially when SI occurs in the context of other risk factors. One known risk for suicide is occupation [2], and the health care workforce is an "at-risk" group [3–5]. Substance use, intense affective states, untreated depression and suicidal thoughts and behaviors are highly prevalent among those who learn and work in health care settings, including students, physicians, nurses and other members of the health care workforce. Each of these conditions, in turn, increases the risk for suicide [6]. However, most health care trainees and workers struggling with mental health concerns do not seek the support they need [7,8].

The American Foundation for Suicide Prevention's (AFSP) Interactive Screening Program (ISP) was developed to screen medical students, trainees, health staff and physicians for distress and suicide risk, to engage those at risk and to offer a confidential way for them to connect with mental health services [9,10]. Individuals are invited to complete a brief, web-based, anonymous stress and depression questionnaire, after which they receive a personalized response from a mental-health-trained counselor. An evaluation of six medical schools using the ISP reported that 98% of 1413 participants (medical students, residents and faculty physicians) were designated as having high or moderate distress, yet only 5% were receiving counseling or therapy [9]. A report on nurses using the ISP found similarly alarming rates of high distress and insufficient mental health treatment [11]. Thus, there remains an urgent need to identify health care workers at risk and connect them with appropriate resources.

There are limited existing studies identifying the risk factors for suicidal thoughts and behaviors among health care trainees and staff. This report describes suicidal thoughts and behaviors and mental health treatment of health care students, trainees, staff and faculty who participated in the UC San Diego screening program from 1 May 2009 through 14 June 2024. Previous reports from this institution have documented high rates of depression, burnout and suicidal ideation among medical students, house staff, faculty and nurses, and low rates of mental health care even among those at highest risk [12–15]. Over time, the program has dramatically increased participation, expanded services to additional health care workers and has weathered the COVID-19 storm. In this report, we explore differences in the frequency of suicidal thoughts and behaviors and the utilization of mental health resources among various sub-groups in our health care trainee and worker population who completed the screening questionnaire. We provide a novel examination of a broad range of predictors for suicidal thoughts and behaviors among health care trainees and workers, including demographics, professional role, intense affective states and maladaptive coping behaviors. Our ultimate goal is to identify actionable targets for suicide prevention among the vulnerable health care community.

2. Materials and Methods

2.1. Overview

The AFSP's ISP has been the key component of UC San Diego's health care workforce suicide prevention program since 2009. The program's initial target audience included all faculty physicians, residents and medical students. In the second year of the program, 2010, it expanded to include pharmacy students. In 2016, there was a broader expansion that included nursing staff and the entire health system staff, from health professionals to support personnel. Email invitations describing the program were sent at least annually to health students, trainees, staff and faculty. The invitations assured recipients of its confidentiality, encouraged individuals to participate in the anonymous web-based screen and provided links to the Healer Education Assessment and Referral (HEAR) program website and the screening tool [10]. A Master's-level program counselor reviewed all questionnaire responses and directly responded to the participants with a customized response based on the level of distress, depression and/or suicide risk indicated by the participants' survey responses [10,16]. The UC San Diego Institutional Review Board (IRB) determined the project to be Not Human Subject Research and excluded the study from IRB review and waived the need for participant informed consent.

2.2. Participants

UC San Diego Health-affiliated physicians, nurses, trainees, students and other staff (e.g., pharmacists, social workers, allied health, hospital staff) who completed the online Stress and Depression Questionnaire between 1 May 2009 and 14 June 2024 (n = 5898) were included in our program evaluation. It is important to note that the HEAR Program was primarily developed as an outreach and education effort to destigmatize help-seeking and prevent suicide, and therefore those who chose to participate did so not for the purpose of research participation, but out of personal interest for services that the program provided.

2.3. Instrument

The HEAR Stress and Depression questionnaire contains the 9-item Patient Health Questionnaire (PHQ-9) [17]; measures of intense affective states (worrying, irritability, anxiety, loneliness, anger, etc.) that have been linked to depression with suicidal ideation; alcohol and drug use; disordered eating behaviors; current suicidal thoughts, behaviors, and past suicide attempts; self-harm; current psychiatric treatment; and age, gender, race or ethnicity. In order to optimize the anonymity of the questionnaire for respondents who were concerned, demographic questions were optional. A final optional item asked participants to provide an email address, which would be encrypted to facilitate anonymous communication with the program counselors through the website. All resulting data used for analysis were de-identified.

2.3.1. Suicidal Thoughts and Behaviors

Participants were asked questions including "during the last two weeks, how often have you...had thoughts about taking your own life? Planned ways of taking your life? Done things to hurt yourself?" Participants were asked to select a response from a four-point scale (0—not at all, 1—some of the time, 2—a lot of the time, 3—most or all the time). For our purposes, respondents were considered as currently having suicidal thoughts and behaviors if they gave a rating of 1 or higher (i.e., at least some of the time) on any of these three items, or on item 9 of the PHQ-9 ("having thoughts that you would be better off dead or thoughts of physically harming yourself" in the last two weeks) [18]. Additionally, respondents were asked if they had ever made a lifetime suicide attempt.

2.3.2. Depression Symptoms and Severity

Participants completed the nine-item Patient Health Questionnaire depression scale (PHQ-9) [17,19]. The PHQ-9 items mirror the Diagnostic and Statistical Manual, 5th edition (DSM-5) criteria for major depression [20]. Participants were asked to select a response from a 4-point scale (0—not at all, 1—some of the time, 2—a lot of the time, 3—most or all the time) that best describes how they felt during the past two weeks [17]. The severity of depression symptoms was operationalized as the sum of scores on the first eight items (PHQ-8); the ninth item evaluating thoughts of self-harm was excluded here because it was incorporated into the suicidal behaviors outcome as described above. The PHQ-8 has been found to be a valid and reliable measure of depression severity and has been found to be comparable to the PHQ-9 as a diagnostic measure for DSM-IV major depression [17]. Data from a representative sample of nearly 200,000 individuals in the United States support the value of the PHQ-8 in population studies [21].

2.3.3. Associated Intense Affective States

Participants were asked to rate on a four-point scale (0—not at all, 1—some of the time, 2—a lot of the time, 3—most or all the time) how often they experienced the following intense affective states over the past four weeks: "feeling nervous or worrying a lot; becoming easily annoyed or irritable; feeling your life is too stressful; having arguments or fights; feeling intensely anxious or having anxiety attacks; feeling intensely lonely; feeling intensely angry; feeling hopeless; feeling desperate; feeling out of control". Each of these affective states has been found to signal suicidal crisis in depressed patients [22]. Responses were transformed into binary variables reflecting low ("not at all" or "some of the time") versus high ("a lot of the time" or "most or all of the time") levels of each affective state.

2.3.4. Alcohol, Substance Use and Disordered Eating Behaviors

Participants were asked if they had engaged in or experienced the following over the past four weeks: "drinking alcohol (including beer or wine) more than usual; using drugs other than alcohol (marijuana, cocaine, etc.); feeling that you can't control what or how much you eat". Response options were given on a four-point scale (0—not at all, 1—some of the time, 2—a lot of the time, 3—most or all of the time). Responses were transformed into binary variables reflecting low ("not at all" or "some of the time") versus high ("a lot of the time" or "most or all of the time") levels of each behavior.

2.3.5. Current Mental Health Treatment

Participants were asked if they were currently taking prescribed medications for anxiety, depression or stress, and if they were receiving counseling or therapy. Responses were combined into a single binary item reflecting whether participants were receiving any mental health treatment or no treatment.

2.4. Procedure

Individuals who participated in the interactive screening program (ISP) created an anonymous online account to complete the survey. Following procedures previously described [16,23], once participants completed and submitted their surveys, a computer program automatically generated a PHQ-9 score and used this, along with responses to other items, to classify respondents into one of three tiers. Criteria for Tier 1 (high risk) included current suicidal thoughts and behaviors; a PHQ-9 score of 15 or higher with feelings of intense anxiety, anger, hopelessness, desperation, or feeling out of control "a lot of the time" or "most of the time" or feelings of nervousness, annoyance, stress, loneliness, or having arguments "most of the time"; and a PHQ-9 score of 10–14 with a history of prior suicide attempts, active problems related to alcohol or drug use, disordered eating behaviors or indications that current problems were making it somewhat difficult to function. Criteria for Tier 2 (moderate risk) included a PHQ-9 score of 10–14 without a history of suicide attempts or current suicidal thoughts and behaviors, problems related to alcohol or drug use or eating behavior or an indication that current problems were making it somewhat difficult to function. Respondents who did not meet any of these criteria were designated as Tier 3 (low risk). Tier classification determined the recommendations for further follow-up, evaluation and support provided to participants. Tier 1 designation is included in Table 1 for descriptive purposes, but the tier variable was not included in analyses in the current manuscript.

Table 1. Descriptive data for the HEAR Interactive Screening Program Stress and Depression Questionnaire, 1 May 2009 to 14 June 2024 (n = 5898).

	N	%
Depression severity		
PHQ-8 ≥ 10	2284	38.72
Maladaptive coping behaviors (occurring a lot or most or all the time over the past four weeks)		
drinking alcohol more than usual	399	6.77
using non-prescription drugs other than alcohol	74	1.25
unable to control eating	1018	17.26
Intense affective states (occurring a lot or most or all the time over the past four weeks)		
nervous	3045	51.63
annoyed	2500	42.39
stressed	2977	50.48
fighting	854	14.48
anxious	1552	26.32
lonely	1419	24.06
angry	772	13.09
hopeless	1165	19.75
desperate	860	14.58
out of control	1082	18.34
Suicidality		
wish to be dead (PHQ-9 item 9 scored as occurring some, a lot, most or all the time over the past 4 weeks)	936	15.87
suicidal thoughts occurring some, a lot, most or all the time over the past two weeks	613	10.39
suicide plans occurring some, a lot, most or all the time over the past two weeks	247	4.19
suicide attempts over the past two weeks	133	2.26
current suicidal thoughts and/or behaviors (endorse any wishes to be dead, thoughts, plans or attempts over the past two to four weeks)	1071	18.16
lifetime suicide attempts	343	5.82
designated tier 1 (high risk) *	3015	51.11
Current mental health treatment		
medication for depression, anxiety or stress	1176	19.94
mental health counseling or psychotherapy	801	13.58
medications and/or therapy	1580	26.79

* Tier 1: Current suicidal thoughts and behaviors; a PHQ-9 score of 15 or higher with feelings of intense anxiety, anger, hopelessness, desperation or feeling out of control "a lot of the time" or "most of the time" or feelings of nervousness, annoyance, stress, loneliness or having arguments "most of the time"; a PHQ-9 score of 10–14 with a history of prior suicide attempts, problems related to alcohol or drug use, disordered eating behaviors or indications that current problems were making it somewhat difficult to function.

2.5. Statistical Approach

Descriptive statistics were used to characterize the study sample. Separate binary logistic regression models were used to test the associations between four families of predictors (demographics, high-risk indicators, maladaptive coping behaviors and intense affective states) and two outcomes (current suicidal thoughts and behaviors, currently receiving mental health treatment). To reduce the potential for confounding, demographic predictors were included as covariates in models testing other families of predictors. Stata 17.0 (StataCorp LLP, College Station, TX, USA) was used for all analyses. Given the number of significance tests planned a priori, a family-wise alpha correction was used to adjust the alpha level for statistical significance to $p < 0.0125$.

3. Results

A total of 5898 participants completed the ISP questionnaire between 1 May 2009 and 14 June 2024. The mean age was 37 years, with 31.5% over the age of 40. Most respondents were female (70.7%). Approximately half identified as non-Hispanic White (50.6%), 17.9% as Asian or Pacific Islander, 10.9% as Latino, 2.5% as Black and 18.2% as "other" (includes American Indian or Alaskan native; multiracial; prefer not to answer). Almost one quarter of the participants were nurses (22.3%), while 16.8 % and 14.6% were residents and fellows, 11.5% medical students, 6.3% faculty or staff physicians, 5.26% pharmacy students and 38.8% "other" (PhD faculty; other faculty; pharmacists; other clinical and nonclinical staff, prefer not to answer; and no answer).

Assessing depression severity, the average PHQ-8 score was 8.6, which falls in the mild depression range. Over a third (38.7%) had a PHQ-8 score > 10 (at least moderately severe). The most frequently endorsed intense affective states were nervousness (51.6%), stressed (50.5%), and annoyed (42.4%). More than one quarter endorsed anxiety (26.3%) and almost that many felt intensely lonely (24.1%), while 19.8% felt hopeless and 14.6% desperate. Just over one quarter of all participants (26.8%) were receiving counseling, therapy or medication for depression, anxiety or stress at the time of completing the screening questionnaire. Detailed descriptive clinical and treatment data are shown in Table 1.

Table 2 provides data on the frequencies of current suicidal thoughts and behaviors, and designation as Tier 1 (high risk) by demographics, role in the health care system and depression severity. Of note, more than 50% of females (53.1%), Hispanics (58.0%), Asians/Pacific Islanders (55.8%), nurses (58.4%) and "other" (51.9%) were categorized as high risk. Fewer participants (but still a considerable number) endorsed current suicidal thoughts and/or behaviors, with 18.4% of those under 40 years of age, 19.5% males, 20.8% Asians/Pacific Islanders, 19.6% nurses, and 36% of those with a PHQ-8 score ≥ 10.

Table 2. Suicidal thoughts, behaviors and tiers by demographics, role and depression severity.

	Thoughts *N* = 613		**Plans** *N* = 247		**Actions** *N* = 133		**PHQ-9 Item 9** *N* = 936		**Current Suicidal Thoughts and/or Behaviors *** *N* = 1071		**Lifetime Attempts** *N* = 343		**Rated Tier 1 **** *N* = 3015	
	N	%	*N*	%	*N*	%	*N*	%	*N*	%	*N*	%	*N*	%
Age														
age < 40 years	366	10.54	129	3.72	87	2.51	569	16.39	638	18.39	212	6.11	1819	52.41
age ≥ 40 years	178	9.59	89	4.80	30	1.62	257	13.85	306	16.49	102	5.50	888	47.84

Table 2. *Cont.*

	Thoughts *N* = 613		**Plans** *N* = 247		**Actions** *N* = 133		**PHQ-9 Item 9** *N* = 936		**Current Suicidal Thoughts and/or Behaviors *** *N* = 1071		**Lifetime Attempts** *N* = 343		**Rated Tier 1 **** *N* = 3015	
Gender														
female	398	9.55	155	3.72	94	2.25	636	15.3	723	17.34	254	6.14	2215	53.13
male	188	12.1	78	5.02	33	2.12	259	16.7	303	19.49	72	4.66	691	44.44
Race														
Black	17	11.64	8	5.48	6	4.11	21	14.38	29	19.86	16	10.96	79	54.11
White	280	9.39	102	3.42	52	1.74	412	13.9	482	16.17	135	4.56	1395	46.80
Hispanic	74	11.5	32	4.99	15	2.34	116	18.1	127	19.81	48	7.58	372	58.03
Asian or Pacific Islander	116	11.0	49	4.64	30	2.84	200	19	219	20.76	77	7.35	589	55.83
other	126	11.72	56	5.21	30	2.79	187	17.4	214	19.91	67	6.23	580	53.95
Role														
medical student	66	9.72	23	3.39	16	2.36	81	12	96	14.14	16	2.36	264	38.88
pharmacy student	26	8.39	15	4.84	10	3.23	52	16.8	57	18.39	16	5.18	146	47.10
house staff	83	9.62	16	1.85	14	1.62	121	14	138	15.99	33	3.82	421	48.78
nursing	142	10.8	60	4.57	31	2.36	231	17.7	257	19.56	114	8.76	766	58.38
physician	31	8.38	8	2.16	4	1.08	42	11.4	51	13.78	2	5.41	150	40.54
other	256	11.2	120	5.25	54	2.36	394	17.3	454	19.85	155	6.87	1224	53.53
Depression severity														
PHQ-8 < 10	118	3.27	46	1.27	33	0.91	182	5.04	251	6.95	102	2.82	995	27.53
PHQ-8 ≥ 10	495	21.67	201	8.8	100	4.38	754	33.01	820	35.9	241	10.55	2020	88.44

* Thoughts, plans, actions and/or PHQ item 9. ** Current suicidal thoughts and behaviors; a PHQ-9 score of 15 or higher with feelings of intense anxiety, anger, hopelessness, desperation or feeling out of control "a lot of the time" or "most of the time" or feelings of nervousness, annoyance, stress, loneliness or having arguments "most of the time"; a PHQ-9 score of 10–14 with a history of prior suicide attempts, problems related to alcohol or drug use, disordered eating behaviors or indications that current problems were making it somewhat difficult to function.

Table 3 provides data on the frequencies of current mental health treatment (current medications for depression, anxiety and/or stress; current mental health counseling or psychotherapy; current medications and/or therapy) by demographics, role in the health care system and depression severity. Of note, only approximately one third of participants (35.9%) with a PHQ-8 score ≥ 10 reported current mental health treatment with medication and/or therapy. While 31.1% of Non-Hispanic White-identifying health care workers reported current mental health treatment, only 18.0% of Asian or Pacific Islander-identifying health care workers reported current mental health treatment.

Table 3. Current mental health treatment by demographics, role, and depression severity.

	Current Medication for Depression, Anxiety and/or Stress		**Current Mental Health Counseling or Psychotherapy**		**Current Medications and/or Therapy**	
	N	%	*N*	%	*N*	%
Demographics						
% age < 40 years	608	17.52	463	13.34	857	24.70
% age ≥ 40 years	463	24.95	272	14.66	585	31.52
% female	903	21.66	592	14.2	1198	28.74
% male	233	14.98	179	11.51	329	21.16
% Black/African American	30	20.55	18	12.33	37	25.34

Table 3. *Cont.*

	Current Medication for Depression, Anxiety and/or Stress		Current Mental Health Counseling or Psychotherapy		Current Medications and/or Therapy	
% White	712	23.88	438	14.69	926	31.06
% Hispanic	154	24.02	106	16.54	202	31.51
% Asian or Pacific Islander	112	10.62	115	10.9	190	18.01
% other	168	15.63	124	11.53	225	20.93
Role						
% medical student	75	11.05	98	14.43	137	20.18
% pharmacy student	34	10.97	35	11.29	53	17.1
% house staff	142	16.45	61	7.07	173	20.05
% nursing	348	26.52	211	9.23	451	34.38
% physician	64	17.3	37	10	85	22.97
% other	490	21.43	352	15.39	657	28.73
Depression Severity						
$ PHQ-8 < 10	512	14.17	419	11.59	761	21.06
% PHQ-8 ≥ 10	664	29.07	382	16.73	819	35.86

3.1. Prediction of Current Suicidal Thoughts and Behaviors

Nearly one in five participants (18.2%) endorsed at least one item reflecting current suicidal thoughts and behaviors. The full model of the association between demographic predictors and current suicidal thoughts and behaviors is shown in Supplementary Table S1. There was a significant inverse association with age [odds ratio (OR) = 0.98 (95% ci 0.97, 0.99)], such that each additional year of respondent age was associated with a 2% reduction in the likelihood of endorsing current thoughts or behaviors. Current thoughts and behaviors were also 20% less likely among respondents who identified as female compared with those who identified as male [OR = 0.80 (0.68, 0.94)]. In terms of racial/ethnic background, current thoughts and behaviors were 38% more common among those who identified as Asian or Pacific Islander [OR = 1.38 (1.14, 1.68)] and 45% more common among those who identified as being from other or multiple backgrounds [OR = 1.45 (1.15, 1.82)] relative to those who identified as non-Hispanic White. There were no significant differences between physicians and any other health care roles.

Table 4 summarizes the associations between predictors of interest and current suicidal thoughts and behaviors in the three additional models. In the depression model, both predictors (PHQ-8 score and history of lifetime suicide attempts) were significantly associated with current thoughts and behaviors. Each additional point on the PHQ-8 scale predicted a 23% increase in the likelihood of current suicidal thoughts and/or behaviors. Similarly, those who reported having made a lifetime suicide attempt were 217% more likely to also endorse current thoughts and behaviors. In the model of the association between maladaptive coping behaviors and current suicidal thoughts and behaviors, all hypothesized predictors were significantly associated with suicidal thoughts and behaviors. More specifically, the endorsement of drinking more than usual, using non-prescription drugs other than alcohol and having difficulty controlling eating behaviors was associated with 107%, 161% and 121% greater odds of current suicidal thoughts and behaviors, respectively.

The model of the association between intense affect and current suicidality indicated that some affective states were stronger predictors of suicidality than others. Hopelessness and loneliness exhibited the strongest associations with suicidal thoughts and behaviors. Individuals who endorsed these states were 204% and 148%, respectively, more likely to also endorse current suicidality, compared with those who did not endorse those states. Additionally, the endorsement of stress and nervousness predicted 87% and 36% greater likelihood of current suicidality. In contrast, annoyance, having arguments or fights, anxiety, desperation and feeling out of control were not significantly associated with current suicidality.

Table 4. Associations between clinical predictors and current suicidal thoughts and behaviors.

Predictor	Odds Ratio	95% Confidence Interval	Standard Error	z-Score
		Model: depression		
PHQ-8 score	1.23 *	1.21, 1.25	0.01	25.83
Lifetime suicide attempt	3.17 *	2.41, 4.18	0.45	8.23
		Model: maladaptive coping		
Drinking more than usual	2.07 *	1.62, 2.64	0.26	5.81
Other substance use	2.61 *	1.57, 4.34	0.68	3.69
Eating out of control	2.21 *	1.86, 2.62	0.19	9.02
		Model: intense affective states		
Nervous	1.36 *	1.08, 1.71	0.16	2.66
Annoyed	1.16	0.95, 1.42	0.12	1.44
Stress	1.87 *	1.49, 2.35	0.22	5.41
Fighting	1.30	1.03, 1.62	0.15	2.25
Anxious	1.09	0.88, 1.33	0.11	0.78
Lonely	2.48 *	2.04, 3.01	0.25	9.17
Angry	0.99	0.78, 1.26	0.12	−0.07
Hopeless	3.04 *	2.41, 3.83	0.36	9.45
Desperate	1.38	1.07, 1.78	0.18	2.52
Out of control	1.07	0.86, 1.33	0.12	0.63

Note: * indicates $p < 0.0125$. All models included demographic covariates (age, gender, race/ethnicity and position). Lifetime suicide attempts were coded as 0 = no attempts, 1 = one or more attempts. Predictors in the maladaptive coping model were all coded as 0 (not at all; some of the time) or 1 (a lot of the time; most or all the time). Predictors in the intense affective states model were treated as continuous variables.

3.2. Predictors of Mental Health Treatment

The associations between demographic predictors and the odds of receiving mental health treatment are shown in Supplemental Table S2. Analyses indicated that women were 42% more likely than men to be in treatment [OR = 1.42 (1.22, 1.66)]. Respondents who identified as Asian or Pacific Islander were 47% less likely to be in treatment compared to those who identified as non-Hispanic White [OR = 0.53 (0.44, 0.64)]; no other racial or ethnic groups differed significantly from the non-Hispanic White group. In terms of position, nurses were 58% more likely than physicians to be receiving mental health care [OR = 1.58 (1.18, 2.14)]. No other position groups were significantly different from physicians. Age was also not significantly associated with treatment status.

Table 5 summarizes the three additional models predicting the likelihood of mental health treatment. Each model included age, gender, racial/ethnic background, and role as covariates. In the depression and risk model, each additional point on the PHQ-8 was associated with 8% greater odds of receiving mental health treatment. Respondents who reported lifetime suicide attempts were 76% more likely to be in treatment compared with those who did not. Current suicidal thoughts and behaviors were not significantly associated with treatment status. In the maladaptive coping model, difficulty controlling eating behaviors was associated with an 86% greater likelihood and drinking more than usual with a 50% greater likelihood of receiving mental health care. Other substance use was unrelated to treatment status.

Table 5. Associations between clinical predictors and current mental health treatment status.

Predictor	Odds Ratio	95% Confidence Interval	Standard Error	z-Score
		Model: depression		
PHQ-8 score	1.08 *	1.06, 1.09	0.01	11.36
Lifetime suicide attempt	1.76 *	1.32, 2.35	0.26	3.84
Current suicidality	1.14	0.94, 1.38	0.11	1.29
		Model: maladaptive coping		
Drinking more than usual	1.50 *	1.19, 1.89	0.18	3.40
Other substance use	1.80	1.08, 3.00	0.47	2.25
Eating out of control	1.86 *	1.59, 2.18	0.15	7.66
		Model: intense affective states		
Nervous	1.25 *	1.05, 1.48	0.11	2.53
Annoyed	1.14	0.97, 1.33	0.09	1.58
Stress	1.30 *	1.10, 1.54	0.11	3.05
Fighting	0.85	0.69, 1.04	0.09	−1.57
Anxious	1.59 *	1.34, 1.90	0.14	5.20
Lonely	1.23	1.03, 1.47	0.11	2.30
Angry	0.80	0.64, 1.00	0.09	−1.99
Hopeless	0.86	0.69, 1.08	0.10	−1.29
Desperate	1.36	1.06, 1.74	0.17	2.46
Out of control	1.16	0.96, 1.42	0.12	1.51

Note: * indicates $p < 0.0125$. All models included demographic covariates (age, gender, race/ethnicity, and position). Lifetime suicide attempt was coded as 0 = no attempts, 1 = one or more attempts; current suicidality was coded as 0 = no, 1 = yes. Predictors in the maladaptive coping model were all coded as 0 (not at all; some of the time) or 1 (a lot of the time; most or all of the time). Predictors in the intense affective states model were treated as continuous variables.

In the model of intense affective states, those who endorsed anxiety were 59% more likely to be receiving mental health treatment. Respondents who endorsed stress had 30% greater odds of being in treatment compared with those who did not. Similarly, endorsement of nervousness was associated with 25% greater odds of being in treatment. Endorsement of other affective states was not associated with the likelihood of being in mental health treatment.

4. Discussion

In this report, we aimed to provide a comprehensive evaluation of suicidal thoughts and behaviors among health care students, trainees, and workers over a 15-year period. Our findings highlight not only the alarming presence of suicidal thoughts and behaviors among health care workers and trainees, but also the concerningly low rates of mental health treatment-seeking within this population. Through examining the associations between suicidal thoughts and behaviors and demographic information, health care role, depression severity, intense affective states and maladaptive coping behaviors, we have re-confirmed known risk factors and identified new predictors to identify health care workers at risk for suicide. We found that health care workers as a group had low rates of mental health treatment, with certain subgroups, including those identifying as Asian or Pacific Islander, males and physicians, even less likely to seek mental health treatment. Overall, the pattern of findings suggests that health care workers' ability and/or willingness to access mental health care may be substantially limited by sociocultural and demographic factors even when a clinical need exists. These results have critical implications for the ongoing need to address the mental health crisis in health care workers and trainees, especially among those with identifiable risk factors for current suicidal thoughts and behaviors.

We found that almost one fifth of the health care workforce (18.2%) who participated in UC San Diego's ISP screening were struggling with current suicidal thoughts and behaviors. It is well established that health care professionals are disproportionately faced with mental health challenges [24,25], which are influenced by grueling occupational hours and exposure to traumatic workplace events. Echoing previous works in the literature, suicidal thoughts and behaviors were associated with higher depression severity, a history of lifetime suicide attempts, male gender and maladaptive coping behaviors such as misuse of alcohol and drugs and disordered eating behaviors [26–28]. In a cohort study evaluating data from the National Violent Death Reporting System in the United States, A review of data from the National Violent Death Reporting System found that health care professionals who died by suicide were more likely to have Asian or Pacific Islander ancestry compared with individuals in the general population who died by suicide [29]. Consistent with this, we found that Asian or Pacific Islander health care workers were more likely to be experiencing current suicidal thoughts or behaviors than their non-Hispanic White counterparts, but less likely to be receiving mental health care. We identified several intense affective states to be associated with current suicidal thoughts and behaviors: hopelessness, loneliness, stress and nervousness. While hopelessness and loneliness have previously been established to be linked to a suicidal crisis [12,30], we are unaware of prior studies identifying the intense affective states of stress and nervousness as additional risk factors. Recognizing intense affective states among health care workers may help direct attention and support to those at risk for experiencing current suicidal thoughts and behaviors. Online screening tools and peer reports are potential interventions to identify health care trainees and workers with concerning intense affective states or other predictors of suicidal thoughts and behaviors [31]. The anonymous encryption of the ISP overcomes issues associated with psychological safety and may enhance acceptability and access to those who might not have otherwise sought treatment [23,32].

Although over half the participants rated themselves as nervous (51.6%) and/or stressed (50.5%), depression severity scores were high and most participants were classified as high risk (51.1%), only about a quarter (26.8%) were receiving any mental health treatment. Our finding that the majority of health care students and providers were not receiving mental health care was no surprise. It is well known that despite their knowledge and resources, health care workers are reluctant to seek mental health care [32]. One of the most well-established and effective methods to prevent suicide is the treatment of depression [33], yet the majority of physicians and nurses with depression do not seek professional care [15,34] and large United States studies have found that only a minority of individuals who die by suicide had recently been in psychiatric care [35–37]. One reason for under-treatment among health care professionals has been attributed to intrusive questions regarding mental health treatment and history used by licensure and accreditation boards. These stigmatizing questions have resulted in many avoiding treatment for mental health conditions, sometimes leading to self-medication through substance use [38,39].

In the current study, it was somewhat reassuring to find past suicide attempts and high depression symptom severity to be associated with receiving mental health treatment, as well as endorsements of high levels of stress, nervousness and anxiety. However, it was concerning that current suicidal thoughts and behaviors and feelings of helplessness and desperation were not. To our knowledge, these important correlates of mental health treatment in health care workers have not been previously reported. This study is also consistent with previous studies in the general population [40], in that females were more likely to receive treatment than males, which may at least partially explain why nurses—predominantly (86.6%) female—were more likely than physicians to receive treatment. We are not aware of previous studies reporting that Asian/Pacific Islander health care workers were less likely than White health care workers to receive mental health care, although this mimics health care disparities observed in community populations [41,42]. More research is needed to understand the specific barriers for mental health service usage among minoritized groups in the health care worker population, but possibilities include cultural and community contributions to mental health stigma and mismatch between cultural needs and available services [43]. Potential interventions to address cultural mental health disparities include adapting assessment procedures to reflect cultural variations in symptom expression, employing language-proficient and cultural humility-trained providers and decreasing stigma and professional consequences for seeking treatment.

This study has several important limitations. As the sample was limited to one university-based, academic medical center in southern California, demographic representation may not reflect the broader national health care workforce. Not all health care students, trainees and professionals took this screening. Participants opted to complete the depression and stress screening, which may have introduced a selection bias by attracting individuals who were distinct from peers and had pre-existing concerns for their mental health. Additionally, the ISP questionnaire is not designed to be a research tool but rather a screening instrument to identify individuals who would benefit from referral to mental health treatment. A wider and perhaps more representative and impactful utilization of this screening and engagement tool might be to include it in initial orientation and onboarding procedures. Underrepresented groups such as Black/African American or gender non-binary individuals had small sample sizes, which may have masked significant associations. Program participants also may have chosen not to complete demographic items in order to protect their identity, and therefore findings based on demographic data need to be further confirmed with prospective studies. Future studies could also employ broader sampling strategies by distributing the screening tool to health care trainees and workers across multiple institutions. Our analysis of current suicidal thoughts and behaviors did account for the intent, severity or immediacy of suicidal thoughts and behaviors, which would help better identify and target the most at-risk population for death by suicide.

This study also has several strengths. It uses a large sample of health care learners and professionals and takes advantage of the AFSP's Interactive Screening Program (ISP), an evidence-based, innovative program that has been widely adopted across more than 200 institutions of higher education, medical and professional degree schools, organizations and workplaces, and has successfully connected over 280,000 individuals to professional help [44]. Our results helped identify actionable targets for suicide prevention among the health care community.

Comparing features associated with suicide risk to those associated with mental health care is one way to identify unmet needs. To that end, identifying as male and as Asian/Pacific Islander were independently associated with increased risk for suicidal thoughts and/or behaviors. However, Asians/Pacific Islanders were less likely than non-Hispanic Whites, and males less likely than females, to receive mental health treatment. Individuals with high levels of intense affective states of nervousness, stress, loneliness and hopelessness were at increased risk for suicidal thoughts and behaviors, but loneliness and hopelessness were not predicters of current treatment. A qualitative study of medical residents' descriptions of stressors in the workplace triangulates the psychological impact of the loneliness that residents face when relocating for training. This finding suggests a need for structured socialization activities to reduce risk. Similarly, taking non-prescribed drugs was associated with suicidal thoughts and/or behaviors, but not with treatment. And perhaps most surprising, current thoughts and/or behaviors were not related to treatment. These features—being a health care worker who identifies as male and/or Asian/Pacific Islander, experiences intense loneliness and/or hopelessness, takes non-prescription drugs and endorses recent suicidal thought and behaviors—may help identify high-risk individuals who require enhanced methods of outreach, identification, acceptance and accessibility of treatment.

5. Conclusions

This program documented high rates of suicidal thoughts and behaviors, validated known risk factors, uncovered new risk factors and revealed suboptimal rates of mental health care utilization in medical students, physician trainees, attending physicians, nurses and others in the health care workforce. In all, almost 6000 unique individuals participated in this screening program's online survey. We now know that the adage "physician heal thyself" can and should be extended to the entire health care family. Future research is indicated to test strategies for earlier engagement in mental health treatment for vulnerable populations within the health care workforce. The implementation of interventions such as systematized, anonymous screenings and streamlining processes to receive mental health support may encourage health care trainees and staff to prioritize and care for their mental health. Only then will health care learners and providers be able to experience the joy the practice of health care is meant to provide, and to deliver the highest level of care to their patients.

Supplementary Materials: The following supporting information can be downloaded at: https://www.mdpi.com/article/10.3390/jcm14020574/s1, Table S1: Association between demographic factors and current suicidality; Table S2: Association between demographic factors and receiving mental health treatment.

Author Contributions: Conceptualization, S.Z. (Sijia Zhang), S.Z. (Sidney Zisook), J.D., D.S. and N.D.; methodology, S.Z. (Sijia Zhang), S.Z. (Sidney Zisook) and N.D.; validation, S.Z. (Sijia Zhang), S.Z. (Sidney Zisook) and N.D.; formal analysis, N.D.; investigation, S.Z. (Sidney Zisook) and D.S.; resources, S.Z. (Sidney Zisook) and D.S.; data curation, S.Z. (Sijia Zhang) and N.D.; writing—original draft preparation, S.Z. (Sijia Zhang), S.Z. (Sidney Zisook), J.D., D.S. and N.D.; writing—review and editing, S.Z. (Sijia Zhang), S.Z. (Sidney Zisook), J.D., D.S. and N.D.; visualization, S.Z. (Sijia Zhang), S.Z. (Sidney Zisook) and N.D.; supervision, S.Z. (Sidney Zisook), J.D., D.S. and N.D.; project administration, S.Z. (Sijia Zhang), S.Z. (Sidney Zisook) and N.D. All authors have read and agreed to the published version of the manuscript.

Funding: This research received no external funding.

Institutional Review Board Statement: Ethical review and approval were waived for this study by the UC San Diego Institutional Review Board due to the determination of this study as Not Human Subject Research.

Informed Consent Statement: Patient consent was waived due to this study was Not Human Subject Research.

Data Availability Statement: The raw data supporting the conclusions of this article belong with the American Foundation for Suicide Prevention.

Acknowledgments: The authors wish to thank the T. Denny Sanford Institute for Empathy and Compassion at the University of California, San Diego for their support of this study and gratefully acknowledge the UC San Diego Health System and Healer Education, Assessment, and Referral (HEAR) Program and the American Foundation for Suicide Prevention (AFSP) for their ongoing efforts to combat burnout, depression and suicide in health care workers, while supporting mental health, wellness and suicide prevention throughout our communities.

Conflicts of Interest: S. Zisook receives research support from Compass Pathways Ltd. None of the other authors have conflicts of interest—financial, personal or other—that may affect the information, research, analysis or interpretation presented in the manuscript.

References

1. McHugh, C.M.; Corderoy, A.; Ryan, C.J.; Hickie, I.B.; Large, M.M. Association between Suicidal Ideation and Suicide: Meta-Analyses of Odds Ratios, Sensitivity, Specificity and Positive Predictive Value. *BJPsych Open* **2019**, *5*, e18. [CrossRef] [PubMed]
2. Peterson, C. Suicide Rates by Industry and Occupation—National Violent Death Reporting System, 32 States, 2016. *MMWR. Morb. Mortal. Wkly. Rep.* **2020**, *69*, 57–62. [CrossRef] [PubMed]
3. Dutheil, F.; Aubert, C.; Pereira, B.; Dambrun, M.; Moustafa, F.; Mermillod, M.; Baker, J.S.; Trousselard, M.; Lesage, F.-X.; Navel, V. Suicide among Physicians and Health-Care Workers: A Systematic Review and Meta-Analysis. *PLoS ONE* **2019**, *14*, e0226361. [CrossRef] [PubMed]
4. Olfson, M.; Cosgrove, C.M.; Wall, M.M.; Blanco, C. Suicide Risks of Health Care Workers in the US. *JAMA* **2023**, *330*, 1161–1166. [CrossRef]
5. Davidson, J.E.; Makhija, H.; Lee, K.C.; Barnes, A.; Richardson, M.G.; Choflet, A.; Ali, T.; Zisook, S. National Incidence of Nurse Suicide and Associated Features. *J. Nurs. Adm.* **2024**, *54*, 649–656. [CrossRef]
6. Turecki, G.; Brent, D.A.; Gunnell, D.; O'Connor, R.C.; Oquendo, M.A.; Pirkis, J.; Stanley, B.H. Suicide and Suicide Risk. *Nat. Rev. Dis. Primers* **2019**, *5*, 74. [CrossRef]
7. Knaak, S.; Mantler, E.; Szeto, A. Mental Illness-Related Stigma in Healthcare: Barriers to Access and Care and Evidence-Based Solutions. *Healthc. Manag. Forum* **2017**, *30*, 111–116. [CrossRef]
8. Mehta, S.S.; Edwards, M.L. Suffering in Silence: Mental Health Stigma and Physicians' Licensing Fears. *AJP Resid. J.* **2018**, *13*, 2–4. [CrossRef]
9. Mortali, M.; Moutier, C. Facilitating Help-Seeking Behavior Among Medical Trainees and Physicians Using the Interactive Screening Program. *J. Med. Regul.* **2018**, *104*, 27–36. [CrossRef]
10. Norcross, W.A.; Moutier, C.; Tiamson-Kassab, M.; Jong, P.; Davidson, J.E.; Lee, K.C.; Newton, I.G.; Downs, N.S.; Zisook, S. Update on the UC San Diego Healer Education Assessment and Referral (HEAR) Program. *J. Med. Regul.* **2018**, *104*, 17–26. [CrossRef]
11. Davidson, J.E.; Accardi, R.; Sanchez, C.; Zisook, S.; Hoffman, L.A. Sustainability and Outcomes of a Suicide Prevention Program for Nurses. *Worldviews Evid.-Based Nurs.* **2020**, *17*, 24–31. [CrossRef] [PubMed]
12. Downs, N.; Feng, W.; Kirby, B.; McGuire, T.; Moutier, C.; Norcross, W.; Norman, M.; Young, I.; Zisook, S. Listening to Depression and Suicide Risk in Medical Students: The Healer Education Assessment and Referral (HEAR) Program. *Acad. Psychiatry* **2014**, *38*, 547–553. [CrossRef] [PubMed]
13. Zisook, S.; Young, I.; Doran, N.; Downs, N.; Hadley, A.; Kirby, B.; McGuire, T.; Moutier, C.; Norcross, W.; Tiamson-Kassab, M. Suicidal Ideation Among Students and Physicians at a U.S. Medical School: A Healer Education, Assessment and Referral (HEAR) Program Report. *Omega* **2016**, *74*, 35–61. [CrossRef]
14. Davidson, J.E.; Zisook, S.; Kirby, B.; DeMichele, G.; Norcross, W. Suicide Prevention: A Healer Education and Referral Program for Nurses. *J. Nurs. Adm.* **2018**, *48*, 85–92. [CrossRef] [PubMed]
15. Zisook, S.; Doran, N.; Moutier, C.; Shapiro, D.; Downs, N.; Sanchez, C.; Accardi, R.; Davidson, J. Supporting Healthcare Workers Well-Being and Suicide Prevention: The HEAR Program May 2009–April 2023. *J. Med. Regul.* **2024**, *110*, 18–32. [CrossRef]
16. Moutier, C.; Norcross, W.; Jong, P.; Norman, M.; Kirby, B.; McGuire, T.; Zisook, S. The Suicide Prevention and Depression Awareness Program at the University of California, San Diego School of Medicine. *Acad. Med.* **2012**, *87*, 320–326. [CrossRef]
17. Kroenke, K.; Spitzer, R.L.; Williams, J.B. The PHQ-9: Validity of a Brief Depression Severity Measure. *J. Gen. Intern. Med.* **2001**, *16*, 606–613. [CrossRef]
18. Louzon, S.A.; Bossarte, R.; McCarthy, J.F.; Katz, I.R. Does Suicidal Ideation as Measured by the PHQ-9 Predict Suicide Among VA Patients? *Psychiatr. Serv.* **2016**, *67*, 517–522. [CrossRef]
19. Kroenke, K. Enhancing the Clinical Utility of Depression Screening. *CMAJ* **2012**, *184*, 281–282. [CrossRef]
20. American Psychiatric. *Association Diagnostic and Statistical Manual of Mental Disorders*, 5th ed.; American Psychiatric Publishing: Arlington, VA, USA, 2013.
21. Kroenke, K.; Strine, T.W.; Spitzer, R.L.; Williams, J.B.W.; Berry, J.T.; Mokdad, A.H. The PHQ-8 as a Measure of Current Depression in the General Population. *J. Affect. Disord.* **2009**, *114*, 163–173. [CrossRef]
22. Hendin, H.; Maltsberger, J.T.; Szanto, K. The Role of Intense Affective States in Signaling a Suicide Crisis. *J. Nerv. Ment. Dis.* **2007**, *195*, 363–368. [CrossRef] [PubMed]

23. Haas, A.; Koestner, B.; Rosenberg, J.; Moore, D.; Garlow, S.J.; Sedway, J.; Nicholas, L.; Hendin, H.; Mann, J.J.; Nemeroff, C.B. An Interactive Web-Based Method of Outreach to College Students at Risk for Suicide. *J. Am. Coll. Health* **2008**, *57*, 15–22. [CrossRef] [PubMed]
24. Schou-Bredal, I.; Bonsaksen, T.; Ekeberg, Ø.; Skogstad, L.; Grimholt, T.K.; Heir, T. A Comparison between Healthcare Workers and Non-Healthcare Workers' Anxiety, Depression and PTSD during the Initial COVID -19 Lockdown. *Public Health Pr. (Oxf)* **2022**, *3*, 100267. [CrossRef] [PubMed]
25. Murthy, V.H. Confronting Health Worker Burnout and Well-Being. *N. Engl. J. Med.* **2022**, *387*, 577–579. [CrossRef]
26. Hawton, K.; Casañas, I.; Comabella, C.; Haw, C.; Saunders, K. Risk Factors for Suicide in Individuals with Depression: A Systematic Review. *J. Affect. Disord.* **2013**, *147*, 17–28. [CrossRef]
27. Smith, A.R.; Zuromski, K.L.; Dodd, D.R. Eating Disorders and Suicidality: What We Know, What We Don't Know, and Suggestions for Future Research. *Curr. Opin. Psychol.* **2018**, *22*, 63–67. [CrossRef]
28. Pospos, S.; Tal, I.; Iglewicz, A.; Newton, I.G.; Tai-Seale, M.; Downs, N.; Jong, P.; Lee, D.; Davidson, J.E.; Lee, S.Y.; et al. Gender Differences among Medical Students, House Staff, and Faculty Physicians at High Risk for Suicide: A HEAR Report. *Depress. Anxiety* **2019**, *36*, 902–920. [CrossRef]
29. Beck, A.T.; Brown, G.; Berchick, R.J.; Stewart, B.L.; Steer, R.A. Relationship between Hopelessness and Ultimate Suicide: A Replication with Psychiatric Outpatients. *Am. J. Psychiatry* **1990**, *147*, 190–195. [CrossRef]
30. Stravynski, A.; Boyer, R. Loneliness in Relation to Suicide Ideation and Parasuicide: A Population-Wide Study. *Suicide Life Threat. Behav.* **2001**, *31*, 32–40. [CrossRef]
31. Daltry, R.; Sibley, S.; MacNamara, L. A Closer Look at the Interactive Screening Program (ISP): Trends in Usage of an Online Screening Program. *J. Coll. Stud. Psychother.* **2021**, *35*, 44–52. [CrossRef]
32. Braquehais, M.D.; Vargas-Cáceres, S. Psychiatric Issues Among Health Professionals. *Med. Clin.* **2023**, *107*, 131–142. [CrossRef] [PubMed]
33. Mann, J.J.; Michel, C.A.; Auerbach, R.P. Improving Suicide Prevention Through Evidence-Based Strategies: A Systematic Review. *Focus* **2023**, *21*, 182–196. [CrossRef] [PubMed]
34. Fond, G.; Lucas, G.; Boyer, L. Untreated Major Depression in Healthcare Workers: Results from the Nationwide AMADEUS Survey. *J. Clin. Nurs.* **2023**, *32*, 7765–7772. [CrossRef] [PubMed]
35. Lee, K.C.; Ye, G.Y.; Choflet, A.; Barnes, A.; Zisook, S.; Ayers, C.; Davidson, J.E. Longitudinal Analysis of Suicides among Pharmacists during 2003-2018. *J. Am. Pharm. Assoc.* **2022**, *62*, 1165–1171. [CrossRef]
36. Ye, G.Y.; Davidson, J.E.; Kim, K.; Zisook, S. Physician Death by Suicide in the United States: 2012-2016. *J. Psychiatr. Res.* **2021**, *134*, 158–165. [CrossRef]
37. Davidson, J.E.; Proudfoot, J.; Lee, K.; Terterian, G.; Zisook, S. A Longitudinal Analysis of Nurse Suicide in the United States (2005-2016) With Recommendations for Action. *Worldviews Evid. Based Nurs.* **2020**, *17*, 6–15. [CrossRef]
38. Melnyk, B.M.; Holod, A.F.; Hsieh, A.P.; Feist, J.C. An Audit of Mental Health Questions on U.S. Nursing Licensure Applications: Evidence to Guide Urgent Action for Change. *Worldviews Evid.-Based Nurs.* **2023**, *20*, 422–430. [CrossRef]
39. Moutier, C.Y.; Myers, M.F.; Feist, J.B.; Feist, J.C.; Zisook, S. Preventing Clinician Suicide: A Call to Action During the COVID-19 Pandemic and Beyond. *Acad. Med.* **2021**, *96*, 624. [CrossRef]
40. Terlizzi, E.P.; Zablotsky, B. Mental Health Treatment Among Adults: United States, 2019. 2020. Available online: https://stacks.cdc.gov/view/cdc/111879 (accessed on 3 January 2025).
41. Misra, S.; Jackson, V.W.; Chong, J.; Choe, K.; Tay, C.; Wong, J.; Yang, L.H. Systematic Review of Cultural Aspects of Stigma and Mental Illness among Racial and Ethnic Minority Groups in the United States: Implications for Interventions. *Am. J. Community Psychol.* **2021**, *68*, 486–512. [CrossRef]
42. Substance Abuse and Mental Health Services Administration [SAMHSA]. Highlights by Race/Ethnicity for the 2023 National Survey on Drug Use and Health. 2023. Available online: https://www.samhsa.gov/data/sites/default/files/NSDUH%202023%20Annual%20Release/2023-nsduh-race-eth-highlights.pdf (accessed on 3 January 2025).
43. Augsberger, A.; Yeung, A.; Dougher, M.; Hahm, H.C. Factors Influencing the Underutilization of Mental Health Services among Asian American Women with a History of Depression and Suicide. *BMC Health Serv. Res.* **2015**, *15*, 542. [CrossRef]
44. Interactive Screening Program. Available online: https://afsp.org/interactive-screening-program/ (accessed on 25 November 2024).

Journal of
Clinical Medicine

MDPI

Article

Music-Based Cognitive Training for Adults with Major Depressive Disorder and Suicide Risk: A Pilot Study

Melissa Tan [1,2,*], Steffi Friyia [1,2], Corene Hurt-Thaut [1], Sakina J. Rizvi [2,3] and Michael H. Thaut [1,4]

1 Music and Health Sciences Research Collaboratory, Faculty of Music, University of Toronto, Toronto, ON M5S 2C5, Canada
2 ASR Suicide and Depression Studies Unit, St. Michael's Hospital, Toronto, ON M5B 1M4, Canada
3 Department of Psychiatry, University of Toronto, Toronto, ON M5T 1R8, Canada
4 Faculty of Medicine, University of Toronto, Toronto, ON M5S 3K3, Canada
* Correspondence: melissac.tan@mail.utoronto.ca

Abstract: Background/Objectives: Cognitive challenges in attention and executive function worsen over time in individuals with major depressive disorder (MDD) and suicidal risk. These difficulties persist beyond acute episodes, with limited targeted treatments available. Neurologic music therapy (NMT) is effective for cognitive rehabilitation in brain injuries and developmental disabilities, suggesting potential benefits for adults with MDD and suicide risk. This pilot study evaluated the feasibility, acceptability, and preliminary effectiveness of short-term NMT on cognitive function in adults with MDD. **Methods**: Adults aged 18+ with MDD and suicidal ideations participated in an 8-week single-arm open label study with 45-min individual in-person NMT sessions using musical attention control training (MACT) and musical executive function training (MEFT). Participants provided feedback on feasibility and acceptability, and pre- and post-intervention assessments included neurocognitive tasks and questionnaires on suicidal ideation, depressive symptoms, and quality of life. **Results**: A total of 18 individuals enrolled, and 10 participants completed the study protocol. Of the participants, 100% were satisfied with their experience with NMT, with 100% noting improvements in attention and 80% in executive function. Participants experienced some improvements in short-term memory (Digit Span Forward Test), cognitive flexibility (Trail Making Test B), and inhibitory control (Stroop Task). Significant reduction in suicidal ideation intensity (Beck Suicidal Scale of Ideation) was observed, as well as significant improvements in quality of life. **Conclusions**: This is the first study using NMT to demonstrate feasibility, acceptability, and effectiveness with respect to cognitive function in adults with MDD and suicide risk, providing preliminary data for future randomized controlled trials.

Keywords: suicide risk; depression; cognition; music-based intervention; neurologic music therapy

1. Introduction

Suicide is a global public health concern, with more than 720,000 people dying annually. It is the fourth leading cause of death for individuals aged 15–29 [1]. Individuals diagnosed with major depressive disorder (MDD) are at higher risk of suicidal behavior [2]. The prevalence of suicide and increased risk among individuals with MDD underscore the urgent need for feasible and acceptable interventions that can effectively address the needs of those at risk.

A critical area where support is needed is cognitive function. Cognitive challenges such as rigidity, impaired problem solving, and dichotomous thinking are common in individuals with suicidal ideation [3]. Research shows that attention, working memory, and inhibition are particularly impaired in those with MDD and a history of suicide attempts, compared to non-attempters and healthy controls [4]. Cognitive dysfunction appears to worsen over time, persisting even when depressive episodes are in remission [5]. While antidepressant pharmacotherapy may have some impact on cognitive function, deficits in concentration and decision making often persist [6–8].

Cognitive functioning may show more specific deficits in individuals with past suicide attempts, such as difficulties with interference control [9], whereas individuals with MDD with no attempt tend to exhibit more general deficits, including challenges with attention, memory, executive functioning, processing speed, and verbal fluency [10]. In individuals with MDD and past suicide attempts, selective attention as well as general attention and memory are impaired compared to non-attempters and healthy controls [9,11]. These impairments can severely impact an individual's daily and occupational functioning [10]. This underscores the importance of targeted interventions to enhance cognitive functioning with the possibility of alleviating depressive symptoms and suicide risk [9–11].

Music-based interventions offer a promising avenue to alleviate cognitive impairments in individuals with MDD and suicide risk. The application of music-based interventions in clinical settings is currently being used to address cognitive function and psychosocial needs in other psychiatric populations that also face similar cognitive dysfunctions due to post-traumatic stress disorder and substance abuse [12,13]. Neurologic music therapy (NMT) has been proven to be effective for cognitive function, addressing areas in attention and perception training, memory training, executive function training, and psychosocial behavior training [14]. Musical attention control training (MACT) and musical executive function training (MEFT) are two techniques that will be explored in the present study.

MACT has been used with various populations, including individuals with ADHD, autism, acquired and traumatic brain injuries, and dementia [14]. A study involving adolescents in secured residential youth care with attention difficulties showed significant improvements in focused, sustained, and alternating attention following participation in MACT, compared to a non-standardized music therapy intervention [15]. Similarly, a pilot study in a forensic psychiatric hospital with patients experiencing psychotic symptoms found that those receiving six weeks of weekly 30-min MACT sessions, in addition to treatment as usual, demonstrated significant improvements in sustained, selective, and alternating attention compared to a control group [16].

MEFT has shown promise for individuals with acquired brain injuries, attention deficit disorders, and neurologic conditions like Parkinson's disease and multiple sclerosis [17]. Participants with traumatic brain injuries who engaged in four 30-min NMT sessions demonstrated significant improvements in cognitive flexibility [18]. Similarly, individuals with traumatic brain injuries who participated in weekly NMT and psychotherapy sessions experienced significant improvements in visual attention, verbal learning, memory, planning, and mental flexibility [19].

There is an urgent need for solutions to improve cognitive functioning in adults with mental health conditions. This pilot study explores the feasibility and acceptability of neurologic music therapy as an adjunctive intervention to support individuals with MDD and suicide risk, as well as assessing the effectiveness on attention and executive function skills.

2. Materials and Methods

2.1. Participant Recruitment

Participants were recruited between July 2023 and April 2024 through three main sources: the Department of Psychiatry at St. Michael's Hospital (Toronto, Ontario), an existing database of individuals who had given consent to be contacted for future studies, and advertisements placed in the community and on Facebook.

All participants met the DSM-V diagnosis for a current major depressive episode (MDE), as confirmed by the mini-international neuropsychiatric interview (MINI), and were experiencing suicidal ideation in the past week (Beck Scale for Suicide Ideation ≥ 10). All participants were required to have more than 12 sessions of psychotherapy for their current depressive episode and, if on medication, were on a stable regimen for at least four weeks; they were required to have not participated in music therapy prior to the study, to have had no private music lessons for a period of at least one year prior to participation, and no presence of cognitive impairment based on self-report and clinician judgment. Participants were excluded if they had impaired or corrected hearing, if there was a presence of active psychosis, and if there was the presence of mood and suicidal symptom severity requiring immediate treatment. Participants were withdrawn if they initiated new psychotropic medication or new psychotherapy treatment during the study.

Participants provided written informed consent prior to participation. The study was approved by the Unity Health Toronto Research Ethics Board (REB#22-280) and was also registered at ClinicalTrials.gov (NCT05694156).

2.2. Study Design

This study utilized a single-arm open label design (see Figure 1). Upon the provision of written informed consent, participants had ten in-person visits: a screening visit to determine eligibility and complete neurocognitive assessments, eight individual music-based cognitive training sessions, and one follow-up visit where they were reassessed (see Figure 2).

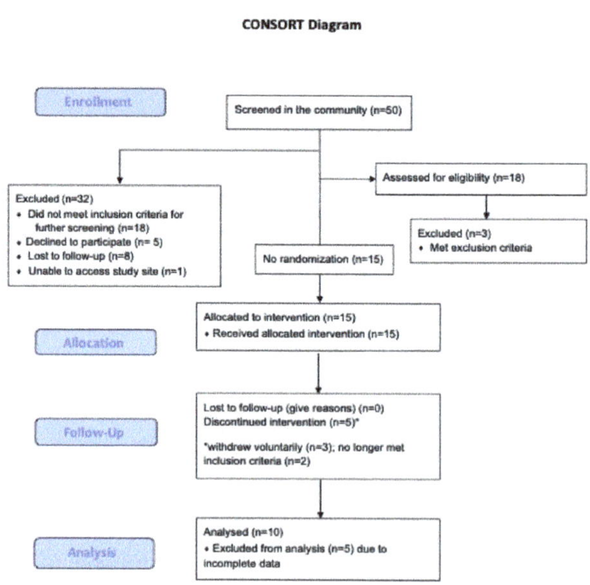

Figure 1. CONSORT study diagram for a single-arm open-label pilot music-based cognitive intervention study involving adults with MDD and suicide risk.

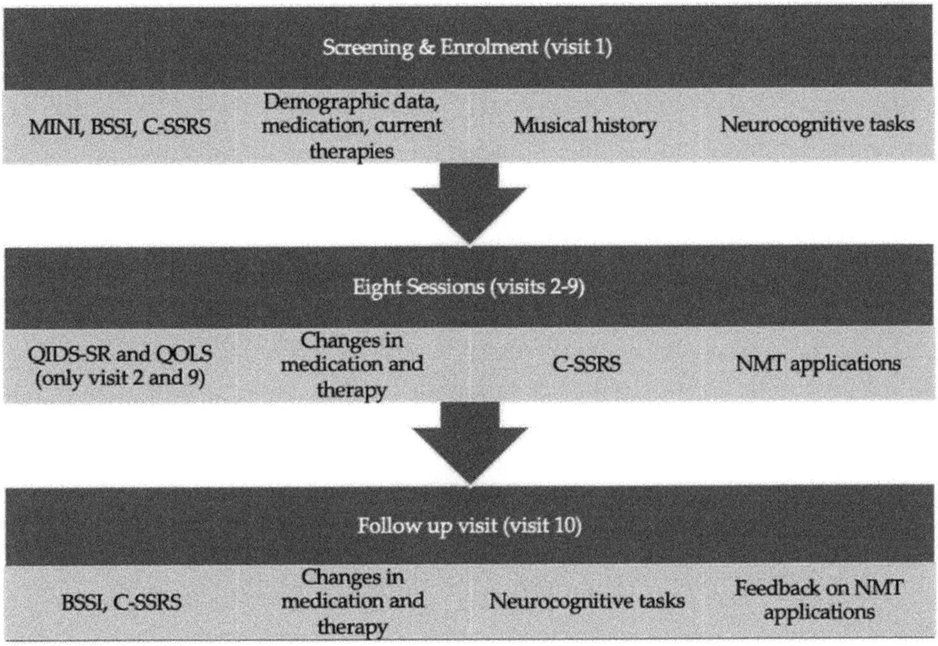

Figure 2. Study design. Abbreviations in order of appearance: mini-international neuropsychiatric interview (MINI); Beck Scale for Suicide Ideation (BSSI); Columbia Suicide Severity Rating Scale (C-SSRS); Quick Inventory of Depressive Symptomatology—Self-Report (QIDS-SR); Quality-of-Life Scale (QOLDS); neurologic music therapy (NMT).

2.2.1. Study Outcome Measures

The feasibility and acceptability of music-based cognitive training sessions were measured by an in-house survey that included both Likert scale questions and open-ended responses (i.e., accessibility, experience, usefulness, relevance, and suggestions for improvement).The Likert scale, rated on a 5-point system, captured key insights on overall satisfaction, ease of incorporating sessions into their weekly schedules, perceptions of improvements in attention and executive function, and the overall helpfulness of the experience.

To assess cognitive function, the following computerized neurocognitive tasks were used: Digit Span Forward and Backward for short-term memory and working memory; Trail Making A and B Tests for processing speed, cognitive flexibility, and set shifting; the Stroop Task for ability to inhibit cognitive interference; and the Go/No-Go Test for inhibitory control. Inquisit Lab was used to administer the Digit Span, Trail Making Tests, and the Stroop Task. E-Prime was used to administer the Go/No-Go Test.

Suicidal ideation severity was assessed using the Beck Scale for Suicide Ideation (BSSI) and the Columbia Suicide Severity Rating Scale (C-SSRS). Depressive symptoms were measured by the Quick Inventory of Depressive Symptomatology—Self-Report (QIDS-SR). Quality of life was assessed using the Quality-of-Life Scale (QOLS).

2.2.2. Procedures

A screening visit (visit 1) was undertaken to conduct a structured diagnostic interview for DSM-V disorders (MINI) and suicidal ideation severity. Demographic data, current medication use, current therapies, and musical history were also collected. The participants completed computerized neurocognitive tasks to assess cognitive functions (i.e., memory, processing speed, cognitive flexibility, and inhibitory control).

Participants were then scheduled for eight in-person individual music-based cognitive training sessions using MACT and MEFT (visits 2–9), which were designed to function as adjunctive therapy. Each session was 45 min, delivered by a licensed psychotherapist (MT) who was also a certified neurologic music therapy fellow (NMT-F) and a certified music therapist (MTA). During the first and last music-based cognitive training sessions (visit 2 and visit 9, respectively), participants completed questionnaires to assess depressive symptoms and quality of life.

Before each of the sessions, and during the follow-up visit (visit 10), the NMT-F or a member of the research staff asked about changes in medication, involvement in psychotherapy, and administered the C-SSRS. After each of the eight music-based cognitive training sessions, the NMT-F completed a post-session form. This documented the music-based tasks completed during the session, the success of completion, and any additional notes of what occurred during the study visit.

The final visit (visit 10) was conducted by a trained research coordinator, who administered the BSSI, neurocognitive tasks, and collected information about changes in psychotherapy participation and medication. Participants completed an in-house survey to obtain feedback on their experience. The follow-up visit was held after the last music-based cognitive training session (visit 9), either on the same day or the following day.

2.3. *Music-Based Cognitive Training Protocol*

Participants did not have to have prior musical knowledge to participate in music-based cognitive training. All exercises were structured using cognitive NMT applications, specifically musical attention control training (MACT) and musical executive function training (MEFT) (see Figure 3).

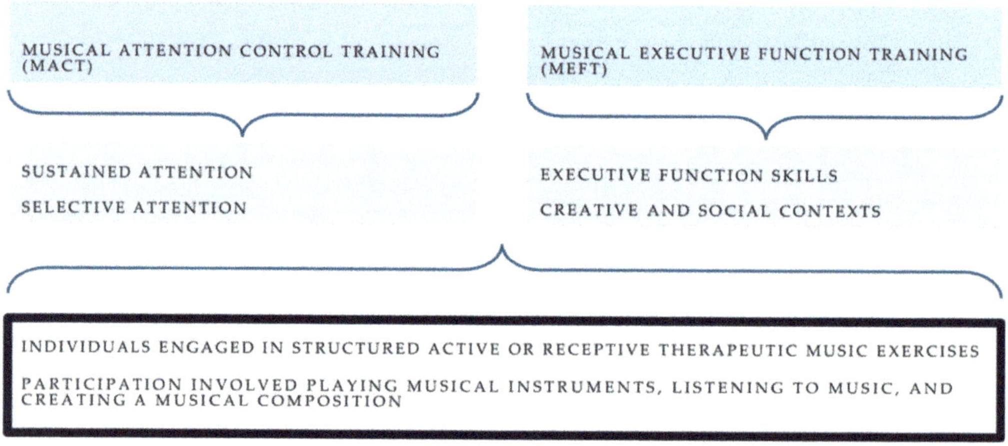

Figure 3. Music-based cognitive intervention schematic. Participants engaged in two NMT applications for cognitive training: MACT and MEFT.

2.3.1. Musical Attention Control Training (MACT)

The exercise protocols derived from MACT consisted of interactive music improvisation exercises between the participant and therapist on various instruments, including the keyboard and various percussion instruments. MACT exercises used structured or receptive therapeutic musical exercises where musical elements cued different responses to practice sustained and selective attention functions. The participant was provided target cues to which they had to respond in predetermined ways. Musical cues included specific melodies, harmonic chords, or instrument changes. Verbal cues included short instructions to prompt a particular musical response. Participant responses to the cues were musical adjustments in playing, i.e., "stop–go", "change in tempo", "change in instrument", "change in pitch register", and "change in loudness".

Selective and sustained auditory attention training required participants to listen to all the musical events and identify a specific target cue among them, responding in a predetermined way. These exercises emphasized on improving the flexibility and adaptability of the auditory attention system by offering a variety of cues and corresponding responses.

2.3.2. Musical Executive Function Training (MEFT)

The exercise protocols derived from MEFT used improvisation and composition exercises to stimulate executive function skills, including organization, problem solving, decision making, reasoning, comprehension, and inhibition, within a social context.

Participants engaged with MEFT exercises that train inhibition where the participant was asked to clap or play an instrument (i.e., handheld percussion) and rest during specific times within a rhythmic pattern (e.g., the participant is instructed to play to a 4-beat rhythm and is instructed to rest on beat 3). The therapist provided verbal cues to encourage the desired musical response. The exercise integrated the opportunity for participants to become self-aware of when they had the desire to respond musically, while simultaneously exercising their ability to inhibit specific musical responses.

Participants also took part in structured musical composition exercises, guided step-by-step through an executive dialogue. This process involved a series of questions and responses to help with decision making, problem solving, reasoning, comprehension, organization, initiation, inhibition, evaluation, analysis, and creativity. The dialogue began with closed-choice questions (e.g., the therapist played different musical options for the participant to choose from) and gradually progressed to open-ended questions, allowing participants to explore musical ideas independently. Compositions were created and performed using percussion and keyboard instruments, integrating the real-time development of both the final product and the process while combining emotional and cognitive components at each stage.

2.4. Statistical Analysis

The feasibility of the pilot study was examined through the evaluation of rates of recruitment, data completion, retention, and feedback survey data. Qualitative content analysis (QCA) was implemented to analyze open-ended responses provided in the feedback survey. Two researchers independently read and coded responses into themes and categories using an inductive approach. Summaries were then compared to establish and finalize themes and categories. Common patterns, insights, and example quotations were then identified, providing a fuller understanding of the participants' experiences.

To assess cognitive and clinical outcomes, paired samples *t*-tests were used to compare results before and after the music-based intervention at baseline and follow-up (visits 1 and 10, respectively). The Wilcoxon signed-rank test was used when normality was not met. Effect sizes were calculated to assess the magnitude of the music-based intervention's impact. Cohen's *d* was used to measure the effect size for the paired samples *t*-test, while the effect size (*r*) was calculated for the Wilcoxon signed-rank test.

All statistical analyses were conducted in R version 4.4.1.

3. Results

3.1. Participant Description

Of the 50 individuals screened for eligibility, 18 participants were enrolled to the study (see Figure 1). Ten participants completed the study protocol described. Study discontinuations were due to initiating new medication and/or psychotherapy (n = 2), time commitments (n = 2), difficulties in completing the weekly C-SSRS assessment (n = 1) and meeting exclusion criteria at the time of enrollment (n = 3). Two participants withdrew after three sessions, two participants withdrew after one session, and one participant withdrew after six sessions. On average, participants completed the eight session protocol over 10 weeks (rage 8–22 weeks). Participant baseline characteristics are described in Table 1.

Table 1. Baseline characteristics of study participants.

Characteristic	Participants (n = 10)	
	Mean	**SD**
Age, y (range)	41.7 (26–69)	13.57
	N	
Female sex at birth	10	
Gender		
Woman	9	
Non-binary/other [a]	1	
Ethnicity		
South Asian	2	
Latino	1	
White	7	
Marital status		
Never married	7	
Married/domestic partnership	2	
Divorced	1	
Education		
High school graduate	1	
Some college, no degree	3	
Associate degree	2	
Bachelor's degree	1	
Master's degree	3	
Occupation status		
Employed	3	
Unemployed, looking for work	1	
Disabled (permanently/temporarily)	5	
Retired	1	
Lifetime suicide attempt	7	
Number of past suicide attempts [b]		
0	3	
1	2	
≥2	5	
Comorbidities		
Agoraphobia	3	
Antisocial personality disorder	2	
Binge eating disorder	1	
Borderline personality disorder	4	
Generalised anxiety disorder	3	
Obsessive compulsive disorder	1	
Panic disorder	4	
Post traumatic stress disorder	4	
Social anxiety disorder	1	

Table 1. *Cont.*

Characteristic	Participants (n = 10) Mean	SD
Psychotropic medication use at baseline [c]	9	
Antidepressants [d]		
SSRI	2	
SNRI	4	
NDRI	2	
SARI	1	
TCA	1	
Antipsychotics	5	
Anti-epileptic	2	
Anxiolytics and hypnotics		
Benzodiazepines	3	
Nonbenzodiazepine hypnotic	1	
Stimulants	2	
Cannabinoid	1	

[a] Includes genderqueer, gender non-conforming, and neither exclusively man nor woman. [b] Number of past suicide attempts in lifetime with no attempts in the last 3 months. [c] Stable medication of at least four weeks. [d] Antidepressant abbreviations: selective serotonin reuptake inhibitor (SSRI); serotonin-norepinephrine reuptake inhibitor (SNRI); norepinephrine–dopamine reuptake inhibitor (NDRI); serotonin antagonist and reuptake inhibitor (SARI); tricyclic antidepressant (TCA).

3.2. Neurocognitive Tasks Outcomes

Baseline-to-week-10 Digit Span Forward results indicated no significant improvements from pre- ($M = 6.2$; $SD = 1.87$) to post-intervention ($M = 6.8$; $SD = 1.75$) [$t(9) = -1.5$, $p = 0.17$], with a small effect size (Cohen's $d = 0.13$) (see Figure 4a). Digit Span Backward results did not meet the assumption of normality, as assessed via the Shapiro–Wilk test. There were no significant differences on the Digit Span Backward results pre- (median = 5) and post-intervention (median = 5), with $V = 16$, $z = -0.26$, $p = 0.79$, $r = -0.08$ (see Figure 4a). The Trails Making Test A indicated no significant difference between pre- ($M = 0.85$ min, $SD = 0.26$) and post-intervention ($M = 0.91$ min, $SD = 0.31$) [$t(9) = -0.65$, $p = 0.53$] (see Figure 4b). The Cohen's d for Trail Making Test A was 0.22, indicating a small effect size. Similarly, the Trail Making Test B showed no significant difference between pre- ($M = 1.25$ min, $SD = 0.42$) and post-intervention ($M = 1.29$ min, $SD = 0.50$) [$t(9) = -0.20$, $p = 0.84$], with an effect size of d = −0.08. An outlier in the Trails B test, evidenced by a maximum value of 2.48 min, contributed to positive skewness (1.72) and elevated kurtosis (3.23). Without the outlier, the paired t test remained insignificant [$t(8) = 0.61$, $p = 0.56$]; however, the Cohen's d increased to −0.25, indicating a small effect size.

Stroop Task interference mean reaction time ratio for pre- and post-testing was calculated by subtracting incongruent and congruent individual participants' mean correct response reaction time and dividing that difference by the individual participants' mean correct congruent response reaction time [20]. Paired samples t test indicated no significant improvements between pre- ($M = 0.34$, $SD = 0.24$) and post-intervention ($M = 0.27$, $SD = 0.29$) [$t(9) = 0.99$, $p = 0.35$] (see Figure 4c). Cohen's d for Stroop Task interference ratio was −0.28, indicating a small effect size.

The Go/No-go task was analyzed with Wilcoxon signed-rank test for five participants as data were not available for the remaining participants due to software issues. The results indicate no significant difference between pre- and post-intervention for Go trials and No-Go trials (see Figure 4d,e). Go trials revealed non-significant improvements in accuracy from pre- (median = 83.9%) to post-intervention (median = 89.3%), $V = 3$, $z = -0.55$, $p = 0.58$, $r = -0.24$. No meaningful changes were observed in reaction time pre- (median = 162.75ms) and post-intervention (median = 161.46ms), $V = 6$,

$z = -0.24$, $p = 0.81$, $r = -0.12$. Similarly, No-Go trials revealed non-significant improvements in accuracy from pre- (median = 90.18%) to post-intervention (median = 94.64%), $V = 1$, $z = -1.63$, $p = 0.10$, $r = -0.73$. No-Go reaction times showed an increase from pre-intervention (median = 190.12 ms) to post-intervention (median = 208.35 ms). However, this change was not statistically significant, with $V = 7$, $z = 0$, $p = 1$, $r = 0$.

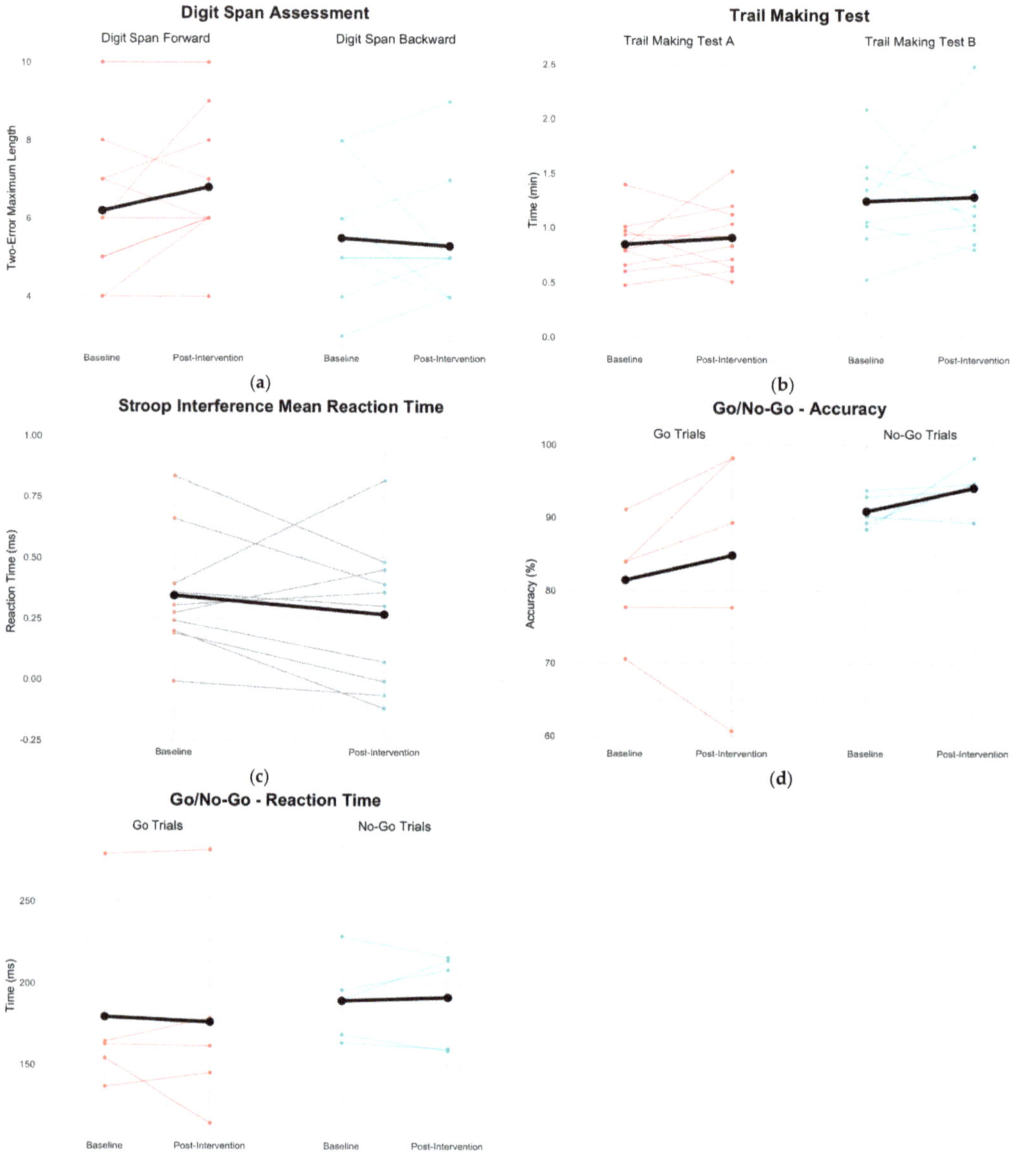

Figure 4. Line graphs represent effects of music-based cognitive intervention at baseline and post-intervention for neurocognitive tasks. Raw scores of each participant and mean scores (black line) are represented: (**a**) Digit Span assessment forward and backward scores of two-error maximum length; (**b**) Trail Making Test A and B (with outlier data) times in minutes; (**c**) Stroop interference mean reaction time in milliseconds; (**d**) Go/No-Go correct responses; (**e**) Go/No-Go reaction time in milliseconds.

3.3. Clinical Outcomes

Assumption of normality was not met for the following tests, as assessed by the Shapiro–Wilk test: BSSI and two domains of the Quality-of-Life Scale, namely, personal development and fulfilment; and recreation.

The Wilcoxon signed-rank test was used to determine if there were improvements in BSSI scores. The results indicated a significant difference between pre- (median = 17) and post-intervention (median = 12.5), $V = 51.5$, $z = -2.40$, $p = 0.02$. BSSI results indicate a significant decrease in intensity of suicidal ideation with a large effect size of $r = -0.76$, suggesting the potential role of the intervention lessening suicidal ideation intensity.

QIDS scores were analyzed using a paired samples t test, resulting in no significant changes between pre- ($M = 18.6$, $SD = 6.26$) and post-intervention ($M = 17$, $SD = 6.57$) [$t(9) = 1.16$, $p = 0.28$]. Cohen's d for QIDS scores was -0.25, indicating a small effect size.

Quality-of-Life Scale results were analyzed across five domains: material and physical well-being; relationship with other people; social community and civic activities; personal development and fulfilment; and recreation. Significant improvements were observed in material and physical well-being (pre-intervention: $M = 7.4$, $SD = 2.8$; post-intervention: $M = 8.5$, $SD = 2.22$; $t(9) = -2.19$, $p = 0.05$; Cohen's $d = 0.44$), relationship with other people (pre-intervention: $M = 15.5$, $SD = 3.72$; post-intervention: $M = 19.2$, $SD = 3.71$; $t(9) = -2.43$, $p = 0.04$; Cohen's $d = 1.0$), and social community and civic activities (pre-intervention: $M = 7.8$, $SD = 2.04$; post-intervention: $M = 10.1$, $SD = 2.42$); $t(9) = -2.91$, $p = 0.02$; Cohen's $d = 1.03$). No significant differences were found in personal development and fulfilment (pre-intervention: median = 16.5; post-intervention: median = 18.5, $V = 13.5$, $z = -1.01$, $p = 0.31$, $r = -0.32$) and recreation (pre-intervention: median = 16.5; post-intervention: median = 19.5, $V = 7.5$, $z = -1.40$, $p = 0.16$, $r = -0.44$). These findings suggest that the intervention may contribute to improvements in quality of life, particularly in the domains of material and physical well-being, relationship with other people, and social community and civic activities (see Table 2). However, due to the absence of a control arm, the impact of receiving concurrent psychotherapy cannot be excluded.

Table 2. Clinical Outcomes at baseline and post music-based cognitive intervention.

Clinical Outcome	Baseline		Post-Intervention		p-Values	Effect Size
	Mean	SD	Mean	SD		
BSSI	19.1	5.84	12.7	7.33	0.02 *	$r = -0.76$
QIDS	18.6	6.26	17	6.57	0.28	$d = -0.25$
Quality of Life Scale						
Material and Physical Well-being	7.4	2.80	8.5	2.22	0.05 *	$d = 0.44$
Relationship with Other People	15.5	3.72	19.2	3.71	0.04 *	$d = 1.00$
Social Community and Civic Activities	7.8	2.04	10.1	2.42	0.017 *	$d = 1.03$
Personal Development and Fulfilment	16.3	5.46	18.5	3.67	0.31	$r = -0.32$
Recreation	16.4	5.52	19.1	3.45	0.61	$r = -0.44$

*: The asterik indicates statistical significance.

3.4. Feasibility and Acceptability

Recruitment for this study was conducted over an eight-month period. During that time, 61 people expressed an interest generated from Facebook advertisements (33%), posters in the community (21%), a database of consent to be contacted for future studies (20%), referrals from the research team (15%), and from the laboratory's website (11%). On average, two participants were enrolled per month over the recruitment period. Among those who started the intervention, the completion rate was 66.7%, while retention rate 55.6%.

Participant feedback of their experience with NMT and music-based cognitive interventions are illustrated in Figure 5. All participants expressed positive statements towards their experience with music-based cognitive training (ranging from somewhat to very satisfied). When asked how manageable it was to fit the sessions into their schedules, 90% reported that it was easy (somewhat or very easy), and 10% expressed neutral thoughts (neither easy nor difficult). All participants noticed improvements in attention after participating in sessions (slightly or much better). Regarding executive function skills, 80% noticed an improvement (slightly or much better), and 20% reported no difference. Participants generally found the sessions helpful, with 60% finding them very or extremely helpful, 30% rating them moderately helpful, and 10% indicating slight helpfulness.

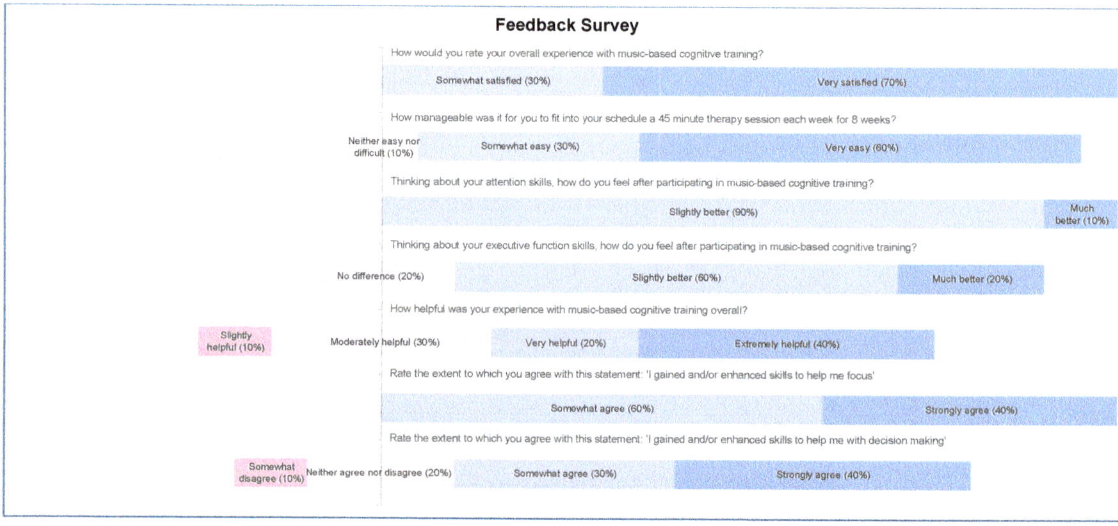

Figure 5. Divergent bar chart of music-based cognitive training feedback survey.

The QCA of open-ended survey questions yielded three central themes: benefits, challenges, and acceptability of participating in music-based cognitive training sessions. Survey questions are listed in Table 3.

Table 3. Open-ended survey questions.

Questions
What was the most beneficial aspect of the study for you?
What was the most challenging aspect of the study for you?
Is there anything else you would like to say about your experience with the study?
If it was available, would you be interested in registering for Neurologic Music Therapy sessions?

The analysis identified several emerging categories within the themes. Among these findings, the most frequently mentioned categories within the theme of benefits were increased focus and enjoyment (see Table 4). Within the theme of challenges, the most cited aspects were musical challenges and transportation barriers (see Table 5). Regarding acceptability, all participants mentioned a continued interest in NMT (see Table 6).

Table 4. Theme: benefits of participating in music-based cognitive training sessions.

Category	No.	Example Quotation
Increased focus	5	"I found it helped my focus" "helped me focus better at home" "Getting stronger at keeping my focus" "my focus got better" "I can focus more and put all my attention in the musical session"
Decision making processes	1	"being able to have a space to make choices and decisions"
Non-judgmental and safe environment	3	"to not be graded based on my results" "The actual study was light-hearted and made me feel safe" "I feel happy the people like me"
Therapeutic alliance	2	"Seeing the same person every week who was encouraging me in-person". "I also actually looked forward to seeing Melissa and doing this activity, which is not that common for me" "Nice people conducting the study".
Receiving feedback	1	"Feedback about how I improved was useful and helped me listen to music in general in other ways"
Enjoyment	6	"was a nice discipline and fun creatively" "It was good to know that I can still enjoy some things". "Getting to participate in an enjoyable activity" "For me was so fun and I love this session its works for my brain". "I knew I would enjoy it once I started!" "I enjoyed it". "I really enjoyed my time, I found it helpful and fun"
Music related benefits	2	"Gaining a little more confidence in my ability to play music". "This was an eye opening experience and I could see how rhythm can help the brain/mind process at a higher level" "I got a keyboard and have decided to try to teach myself basic piano, skills, to help distract myself when feeling dark"
Contributions to research	1	"To potentially help others learn more about depression".
Personal growth	4	"Honestly, using my brain in a different way–getting outside of myself for a period of time". "This study required participation within my comfort zone, it was nice to see others genuinely interested in learning more about what I experience with depression". "I felt better after every session" "It quietened the negative voices" "Helping me find voice was the most beneficial".

Table 5. Theme: challenges of participating in music-based cognitive training sessions.

Category	No.	Example Quotation
Self-criticism	1	"I would be hard on myself"
Musical challenges	2	"All rhythm-based tasks were a challenge"
Transportation barriers	2	"Sometimes getting to the appointment, especially if [public transit] was delayed because I would be late (or too early!) and would be stressed" "The study required transit I would normally not take due to anxiety/fear, but pushed me to attend anyway".
Disclosure of information	1	"Finding the balance between being honest enough for correct information to be gathered while avoiding being committed to a hospital stay".
Depressive symptoms	1	"Because my health issues and depression can keep me from wanting to leave the house, I have had to cancel a few times"

Table 6. Theme: acceptability of music-based cognitive training sessions.

Category	No.	Example Quotation
Integration of flexibility and structure	1	"It was a good mix of structure and creativity".
Access to free services	2	"It would be great to have this as a free program as well because I found it to be really helpful personally" "Yes, if it was financially feasible"
Continued interest in NMT	10	"Yes, if it was financially feasible" "Absolutely. This setting has been a positive way to learn how to focus more and dissociate less". "Definitely yes". "Yes, absolutely" "100 percent I would happily invest time and money into participating"

4. Discussion

The experience of cognitive dysfunction in individuals with suicide risk and MDD is a daily challenge, and there is an increasing need to develop effective interventions to support these individuals [21,22]. Our research provides new insights into addressing cognitive function and reducing suicidal ideations using music-based interventions, specifically two neurologic music therapy applications: MACT and MEFT for cognitive function. The MACT and MEFT protocols utilized in this study were derived from the Oxford Handbook of Neurologic Music Therapy [14]. Adaptions were made based on the participant's progress, which aligns with the protocol's flexibility. Specifically, the music provided by the NMT was tailored and modified based on the participant's task completion, preferences, and sensory needs.

Findings from this study reveal that participating in eight sessions of MACT and MEFT led to a significant improvement in suicidal ideation intensity. This reduction highlights the clinical relevance of the intervention in decreasing the intensity of suicidal ideation, suggesting its potential as a valuable therapeutic approach. Participating in music-based interventions engages and alters the orbitofrontal cortex (OFC), anterior cingulate cortex (ACC), amygdala, ventral striatum, insula, hippocampus, and ventromedial prefrontal cortex (vmPFC) [23]. MACT and MEFT have potential to directly target key functions such as reward processing, cognitive integration, and emotional responses. Similarly, the neurobiological mechanisms involved in suicidal ideation include alterations in the OFC, ACC, and amygdala [24]. This overlap suggests that NMT could modulate the brain regions impacted in suicidal risk, making it a potentially complementary adjunct to other interventions.

Psychological mechanisms may also contribute to the decrease in suicidal ideation intensity. Active engagement in music-based cognitive interventions provides a space for different thought patterns, potentially fostering a sense of accomplishment and self-expression. This aligns with existing literature highlighting the therapeutic benefits of music-based interventions in mental health treatment [25,26]. Additionally, social and environmental factors, such as weekly in-person support, may offer immediate relief by changing the environment and reducing feelings of isolation. Consistent social interaction, a supportive environment, and therapeutic relationships play a crucial role in mitigating suicidal thoughts as they provide a sense of community and belonging [27]. These combined mechanisms may contribute to the reduction in suicidal ideation intensity and offer a sense of belonging, underscoring the potential of NMT applications for mental health.

Depressive symptoms, as measured by the QIDS, remained within the severe range from baseline to post-intervention. The absence of significant improvements in depressive symptoms, in contrast to the observed reduction in suicidal ideation intensity, may be attributed to several factors. The music-based intervention was primarily designed to enhance functional aspects of cognition rather than directly target depressive symptoms. This focus on cognitive function may explain the lack of significant change in depressive symptoms and suggests that the intervention may target mechanisms specifically related to suicidal ideation, rather than general depressive symptoms. Additionally, the intervention's duration of eight sessions may have been insufficient to elicit notable changes in depressive symptoms. Therefore, longer intervention periods should investigate the impacts of extended music-based interventions on depressive symptoms [28]. Previous research using music-based interventions to address depressive symptoms indicates an improvement in depressive symptoms; however, generalizability of the results is difficult, and caution is necessary when interpreting results [28–30]. While depressive symptoms encompass a range of emotional and physical experiences, suicidal ideation is a more specific acute onset of psychological distress. These findings highlight that depressive symptoms and suicidal ideations may not always be related, challenging common assumptions and conceptualizations of their relationship [31]. This suggests that more distinct music-based interventions may be needed to address depressive symptoms. However, the reduction in suicidal ideation intensity observed in this study suggests that NMT applications may have a more immediate effect on alleviating acute distress, even if there were no significant impacts on depressive symptoms.

There was also a significant improvement on the Quality-of-Life Scale, specifically in the domains of material and physical wellbeing, relationship with other people, and social community and civic activities. This improvement is particularly relevant for individuals experiencing suicidal ideation, who frequently experience feelings of isolation and hopelessness. An increase in quality of life may help mitigate suicide risk and enhance coping mechanisms, increase motivation for continued therapeutic engagement, and enhance social integration for this clinical population [32]. Previous research has demonstrated that music-based interventions can enhance quality of life and offer a sense of connection and belonging [30,33,34]. The in-person delivery of the intervention may have contributed to enhancing social integration and community, contributing to improvements in quality of life. Exploring the potential of group sessions versus individual sessions could be valuable as group settings might further enhance social integration and community, providing additional support.

The feasibility of this study was demonstrated through several key findings. Recruitment was conducted through a multi-faceted approach reaching different segments of the clinical population. Facebook advertisements was the most successful channel, indicating that social media is a powerful tool. Expanding to other platforms could further increase reach. In combination with community posters, which were the second most effective channel, combining this with digital posters through local online community groups might enhance recruitment. This study had a good retention rate of 55.6%, with ten out of eighteen enrolled participants completing the study. This higher retention rate, compared to what is noted in suicide research, may be attributed to the novelty of music-based interventions, which could have enhanced participation motivation and adherence [35]. Notably, 100% of the participants were satisfied with their experience, and everyone expressed continued interest in NMT sessions.

Participants reported notable improvements in their cognitive abilities, with 100% indicating enhanced attentional skills and 80% noting better executive function skills. This increased self-efficacy in cognitive abilities suggests a promising potential for future growth in these areas, as well as psychological progress and overall confidence [36]. Despite these positive self-reports, standardized assessments did not show significant improvements.

Although significance was not reached, raw mean scores showed improvements in auditory attention, short-term memory, mental flexibility and set shifting, interference control, and inhibition. This discrepancy could be due to the lack of established best practice for assessing cognitive performance in individuals with MDD. Current assessments fail to provide a comprehensive picture and may not be sensitive enough to capture incremental changes or improvements [6,37].

It is important to recognize the limitations of this study. As this was a pilot study that was underpowered for statistical tests, effect sizes provide some insight as to what may be achieved in a powered study. The MACT and MEFT applications used in this study were specifically designed to address impaired neurocognitive mechanisms, such as short-term memory, auditory attention, mental flexibility and set-shifting, cognitive control, problem solving, and decision making, through structured tasks that paralleled these functions through music. However, it is important to note that cognitive assessments were evaluated only at baseline and post-intervention, which introduces the potential for confounding variables to influence participant performance. Post-intervention assessments were conducted either on the same day or the following day after the last music-based cognitive training session. This timing could be a limitation regarding the retention of cognitive improvements, as immediate post-intervention assessments may not accurately reflect the long-term cognitive benefits of the NMT interventions. Future studies should consider re-assessment one week later to better understand the lasting effects and to determine if cognitive improvements are sustained over time.

While our findings indicate a significant reduction in suicidal ideation intensity after MACT and MEFT, which are evidence-based standardized interventions [14], it is important to consider the possibility that other factors that may have influenced these results. Suicidal ideation can fluctuate over short periods, and improvements may be partially attributed to such fluctuations [38,39]. Additionally, the therapeutic setting and the interaction with the therapist may have contributed to improvements in suicidal ideation, independent of NMT itself [26].

Due to the small sample size and the inclusion of participants with a stable medication regimen and more than 12 psychotherapy sessions for their current depressive episodes, previous treatments and co-morbidities were not evaluated in the analysis. Future studies with larger sample sizes and more detailed medical histories could further explore the potential impact of these factors.

Additionally, the dosage of the therapy, consisting of only eight sessions of 45 min each, may not have been sufficient to observe significant changes in cognition. While NMT lacks specific guidelines for dosage of cognitive interventions like MACT and MEFT, there are recommendations for applications in the sensorimotor and speech and language domains, such as rhythmic auditory stimulation (RAS), melodic intonation therapy (MIT), and rhythmic speech cueing (RSC), which include specific session durations and frequencies. These recommendations vary depending on specific aims and diagnostics; however, they generally suggest multiple sessions per week (3–5 sessions), lasting between 30 and 60 min, over a period of 3–11 weeks [14,40–42]. These guidelines could serve as indicators for MACT and MEFT interventions, suggesting that longer and more frequent sessions might be necessary to produce measurable cognitive improvements. Implementing an at-home program could provide more frequent and sustained engagement, potentially leading to more significant cognitive changes. This approach would allow participants to integrate and transfer applications learned during sessions into their daily routines, thereby enhancing the potential for long-term cognitive benefits.

This study recruited only participants assigned female at birth, which limits the generalisability of the findings to other populations. Although this was not the intention, the recruitment methods used, such as Facebook and community posters, may have inadvertently favored individuals assigned female at birth who are active on social media or engaged in community activities. These limitations should be considered when interpreting the results.

It is crucial to acknowledge the challenges participants faced in attending sessions, including transportation barriers and symptoms of depression that hindered their willingness to leave the house. These obstacles highlight the necessity for flexible intervention delivery methods. An online option may warrant further exploration, as it could enhance accessibility, participation, and retention. Investigating whether similar outcomes for both suicidal ideation and cognitive function can be achieved in an online format would provide valuable insights into the effectiveness of music-based cognitive interventions across diverse settings.

5. Conclusions

This pilot intervention study used an innovative approach integrating mental health, neurorehabilitation, and music. Using neurologic music therapy applications (i.e., MACT and MEFT) provided valuable insights into its feasibility and acceptability with individuals with MDD and suicide risk. MACT and MEFT have often been used with other clinical populations (e.g., acquired and traumatic brain injury) and have shown improvements in cognitive function [19,43]. This study demonstrates that these applications can also be successfully implemented for individuals with mental health challenges, specifically depression and suicidal risk. The in-person protocol enabled participants to engage with the music in real time, though it restricted participation to those who could physically access the study site. A robust safety protocol was in place, and no high-risk incidents or adverse events occurred. However, the study's small sample size and single-arm design limit the broader applicability of the results. Additionally, while the broad inclusion criteria reflected real-world conditions of this clinical population, it also increased variability, making it harder to identify specific outcomes for different subgroups.

Future research should utilize a randomized control paradigm and include a neuroimaging component to understand further the efficacy and underlying neural mechanisms of cognitive training with MACT and MEFT with this clinical population. Additionally, exploring neurodiversity and sensory profiles within this clinical population would yield valuable insights and enable us to explore the broader implications of MACT and MEFT applications. These approaches may uncover specific cognitive and neural patterns that contribute to vulnerability and resilience in affected individuals.

In conclusion, the present pilot study demonstrates that eight individual music-based cognitive sessions completed within a 10-week period is a feasible and acceptable therapy. Furthermore, improvements in self-reported increased confidence in attentional and executive function skills, suicidal ideation intensity, and overall quality of life were observed, therefore supporting the potential of NMT interventions as an effective therapy for individuals with MDD and suicide risk. The substantial reduction in intensity of suicidal ideation is particularly promising, highlighting the intervention's profound impact, while the initial cognitive improvements, though modest, pave the way for further exploration and enhancement.

Author Contributions: Conceptualization, M.T., C.H.-T., S.J.R., and M.H.T.; methodology, M.T., S.J.R., and M.H.T.; validation, C.H.-T., S.J.R., and M.H.T.; formal analysis, M.T. and S.F.; investigation, M.T.; data curation, M.T. and S.F.; writing—original draft preparation, M.T.; writing—review and editing, S.F., C.H.-T., S.J.R., and M.H.T.; visualization, M.T. and S.F.; supervision, S.J.R. and M.H.T.; project administration, M.T. and S.F. All authors have read and agreed to the published version of the manuscript.

Funding: This research received no external funding.

Institutional Review Board Statement: This study was conducted in accordance with the Declaration of Helsinki and approved by the Research Ethics Board of Unity Health Toronto (REB#22-280; approved 21 April 2023).

Informed Consent Statement: Informed consent was obtained from all participants involved in this study.

Data Availability Statement: The raw data supporting the conclusions of this article will be made available by the authors on request.

Acknowledgments: The authors acknowledge the study participants.

Conflicts of Interest: The authors declare no conflicts of interest.

References

1. World Health Organization. Suicide. World Health Organization 2024. Available online: https://www.who.int/news-room/fact-sheets/detail/suicide (accessed on 1 May 2024).
2. Cai, H.; Xie, X.M.; Zhang, Q.; Cui, X.; Lin, J.X.; Sim, K.; Ungvari, G.S.; Zhang, L.; Xiang, Y.T. Prevalence of suicidality in major depressive disorder: A systematic review and meta-analysis of comparative studies. *Front. Psychiatry* **2021**, *12*, 690130. [CrossRef]
3. Rutter, S.B.; Cipriani, N.; Smith, E.C.; Ramjas, E.; Vaccaro, D.H.; Martin Lopez, M.; Calabrese, W.R.; Torres, D.; Campos-Abraham, P.; Llaguno, M.; et al. Neurocognition and the suicidal process. In *Behavioral Neurobiology of Suicide and Self Harm*; Springer: Cham, Switzerland, 2020; pp. 117–153.
4. Keilp, J.G.; Gorlyn, M.; Russell, M.; Oquendo, M.A.; Burke, A.K.; Harkavy-Friedman, J.; Mann, J.J. Neuropsychological function and suicidal behavior: Attention control, memory and executive dysfunction in suicide attempt. *Psychol. Med.* **2013**, *43*, 539–551. [CrossRef]
5. McIntyre, R.S.; Soczynska, J.Z.; Woldeyohannes, H.O.; Alsuwaidan, M.T.; Cha, D.S.; Carvalho, A.F.; Jerrell, J.M.; Dale, R.M.; Gallaugher, L.A.; Muzina, D.J.; et al. The impact of cognitive impairment on perceived workforce performance: Results from the International Mood Disorders Collaborative Project. *Compr. Psychiatry* **2015**, *56*, 279–282. [CrossRef]
6. Coles, A.S.; Lee, Y.; Subramaniapillai, M.; McIntyre, R.S. Cognitive deficits in major depression: From mechanisms to management. In *Major Depressive Disorder*; Elsevier: Amsterdam, The Netherlands, 2020; pp. 51–62.
7. Culpepper, L.; Lam, R.W.; McIntyre, R.S. Cognitive impairment in patients with depression: Awareness, assessment, and management. *J. Clin. Psychiatry* **2017**, *78*, 1383–1394. [CrossRef]
8. Trivedi, M.H.; Greer, T.L. Cognitive dysfunction in unipolar depression: Implications for treatment. *J. Affect. Disord.* **2014**, *152–154*, 19–27. [CrossRef]
9. Keilp, J.G.; Gorlyn, M.; Oquendo, M.A.; Burke, A.K.; Mann, J.J. Attention deficit in depressed suicide attempters. *Psychiatry Res.* **2008**, *159*, 7–17. [CrossRef]
10. Millan, M.J.; Agid, Y.; Brüne, M.; Bullmore, E.T.; Carter, C.S.; Clayton, N.S.; Connor, R.; Davis, S.; Deakin, B.; DeRubeis, R.J.; et al. Cognitive dysfunction in psychiatric disorders: Characteristics, causes and the quest for improved therapy. *Nat. Rev. Drug Discov.* **2012**, *11*, 141–168. [CrossRef]
11. Keilp, J.G.; Beers, S.R.; Burke, A.K.; Melhem, N.M.; Oquendo, M.A.; Brent, D.A.; Mann, J.J. Neuropsychological deficits in past suicide attempters with varying levels of depression severity. *Psychol. Med.* **2014**, *44*, 2965–2974. [CrossRef]
12. Hakvoort, L.; de Jong, S.; van de Ree, M.; Kok, T.; Macfarlane, C.; de Haan, H. Music therapy to regulate arousal and attention in patients with substance use disorder and posttraumatic stress disorder: A feasibility study. *J. Music Ther.* **2020**, *57*, 353–378. [CrossRef]
13. Wang, C.C.; Emrich, M.; Rives, H.; Ovalles, A.; Wright, D.; Wyka, K.; Difede, J. Music Interventions for Posttraumatic Stress Disorder: A Systematic Review. *J. Mood Anxiety Disord.* **2024**, *6*, 100053. [CrossRef]
14. Thaut, M.H.; Hoemberg, V. (Eds.) *Handbook of Neurologic Music Therapy*; Oxford University Press: Oxford, UK, 2014; pp. 150–160, 257–269.
15. Abrahams, T.P.; van Dooren, J.C. Musical Attention Control Training (MACT) in secure residential youth care: A randomised controlled pilot study. *Arts Psychother.* **2018**, *57*, 80–87. [CrossRef]
16. Van Alphen, R.; Stams, G.J.J.M.; Hakvoort, L. Musical attention control training for psychotic psychiatric patients: An experimental pilot study in a forensic psychiatric hospital. *Front. Neurosci.* **2019**, *13*, 570. [CrossRef]
17. Hegde, S. Neurologic music therapy targeting cognitive and affective functions. In *The Oxford Handbook of Music and the Brain*; Thaut, M.H., Hodges, D.A., Eds.; Oxford University Press: Oxford, UK, 2018; pp. 738–759.

18. Thaut, M.H.; Gardiner, J.C.; Holmberg, D.; Horwitz, J.; Kent, L.; Andrews, G.; Donelan, B.; McIntosh, G.R. Neurologic Music Therapy Improves Executive Function and Emotional Adjustment in Traumatic Brain Injury Rehabilitation. *Ann. N. Y. Acad. Sci.* **2009**, *1169*, 406–416. [CrossRef]
19. Gardiner, J.C.; Horwitz, J.L. Neurologic music therapy and group psychotherapy for treatment of traumatic brain injury: Evaluation of a cognitive rehabilitation group. *Music Ther. Perspect.* **2015**, *33*, 193–201. [CrossRef]
20. Barzykowski, K.; Wereszczyński, M.; Hajdas, S.; Radel, R. An Inquisit-web protocol for calculating composite inhibitory control capacity score: An individual differences approach. *MethodsX* **2021**, *8*, 101530. [CrossRef]
21. Linskens, E.J.; Venables, N.C.; Gustavson, A.M.; Sayer, N.A.; Murdoch, M.; MacDonald, R.; Sultan, S. Population- and community-based interventions to prevent suicide. *Crisis* **2022**, *44*, 330–340. [CrossRef]
22. Purebl, G.; Schnitzspahn, K.; Zsák, É. Overcoming treatment gaps in the management of depression with non-pharmacological adjunctive strategies. *Front. Psychiatry* **2023**, *14*, 1268194. [CrossRef]
23. Blood, A.J.; Zatorre, R.J. Intensely pleasurable responses to music correlate with activity in brain regions implicated in reward and emotion. *Proc. Natl. Acad. Sci. USA* **2001**, *98*, 11818–11823. [CrossRef]
24. Vieira, R.; Faria, A.R.; Ribeiro, D.; Picó-Pérez, M.; Bessa, J.M. Structural and functional brain correlates of suicidal ideation and behaviors in depression: A scoping review of MRI studies. *Prog. Neuro-Psychopharmacol. Biol. Psychiatry* **2023**, *126*, 110799. [CrossRef]
25. McCaffrey, T.; Edwards, J. "Music therapy helped me get back doing": Perspectives of music therapy participants in mental health services. *J. Music Ther.* **2016**, *53*, 121–148. [CrossRef]
26. Foster, A.; Alderman, M.; Safin, D.; Aponte, X.; McCoy, K.; Caughey, M.; Galynker, I. Teaching suicide risk assessment: Spotlight on the therapeutic relationship. *Acad. Psychiatry* **2021**, *45*, 257–261. [CrossRef] [PubMed]
27. Wang, X.; Huang, W.; Liu, S.; He, C.; Wu, H.; Cheng, L.; Deng, S. Music therapy for depression: A narrative review. *Brain-X* **2024**, *2*, e72. [CrossRef]
28. Aalbers, S.; Spreen, M.; Bosveld-van Haandel, L.; Bogaerts, S. Evaluation of client progress in music therapy: An illustration of an N-of-1 design in individual short-term improvisational music therapy with clients with depression. *Nord. J. Music Ther.* **2017**, *26*, 256–271. [CrossRef]
29. Aalbers, S.; Spreen, M.; Pattiselanno, K.; Verboon, P.; Vink, A.; van Hooren, S. Efficacy of emotion-regulating improvisational music therapy to reduce depressive symptoms in young adult students: A multiple-case study design. *Arts Psychother.* **2020**, *71*, 101720. [CrossRef]
30. Braun Janzen, T.; Al Shirawi, M.I.; Rotzinger, S.; Kennedy, S.H.; Bartel, L. A pilot study investigating the effect of music-based intervention on depression and anhedonia. *Front. Psychol.* **2019**, *10*, 1038. [CrossRef]
31. Keilp, J.G.; Grunebaum, M.F.; Gorlyn, M.; LeBlanc, S.; Burke, A.K.; Galfalvy, H.; Oquendo, M.A.; Mann, J.J. Suicidal ideation and the subjective aspects of depression. *J. Affect. Disord.* **2012**, *140*, 75–81. [CrossRef]
32. Büsselmann, M.; Nigel, S.; Otte, S.; Lutz, M.; Franke, I.; Dudeck, M.; Streb, J. High quality of life reduces depression, hopelessness, and suicide ideations in patients in forensic psychiatry. *Front. Psychiatry* **2020**, *10*, 1014. [CrossRef]
33. Grocke, D.; Bloch, S.; Castle, D. The effect of group music therapy on quality of life for participants living with a severe and enduring mental illness. *J. Music Ther.* **2009**, *46*, 90–104. [CrossRef]
34. Raglio, A.; Attardo, L.; Gontero, G.; Rollino, S.; Groppo, E.; Granieri, E. Effects of music and music therapy on mood in neurological patients. *World J. Psychiatry* **2015**, *5*, 68. [CrossRef]
35. Rodwin, A.H.; Shimizu, R.; Travis, R., Jr.; James, K.J.; Banya, M.; Munson, M.R. A systematic review of music-based interventions to improve treatment engagement and mental health outcomes for adolescents and young adults. *Child Adolesc. Soc. Work J.* **2023**, *40*, 537–566. [CrossRef]
36. Bandura, A. Perceived self-efficacy in cognitive development and functioning. *Educ. Psychol.* **1993**, *28*, 117–148. [CrossRef]
37. Lam, R.W.; Kennedy, S.H.; McIntyre, R.S.; Khullar, A. Cognitive dysfunction in major depressive disorder: Effects on psychosocial functioning and implications for treatment. *Can. J. Psychiatry* **2014**, *59*, 649–654. [CrossRef] [PubMed]
38. Kivelä, L.; van der Does, W.A.; Riese, H.; Antypa, N. Don't miss the moment: A systematic review of ecological momentary assessment in suicide research. *Front. Digit. Health* **2022**, *4*, 876595. [CrossRef] [PubMed]
39. Bryan, C.J.; Butner, J.E.; May, A.M.; Rugo, K.F.; Harris, J.A.; Oakey, D.N.; Rozek, D.C.; Bryan, A.O. Nonlinear change processes and the emergence of suicidal behavior: A conceptual model based on the fluid vulnerability theory of suicide. *New Ideas Psychol.* **2020**, *57*, 100758. [CrossRef]
40. Braun Janzen, T.; Koshimori, Y.; Richard, N.M.; Thaut, M.H. Rhythm and music-based interventions in motor rehabilitation: Current evidence and future perspectives. *Front. Hum. Neurosci.* **2022**, *15*, 789467. [CrossRef]
41. Ghai, S.; Ghai, I.; Schmitz, G.; Effenberg, A.O. Effect of rhythmic auditory cueing on parkinsonian gait: A systematic review and meta-analysis. *Sci. Rep.* **2018**, *8*, 506. [CrossRef]

42. Tamplin, J.; Baker, F.A. Therapeutic singing protocols for addressing acquired and degenerative speech disorders in adults. *Music Ther. Perspect.* **2017**, *35*, 113–123. [CrossRef]
43. Jones, C.; Richard, N.; Thaut, M. Investigating music-based cognitive rehabilitation for individuals with moderate to severe chronic acquired brain injury: A feasibility experiment. *NeuroRehabilitation* **2021**, *48*, 209–220. [CrossRef]

Journal of
Clinical Medicine

MDPI

Article

Suicidality in Adolescence: Insights from Self-Reports on Depression and Suicidal Tendencies

Marika Orlandi [1,2,*], Erica Casini [2], Diletta Cristina Pratile [1], Chiara Iussi [1], Cecilia Ghiazza [1], Renato Borgatti [1,2] and Martina Maria Mensi [1,2]

[1] Department of Brain and Behavioral Sciences, University of Pavia, 27100 Pavia, Italy
[2] Child Neurology and Psychiatry Unit, IRCCS Mondino Foundation, via Mondino 2, 27100 Pavia, Italy
* Correspondence: marika.orlandi@mondino.it

Abstract: Background and Objectives. Suicide represents a primary global health concern, particularly among young individuals aged 15 to 29. Clinicians are actively engaged in efforts to prevent suicide and implement timely interventions. This study aimed to evaluate the effectiveness of self-reported measures in differentiating between adolescents exhibiting suicidal ideation (SI) only and those at risk or with a previous history of suicide attempts (SA). **Methods**. Seventy-eight adolescent patients (mean age: 15.53 ± 1.49) were classified into two groups using the Columbia Suicide Severity Rating Scale (C-SSRS). Forty-five patients presented with SI but lacked a prior history of SA, while 33 adolescents had a documented history of either concrete or interrupted SA. Notably, all participants in the SA group also reported SI. Participants completed the Multi-Attitude Suicide Tendency Scale (MAST) and the Beck Depression Inventory-Short Form (BDI-SF) to assess protective and risk factors associated with suicidality, as well as perceived depression. **Results**. Attraction toward life (AL) exhibited a negative correlation with perceived depression in both groups, whereas attraction toward death (AD) was positively correlated with depression in the SA group. In the SI group, scores for repulsion by life (RL) demonstrated a positive correlation with depression. Furthermore, RL scores were significantly higher in the SA group. ROC analysis revealed good accuracy for both assessment tools in differentiating the two groups. **Conclusions**. The BDI-SF and MAST are effective instruments for identifying adolescents at risk for suicide and implementing tailored preventive and therapeutic interventions. The user-friendly nature and adaptability make those self-report measures useful in various settings, allowing administration without clinician involvement.

Keywords: suicide; suicide ideation; suicide attempt; adolescence; self-report; prevention; depression

1. Introduction

In 2024, suicide was the third leading cause of death worldwide among individuals aged 15 to 29 years [1], and the age at which suicidal ideation (SI) or suicide attempts (SA) occur is dropping alarmingly. In fact, recent evidence indicates that children aged 6 to 10 are already seeking mental health support for suicidality-related concerns [2]. Suicidal thoughts and behaviours arise from a complex interplay of social, psychological, socio-cultural, and environmental factors [3,4]. Social factors such as peer rejection, bullying, and academic stress significantly contribute to adolescent suicidality [5,6]. Additionally, exposure to familial conflict, abuse, neglect, a family history of suicidal behaviours, substance abuse, or financial issues further amplifies suicide risk [7,8]. From a psychological perspective, adolescents with poor emotional regulation, impulsivity, and perceived burdensomeness face an increased risk for SI and SA [3,4]. Sociocultural factors, including stigma surrounding mental health, feelings of guilt or shame, and restrictive cultural norms regarding emotional expression, may further elevate suicide risk [9]. Moreover, environmental factors, such as limited access to health care, unsupportive school environments, and exposure to disasters, including hurricanes, earthquakes, accidental fires, armed conflicts, or pandemics, contribute to heightened suicidality risk [10].

The COVID-19 pandemic has profoundly impacted mental health, particularly among young individuals, exacerbating the prevalence of psychiatric disorders and symptoms such as anxiety, depression, post-traumatic stress disorder (PTSD), eating disorders, sleep disturbances, substance use disorders, self-harm, SI, and SA [11–14].

Consequently, clinicians must refine assessment methodologies and enhance preventive and therapeutic interventions. In fact, adolescents often engage in SA as a cry for help, as verbalising distress may be difficult for them [15]. This developmental stage is characterised by frequent crises, emotional maladjustments, impulsivity, and a heightened sense of urgency [16]. Some adolescents may perceive suicide as an escape from personal problems, a way to alleviate psychological distress or shame, or even a means of resolving social or familial conflicts [17,18]. Others may perceive it as a revenge [16]. Survivors of SA frequently encounter stigma and are at an increased risk of future attempts [19,20].

Given that adolescence is a critical period for the early detection, prevention, and intervention of suicidality [21], those risk factors must be addressed. Despite extensive efforts by researchers and clinicians to develop effective suicide prevention strategies, significant gaps remain in the literature [22,23]. Studies have identified inconsistencies in self-reported assessments of SI and behaviours, mainly due to factors such as recall bias, stigma, or differences in question phrasing (e.g., structured interviews vs. self-reports) and time points [24]. To overcome these limitations, previous research has explored the use of brief, structured questionnaires designed to identify key characteristics distinguishing individuals with SI from those with a history of SA, thereby enhancing risk identification and prevention efforts [25]. Additionally, self-report measures have been employed to examine the unique aspects of depression among suicidal adolescents [26]. While depressive disorders are not always present in individuals exhibiting suicidal behaviours, depression remains a significant risk factor for adolescent suicide [27,28].

Given the urgency of early detection, researchers have also considered involving additional caregivers in the screening process. Studies have sought to identify depressive symptoms and other relevant characteristics using tools that do not require clinician supervision [29]. For instance, prior research employed the Multi-Attitude Suicide Tendency Scale (MAST) [30] to investigate correlations between personality traits and suicidal behaviour [31], the presentation of depression in adolescents at risk for suicide [26], and the distinguishing characteristics of SA compared to those experiencing SI only [25].

This study aims to evaluate the efficacy of two brief, cost-effective self-report measures in differentiating between adolescents who experience SI exclusively and those who have a history of SA. We hypothesise that distinct differences will emerge between these two groups and that specific relationships among the questionnaire subscales will help identify adolescents at heightened risk for SA.

2. Materials and Methods

2.1. Study Design

This cross-sectional study was conducted following the REporting of studies Conducted using Observational Routinely collected health Data (RECORD) guidelines (Table S1). The study protocol was approved by the Ethics Committee of Policlinico San

Matteo in Pavia, Italy (P-20200055757), and adhered to the principles of the Declaration of Helsinki and its subsequent amendments [32]. Patients and their caregivers provided written informed consent to participate in the study, with the option to withdraw without justification. All data were pseudonymised and are available in the Zenodo repository [33].

2.2. Participants

The study enrolled 165 help-seeking male and female patients aged 12 to 18 years who were either outpatients or inpatients at the Child Neurology and Psychiatry Unit of the National Neurological Institute IRCSS Mondino Foundation in Pavia, Italy, between May 2020 and October 2022. A total of 87 patients were excluded based on the following criteria: intellectual disability (IQ $\leq$ 70), insufficient comprehension of the Italian language by the patients or their caregivers, absence of SI or SA, and lack of consent to participate in the study. The final study population is illustrated in Figure 1.

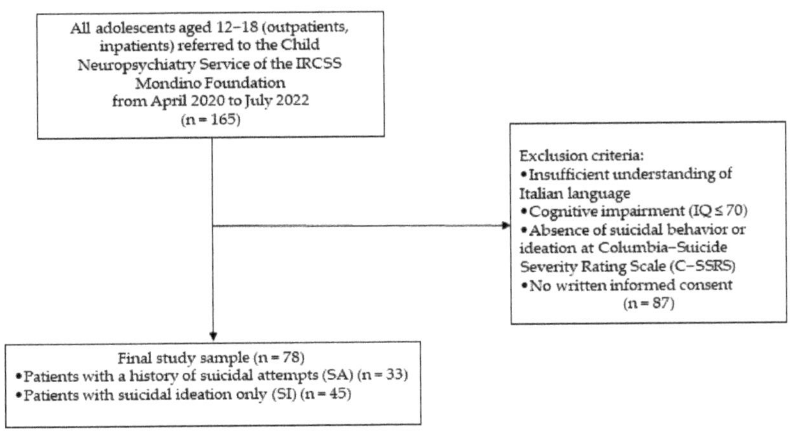

Figure 1. Study population [author's own processing].

Patients were categorised into two groups based on their responses to the Columbia-Suicide Severity Rating Scale (C-SSRS) [34], a semi-structured interview designed to assess the frequency and severity of SI, as well as suicidal behaviour and SA.

The first group comprised patients who exhibited SI but did not provide affirmative responses to any of the suicidal behaviour items in the C-SSRS. Within this group, 53.33% reported a "passive" SI, with an intensity score ranging from 1 ("Wish to be Dead") to 2 ("Non-Specific Active Suicidal Thoughts"), indicating a general desire to die without intent to engage in self-harm. The remaining 46.67% exhibited "active" SI, scoring between 3 ("Active Suicidal Ideation with Any Methods—Not Plan—without Intent to Act") and 5 ("Active Suicidal Ideation with Specific Plan and Intent") on the C-SSRS. "Active" SI denotes a persistent and specific contemplation of self-harm with an anticipated fatal outcome. Only 13.33% of the SI group reported an SI intensity of 5.

The second group comprised patients with a documented history of SA, including either concrete or interrupted attempts. These individuals were assessed using the suicidal behaviour items of the C-SSRS. They reported the ingestion of massive dosages of medications or toxic substances (such as bleach) and defenestration as primary methods to attempt their lives. Severe self-inflicted injuries resulting in severe blood loss, as well as hanging or the use of firearms, were rarely reported. Notably, all patients in the SA group also experienced SI. Specifically, 21.21% of the SA group exhibited "passive" SI (score 1 to 2 on the C-SSRS), while 78.79% reported "active" SI (score 3 to 5), with 48.49% reaching the highest SI severity score of 5.

2.3. Instruments

A child neuropsychiatrist collected sociodemographic and anamnestic data, including socioeconomic status (SES) [35]. SES levels were categorised as follows: low (8–19), middle-low (20–29), middle (30–39), middle-high (40–54), and high (55–66). We assessed social relationships according to four categories: social withdrawal (the participant is unable to function socially or maintain interpersonal relationships), poor social relationships (the participant may have some meaningful interpersonal relationships with peers but struggles with conflict resolution and developing or maintaining age-appropriate intimate relationships), or adequate social relationships (the participant engages in a wide range of social and interpersonal activities and exhibits age-appropriate involvement in intimate relationships). Moreover, academic performance was categorised as excellent (As), good (Bs), sufficient (Cs), poor (Ds and Fs), or school withdrawal (the participant is not attending school).

To exclude individuals with intellectual disabilities, we administered the Wechsler Intelligence Scale for Children-Fourth Edition (WISC-IV) [36], designed for children and adolescents aged 6 years to 16 years and 11 months, or the Wechsler Adult Intelligence Scale-Fourth Edition (WAIS-IV) [37], designed for adolescents and adults aged 16 years to 90 years and 11 months. Given the age overlap at 16 years, the choice between the WISC-IV and WAIS-IV often depends on the context, the individual's cognitive development, and the assessment goals. For this study, to reduce biases, we administered the WAIS-IV to all adolescents from 16 years old.

A trained clinician or psychologist conducted the standardised clinical interview Kiddie Schedule for Affective Disorders and Schizophrenia-Present and Lifetime Version (K-SADS-PL) for DSM-5 [38,39] for the participants and/or their parents or guardians in separate sessions to confirm the psychiatric diagnoses and comorbidities. This semi-structured diagnostic interview assesses both lifetime and current psychopathological disorders in children and adolescents according to DSM-5 criteria, including mood disorders, eating disorders, obsessive-compulsive disorder (OCD), post-traumatic stress disorder (PTSD), mania, autism spectrum disorders, and substance use disorders. All diagnoses were established following DSM-5 criteria [40] and corroborated via the K-SADS-PL.

To assess the characterisation of SI, we employed:

- The Columbia Suicide Severity Rating Scale (C-SSRS) [34].

This semi-structured interview evaluates the severity and intensity of SI using a five-point scale from a generic desire to die to active suicidal ideation with a specific plan and intention. A score of 1 corresponds to the wish to be dead, 2 represents non-specific active suicidal thoughts, 3 denotes active SI with any method (without a specific plan) and without intent to act, 4 signifies active SI with some intent to act but lacking a specific plan, and 5 reflects active SI with a detailed plan and purpose. Additionally, this scale assesses behaviours that may indicate an individual's intention to commit suicide and emphasises previous SA. The C-SSRS examines the occurrence of actual, interrupted, and aborted suicide attempts throughout an individual's lifetime (using a dichotomous response format), the frequency of each type of attempt, preparatory actions (also using a dichotomous response), and the actual and potential lethality associated with suicidal behaviours in the context of concrete attempts.

- The Multi-Attitude Suicide Tendency Scale (MAST) [30].

This 30-item self-report questionnaire evaluates suicide risk and protective factors using a Likert scale from 1 (strongly disagree) to 5 (strongly agree). It comprises four subscales investigating subjective attitudes as mediators of suicidality without differentiating between SI and SA.

(1) Repulsion by Death (RD): RD may be significantly elevated even among individuals exhibiting a pronounced inclination towards self-destructive behaviours. This phenomenon arises from the recognition that death is an unavoidable conclusion to life. RD serves as a substantial deterrent against self-destructive tendencies, potentially influenced by the apprehension of severe repercussions following death. A score equal to or lower than 3 indicates risk, while a higher score is considered a protective factor. The Cronbach's alpha coefficient for this measure was 0.92.

(2) Attraction toward Life (AL): Attraction toward Life (AL) is significantly influenced by an individual's sense of security within interpersonal relationships, including those with family and friends, as well as romantic relationships and self-esteem. This construct generally serves as a deterrent to self-destructive behaviours. A score equal to or lower than 3 indicates risk, while a higher score is considered a protective factor. The reliability of this measure, as indicated by Cronbach's alpha, was 0.85.

(3) Repulsion by Life (RL): RL encompasses experiences of suffering, including the inability to resolve feelings of guilt, the loss of loved ones, experiences of abuse, tendencies toward self-destructive behaviour, and identification with depressed parents. A score of 3 or higher indicates a risk, while a score below 3 is a protective factor. The reliability of this measure, as indicated by Cronbach's alpha, was 0.79.

(4) Attraction to Death (AD): AD arises from a distorted perception of death as reversible and as a potential escape from life's challenges. Death is frequently idealised during adolescence as a mystical union with the universe. For individuals who have experienced the loss of a loved one, this may represent a desire to reunite with the deceased. A score of 3 or higher on the AD scale is associated with an increased risk, while a lower score is a protective factor. The scale's reliability, as measured by Cronbach's alpha, was 0.79.

The reliability of the MAST in distinguishing risk and protective factors in adolescent suicidality has been established in prior research [41–43].

To evaluate the severity of patients' perceived depression, we administered:

- The Beck Depression Inventory-Short Form (BDI-SF) [44]

This 13-item self-report questionnaire employs a 4-point Likert scale (0–3). Higher scores indicate greater severity of depressive symptoms, with the following classifications: scores of 5–7 denote mild symptoms, scores of 8–15 indicate moderate symptoms, and scores of 16 or higher are categorised as severe. The items assess various dimensions of depressive symptoms, including sadness, pessimism, feelings of failure, dissatisfaction, guilt, self-esteem, self-harm, social withdrawal, indecision, self-image, difficulties in work performance, fatigue, and appetite disturbances. The reliability of the questionnaire is supported by a Cronbach's alpha coefficient of 0.91.

2.4. Analysis

The analyses were conducted utilising JASP (Version 0.19.1) [45]. Descriptive statistics were computed for sociodemographic variables. The internal consistency of the questionnaires was assessed using Cronbach's alpha. A paired samples *t*-test was employed to investigate differences between the two groups based on categorical variables. The Mann–Whitney U test assessed differences between the two groups concerning the MAST and BDI-SF scales. This non-parametric test was chosen due to the non-normal distribution of the data, as it does not assume normality and is appropriate for comparing independent samples. Normality was assessed using the Shapiro–Wilk test, confirming that the data did not follow normal distribution. The relationship between the BDI-SF and the MAST scores was examined using Spearman's rank correlation. Bonferroni correction was applied to reduce the probability of type I errors due to multiple testing. Significance levels are reported as p-values, with values below 0.05 considered statistically significant. Finally, receiver operating characteristic (ROC) analyses were conducted with R [46] to quantify the accuracy of these measures in discriminating between the two groups.

3. Results

3.1. Descriptive Analyses

We enrolled 78 adolescents, categorising them into two groups based on the C-SSRS criteria. The SI group comprised 45 participants, while the SA group included 33 participants. Descriptive analyses indicated that the groups were homogeneous in age, ethnicity, family status (presence of separated or divorced parents), and SES. However, a notable difference emerged in gender distribution, with a higher proportion of females in the SA group. Moreover, differences were observed in active and passive SI, with the SA group exhibiting a higher prevalence of active SI (Table 1).

Table 1. Sociodemographic data and diagnoses according to DSM-5 criteria.

	Total (n = 78) n (%)	SI (n = 45) n (%)	SA (n = 33) n (%)	χ^2	df	p
Age (Mean ± SD)	15.53 ± 1.49	15.39 ± 1.66	15.66 ± 1.66	0.81	76	0.209
Gender (female)	69 (88.46)	37 (82.22)	32 (96.97)	4.06	1	0.044
Ethnicity				2.47	4	0.649
Caucasian	67 (85.90)	37 (82.22)	30 (90.91)			
Asian	1 (1.28)	1 (2.22)	0 (0.00)			
African	5 (6.41)	3 (6.67)	2 (6.06)			
Latina	3 (3.84)	2 (4.44)	1 (3.03)			
Mixed	2 (2.56)	2 (4.44)	0 (0.00)			
Separate/divorced parents	26 (33.33)	13 (28.89)	13 (39.39)	0.875	1	0.350
SES [a]				2.33	4	0.675
Low	11 (14.10)	8 (17.78)	3 (9.09)			
Medium-low	10 (12.82)	5 (11.11)	5 (15.15)			
Medium	16 (20.51)	8 (17.78)	8 (24.24)			
Medium-high	17 (21.80)	8 (17.78)	9 (27.27)			
High	7 (8.97)	3 (6.67)	4 (12.12)			
School performances [b]				1.180	4	0.881
Poor	14 (17.95)	7 (15.56)	7 (21.21)			
Sufficient	18 (23.08)	9 (20.00)	9 (27.27)			
Good	26 (33.28)	16 (35.56)	10 (30.30)			
Excellent	14 (17.95)	9 (20.00)	5 (15.15)			
School withdrawal	5 (6.41)	3 (6.67)	2 (6.06)			
Social relations [c]				3.689	2	0.158
Social withdrawal	10 (12.82)	3 (6.67)	7 (21.21)			
Poor	44 (56.41)	26 (57.78)	18 (54.55)			
Adequate	23 (29.49)	15 (33.33)	8 (24.24)			
Risky behaviours [d]	49 (62.82)	21 (46.67)	28 (84.85)	18.235	6	0.006
Active SI	47 (60.26)	21 (46.67)	26 (78.79)	8.202	1	0.004
DSM-5 diagnosis						
Learning disability	2 (2.56)	1 (2.22)	1 (3.03)	2.098	2	0.350
Psychotic disorders [e]	17 (21.79)	6 (13.32)	11 (33.33)	5.625	3	0.131
Bipolar and related	3 (3.84)	2 (4.44)	1 (3.03)	2.834	2	0.242
Depression	46 (58.88)	24 (53.28)	22 (66.66)	10.548	4	0.032
Disruptive mood dysregulation	2 (2.56)	2 (4.44)	0 (0)			
MDD	22 (28.20)	10 (22.2)	12 (36.36)			
Persistent depressive disorder	7 (8.97)	1 (2.22)	6 (18.18)			
Unspecified depressive disorder	15 (19.23)	11 (24.42)	4 (12.12)			

Table 1. *Cont.*

	Total (n = 78) n (%)	SI (n = 45) n (%)	SA (n = 33) n (%)	χ^2	df	*p*
Anxiety	25 (32.00)	15 (33.3)	10 (30.3)	4.962	5	0.420
Specific phobia	1 (1.28)	1 (2.22)	0 (0)			
Social anxiety disorder	3 (3.84)	2 (4.44)	1 (3.03)			
Panic disorder	3 (3.84)	1 (2.22)	2 (6.06)			
GAD	8 (10.25)	3 (6.66)	5 (15.15)			
Unspecified anxiety disorder	10 (12.82)	8 (17.77)	2 (6.06)			
OCD	3 (3.84)	2 (4.44)	1 (3.03)	0.103	1	0.748
Eating disorders	20 (25.6)	14 (31.08)	6 (18.18)	6.859	4	0.144
Personality disorders (PD)	26 (33.28)	9 (19.98)	17 (51.51)	9.194	3	0.027
High risk for PD(s) [f]	23 (29.49)	8 (17.78)	15 (45.46)			
Borderline PD	3 (3.84)	1 (2.22)	2 (6.06)			
Substance use disorders	2 (2.56)	1 (2.22)	1 (3.03)	0.050	1	0.823

Legend. Significance: $p < 0.05$; [a] SES: low (8–19), middle-low (20–29), middle (30–39), middle-high (40–54), high (55–66); [b] school performances: poor (Ds and Fs), sufficient (Cs), good (Bs), excellent (As), school withdrawal; [c] social relations: social withdrawal (the participant is unable to function socially or maintain interpersonal relationships), poor social relationships (the participant may have some meaningful interpersonal relationships with peers but struggles with conflict resolution and developing or maintaining age-appropriate intimate relationships), or adequate social relationships (the participant engages in a wide range of social and interpersonal activities and exhibits age-appropriate involvement in intimate relationships); [d] risky behaviours: non-suicidal self-injury (cutting or other), substance use, attempted suicide, non-suicidal self-injury and substance use, non-suicidal self-injury and attempted suicide, substance use and attempted suicide, all the previous; [e] psychotic disorders: brief psychotic disorder, unspecified schizophrenia spectrum and other psychotic disorder, clinical high risk for psychosis (CHR-P); bipolar and related: cyclothymic disorder, Unspecified Bipolar and Related Disorder; [f] high risk for PD(s): since diagnosing a PD in children and adolescents is not always appropriate, minors who exhibit characteristics of subthreshold PD but do not fully meet the criteria of the DSM-5 are considered at high risk for PD(s); GAD: generalised anxiety disorder; MDD: major depressive disorder; OCD: obsessive-compulsive disorder; ODD: oppositive defiant disorder.

3.2. MAST Differences Between the SI and SA Groups

After applying the Bonferroni correction, the analyses identified a significant difference between the two groups in the RL subscale of the MAST, as shown in Table 2.

Table 2. MAST differences between the two groups.

	SI		SA				
	M	SD	M	SD	t	*p*	Adj *p*
MAST-AL	2.83	0.85	2.45	0.68	2.030	0.023	0.115
MAST-RL	3.28	0.90	3.75	0.55	2.691	0.005	0.025
MAST-AD	3.16	0.82	3.47	0.57	1.896	0.031	0.155
MAST-RD	2.46	1.02	2.12	0.81	1.523	0.066	0.33

Legend: Significance: $p < 0.05$. AL: attraction toward life; RL: repulsion by life; AD: attraction toward death; RD: repulsion by death.

3.3. Differences Between the SI and SA Groups Concerning BDI-SF

The Mann–Whitney U test revealed a statistically significant difference in depression levels between the two groups (U = 404.00, $p = 0.003$; Adj $p = 0.015$). Specifically, the SA group exhibited higher levels of depression ($M_{SA} = 23.97$, SD = 9.69; min 0, max 35; M rank = 49.97) compared to the SI group ($M_{SI} = 16.07$, SD = 11.12; min 0, max 37; M rank = 31.68). The area under the curve (AUC) for the BDI-SF was 0.706, indicating good accuracy (Figure 2).

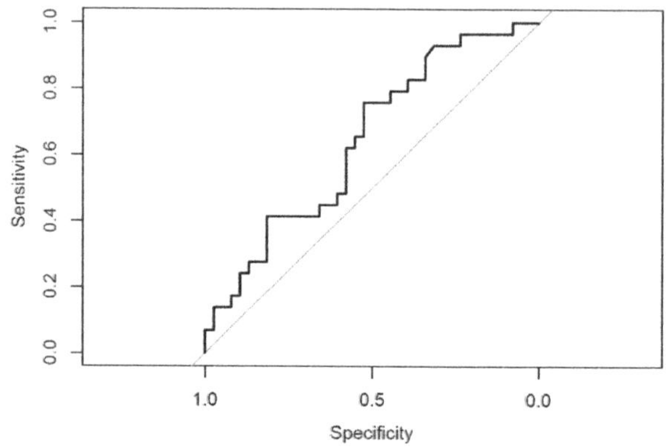

Figure 2. ROC curve illustrating the ability of BDI-SF to differentiate between SI and SA groups [author's own processing].

3.4. Comparison Between the MAST and BDI-SF

Within both groups, higher levels of AL were associated with lower levels of depression. Conversely, elevated AD correlated with increased depression levels, but only in the SA group. Notably, in the SI group, higher RL scores were linked to increased BDI-SF scores (Table 3).

Table 3. Correlations between BDI-SF and MAST.

	BDI-SF					
	SI			SA		
	r	p	Adj p	r	p	Adj p
MAST AL	−0.633	<0.001	<0.001	−0.567	0.001	0.005
MAST RL	0.638	<0.001	<0.001	0.242	0.198	0.99
MAST AD	0.365	0.024	0.12	0.557	0.001	0.005
MAST RD	0.056	0.737	3.685	−0.332	0.073	0.365

Legend: Significance: $p < 0.05$. AL: attraction toward life; RL: repulsion by life; AD: attraction toward death; RD: repulsion by death.

Finally, ROC analyses evaluating the discriminative power of the MAST and BDI-SF in distinguishing between the two groups yielded an AUC of 0.727, which is considered good (Figure 3).

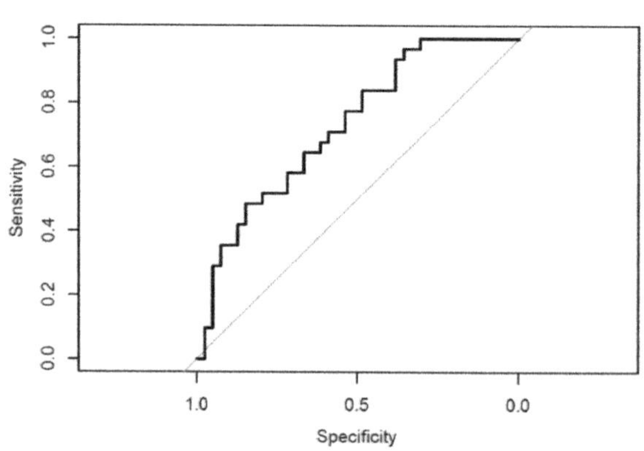

Figure 3. ROC curve illustrating the ability of BDI-SF and MAST to differentiate between SI and SA groups [author's own processing].

4. Discussion

This study aimed to evaluate the effectiveness of two brief and cost-less self-report measures in distinguishing between adolescents exhibiting SI and those at risk or with a previous history of SA. Building upon prior research [25], we first compared MAST subscales across the two groups. Results indicated significant differences in the RL subscale, with higher scores in the SA group, consistent with the findings by Maggiolini et al. [47]. Participants exhibited reduced coping capacity, unsolved guilt, and limited bodily awareness, in line with prior studies highlighting a prevalence of internalising disorders, such as depressive disorders [27,28]. Additionally, they expressed greater social withdrawal [25,47], a factor frequently associated with loneliness, non-suicidal self-injury (NSSI), SI, SA, and deliberate self-harm, with or without suicidal intent [48]. Furthermore, the literature underscores that feelings of loneliness, helplessness, and hopelessness are strongly linked to social withdrawal, depression, and SI or SA [48–50]. Although these constructs were not directly assessed in the present study, they represent critical areas for further research to enhance the understanding of suicide risk factors in adolescents.

The existing literature highlights depression as a significant risk factor in the aetiology of suicidal behaviour among adolescents [27,28]. Individuals experiencing depressive symptoms often express a desire to die or engage in suicidal behaviour, perceiving them as a potential solution to their problems [51]. A previous study [50] identified severe depression as a key predictor of SI in both adolescents and adults.

To further examine the role of depression, we administered the BDI-SF. The results indicated that the SA group reported higher levels of depressive symptoms compared to the SI group. This finding aligns with previous studies [25] and reinforces depression as a specific risk factor for SA. Consequently, the BDI-SF serves a predictive function, facilitating the early identification of at-risk individuals. Timely access to appropriate psychological assessment and treatment may alleviate patients' depressive symptoms and reduce suicide risk.

The comparative analysis of BDI-SF and MAST scores revealed a negative correlation between AL scores and perceived depression in both groups. This finding is consistent with Maggiolini et al., who linked low AL scores to internalising symptoms [47]. AL reflects an individual's positive outlook on life, signifying the pleasantness of their existence and enhancing self-affirmation and interpersonal relationships [52]. Thus, high levels of AL could be considered a protective factor against depression and suicidality.

Furthermore, we interestingly observed that higher AD scores correlated with increased perceived depression levels, but only in the SA group. AD represents a distorted perception of death as reversible and as an escape from life's challenges or a way to reunite with someone deceased. This is in line with previous studies stating that an increased risk of SA accompanies a distorted view of reality and the presence of psychotic features [53].

Moreover, we observed a positive correlation between high RL levels and BDI-SF scores in the SI group, suggesting that higher RL levels are associated with increased depressive symptoms. This could be explained because RL encapsulates profound experiences of trauma, guilt, loss, and self-destructive tendencies. This difference could also be related to the differences in active and passive SI expressed by the two groups. A previous study highlighted that patients with SA show more intense SI severity according to the C-SSRS [25]. This supports the importance of assessing intent and planning, as these factors significantly increase the risk of SA.

Furthermore, a comparison between the two samples revealed differences in the diagnosis of depressive disorders. Despite the higher presence of perceived depression in the SA group, according to BDI-SF, individuals with SI were more frequently diagnosed with depressive disorders, albeit with milder symptoms. Additionally, personality disorder

(PD) features were more prevalent in the SA group, particularly borderline PD traits, such as impulsivity and anxious lability, which have emerged as significant markers for suicidality and SA relapse [54]. This finding is consistent with prior research indicating that individuals with SA may exhibit higher levels of impulsivity than those with SI, particularly under negative emotional states [55]. Another study found that impulsive reactivity to emotional stimuli is strongly linked to SA, even when controlling for psychiatric diagnoses and symptoms [56]. While our findings align with research suggesting that patients with SA exhibit more PD-related symptoms [25], it is essential to note that diagnosing PD at a young age is not always considered accurate. Clinicians should closely monitor adolescents exhibiting high-risk PD traits over time to track symptom trajectories. In light of that, recent research involving adolescents suggests that early onset of symptoms, externalising behaviours, and caregiver-reported internalising symptoms may predispose adolescents to fully developed PDs in adulthood [57]. Our findings support the notion that suicidality is transdiagnostic, cutting across multiple psychiatric conditions [58].

The ROC analysis provided further evidence that the BDI-SF and MAST demonstrated good accuracy in distinguishing between adolescents with SI and those with a history of SA. These results suggest that both tools can serve as reliable initial screening measures, particularly in non-clinical settings where quick, cost-effective assessments are needed. However, depression manifests heterogeneously, making its diagnosis inherently challenging [59]. Suicidality represents a complex construct that includes diverse symptoms and varying degrees of severity [60].

Nevertheless, differentiating between adolescents with SI and those with SA remains complex [61]. Additionally, assessing at-risk adolescents is further complicated by the challenge of identifying factors that facilitate the transition from ideation to attempt. This understanding is crucial for developing timely and effective interventions and preventive strategies.

Our findings suggest that self-reported measures may be valuable early screening tools in non-clinical settings, such as schools. However, effective screening requires a multi-method approach, incorporating multiple instruments and perspectives. Unfortunately, timely access to mental health services remains inconsistent.

The study presents some limitations. First, the sample demonstrates gender heterogeneity, as the SA group comprises primarily female participants. This reflects the literature stating that female adolescents present a higher risk for SA and males for suicide death [62]. Moreover, research shows differences in help-seeking tendencies, with young males asking for help from those they trust (e.g., friends and parents) and adopting self-reliance as the preferred strategy to cope with mental issues. At the same time, females seem to have more confidence in mental health professionals [63]. Second, both groups consist solely of individuals diagnosed with severe neuropsychiatric disorders and do not include a healthy control group. Furthermore, the participants were self-selected; they consented to participate in the study from a larger cohort admitted to our institution. Moreover, the study's cross-sectional design, even if inexpensive and quick to conduct, does not allow for the determination of causality. A final limitation is associated with the use of two self-administered questionnaires, which may result in socially desirable responses, inaccurate self-assessment, or an exaggeration of psychopathological conditions.

5. Conclusions

The study underscores the potential of the MAST and BDI-SF as practical self-report tools for differentiating adolescents with SI from those with or at risk of SA. Their ease of use makes them valuable for early screening, particularly in non-clinical settings. However, given the potential discrepancies between clinician evaluation and self-reported symptoms, it is crucial to integrate various assessment methods. Clinicians should also actively involve important caregivers to develop tailored prevention strategies. Implementing evidence-based screening protocols and multidisciplinary prevention programs may help reduce suicide risk factors and enhance protective ones. Given that suicide is transdiagnostic and recognised as a leading cause of adolescent mortality worldwide, early detection through screening and intervention is essential [64].

The study's strengths are primarily attributed to the user-friendly design of the questionnaires. Surveying varied contexts would yield valuable insights, as suggested by prior research involving the general population [11,12]. The implementation of written questionnaires facilitates expression for individuals reluctant to verbalise their feelings. Additionally, the reliability of C-SSRS further enhances the robustness of the study [65]. Nevertheless, considering the complex nature of suicide risk factors, future research should expand these preliminary findings by investigating a larger, more heterogeneous sample, including a control group. Future studies could also incorporate clinical observations and explore additional risk factors such as loneliness, helplessness, and hopelessness.

Supplementary Materials: The following supporting information can be downloaded at: https://www.mdpi.com/article/10.3390/jcm14041106/s1. Table S1. The RECORD statement—checklist of items, extended from the STROBE statement, that should be reported in observational studies using routinely collected health data [66].

Author Contributions: M.O.: Conceptualization, data curation, formal analysis, investigation, project administration, writing—original draft, writing—review and editing; E.C.: formal analysis, writing—review and editing; D.C.P. data curation, writing—review and editing; C.I.: data curation, project administration; C.G. project administration; R.B.: methodology, supervision; M.M.M.: conceptualization, methodology, supervision. All authors have read and agreed to the published version of the manuscript.

Funding: This research was funded by Ministero della Salute [Ricerca Corrente 2025–2027].

Institutional Review Board Statement: The present study, which involves human participants, was approved by the Ethics Committee of Policlinico San Matteo in Pavia, Italy (P-20200055757, approval date 1 July 2020) and conducted following the declaration of Helsinki and its later amendments [32].

Informed Consent Statement: Informed consent was obtained from all subjects involved in the study. Written informed consent to publish this paper has been obtained from the patients. Written informed consent was provided by the participant's legal guardian/next of kin.

Data Availability Statement: The data underlying this article are available upon reasonable request in Zenodo (10.5281/zenodo.10355718) [33].

Conflicts of Interest: The authors declare no conflicts of interest.

References

1. World Health Organization Suicide. Available online: https://www.who.int/news-room/fact-sheets/detail/suicide (accessed on 25 January 2025).
2. Lo, C.B.; Bridge, J.A.; Shi, J.; Ludwig, L.; Stanley, R.M. Children's Mental Health Emergency Department Visits: 2007–2016. *Pediatrics* **2020**, *145*, e20191536. [CrossRef] [PubMed]
3. Holman, M.S.; Williams, M.N. Suicide Risk and Protective Factors: A Network Approach. *Arch. Suicide Res.* **2022**, *26*, 137–154. [CrossRef]
4. Turecki, G.; Brent, D.A.; Gunnell, D.; O'Connor, R.C.; Oquendo, M.A.; Pirkis, J.; Stanley, B.H. Suicide and Suicide Risk. *Nat. Rev. Dis. Primers* **2019**, *5*, 74. [CrossRef]
5. Esposito, C.; Bacchini, D.; Affuso, G. Adolescent Non-Suicidal Self-Injury and Its Relationships with School Bullying and Peer Rejection. *Psychiatry Res.* **2019**, *274*, 1–6. [CrossRef]
6. Steare, T.; Gutiérrez Muñoz, C.; Sullivan, A.; Lewis, G. The Association between Academic Pressure and Adolescent Mental Health Problems: A Systematic Review. *J. Affect. Disord.* **2023**, *339*, 302–317. [CrossRef]

7. Eslava, D.; Martínez-Vispo, C.; Villanueva-Blasco, V.J.; Errasti, J.M.; Al-Halabí, S. Family Conflict and Suicidal Behaviour in Adolescence: The Mediating Role of the Assertive Interpersonal Schema. *Sustainability* **2023**, *15*, 5149. [CrossRef]
8. Wagner, B.M.; Silverman, M.A.C.; Martin, C.E. Family Factors in Youth Suicidal Behaviors. *Am. Behav. Sci.* **2003**, *46*, 1171–1191. [CrossRef]
9. Carpiniello, B.; Pinna, F. The Reciprocal Relationship between Suicidality and Stigma. *Front. Psychiatry* **2017**, *8*, 35. [CrossRef]
10. Liu, X.-Q.; Wang, X. Adolescent Suicide Risk Factors and the Integration of Social-Emotional Skills in School-Based Prevention Programs. *World J. Psychiatry* **2024**, *14*, 494–506. [CrossRef]
11. Mensi, M.M.; Iacopelli, M.; Orlandi, M.; Capone, L.; Rogantini, C.; Vecchio, A.; Casini, E.; Borgatti, R. Psychiatric Symptoms and Emotional Impact of the COVID-19 Pandemic on Italian Adolescents during the Third Lockdown: A Cross-Sectional Cohort Study. *Sci. Rep.* **2022**, *12*, 20901. [CrossRef]
12. Mensi, M.M.; Capone, L.; Rogantini, C.; Orlandi, M.; Ballante, E.; Borgatti, R. COVID-19-Related Psychiatric Impact on Italian Adolescent Population: A Cross-Sectional Cohort Study. *J. Community Psychol.* **2021**, *49*, jcop.22563. [CrossRef] [PubMed]
13. Tavano, S.; Caini, S.; Sforzi, I.; Silvestri, C.; Voller, F.; Pisano, T. Mental Health of Children and Adolescents before and during the COVID-19 Pandemic: How Did the Lockdown Modify Psychiatric Emergencies in Tuscany, Italy? *J. Clin. Med.* **2023**, *12*, 4154. [CrossRef] [PubMed]
14. Guessoum, S.B.; Lachal, J.; Radjack, R.; Carretier, E.; Minassian, S.; Benoit, L.; Moro, M.R. Adolescent Psychiatric Disorders during the COVID-19 Pandemic and Lockdown. *Psychiatry Res.* **2020**, *291*, 113264. [CrossRef] [PubMed]
15. Giampieri, E.; Clerici, M. Il Suicidio Oggi. Implicazioni Sociali e Psicopatologiche. [Suicide Nowadays. Social and Psychopathological Implications]. In *Suicidio E Psicobiologia*; Springer: Berlin/Heidelberg, Germany, 2013; pp. 97–103.
16. Pietropolli Charmet, G.; Piotti, A. *Il Tentativo Di Suicidio in Adolescenza. [Suicidal Attempt in Adolescence]*; Raffaello Cortina Editore: Milano, Italy, 2009.
17. Tezanos, K.M.; Pollak, O.H.; Cha, C.B. Conceptualizing Death: How Do Suicidal Adolescents View the End of Their Lives? *Suicide Life Threat. Behav.* **2021**, *51*, 807–815. [CrossRef]
18. Piotti, A.; De Monte, G. *Quando La Scuola Viene Ferita: Interventi Dopo Il Suicidio Di Uno Studente*, 2017th ed.; FrancoAngeli: Milan, Italy, 2017.
19. Mayer, L.; Rüsch, N.; Frey, L.M.; Nadorff, M.R.; Drapeau, C.W.; Sheehan, L.; Oexle, N. Anticipated Suicide Stigma, Secrecy, and Suicidality Among Suicide Attempt Survivors. *Suicide Life Threat. Behav.* **2020**, *50*, 706–713. [CrossRef]
20. Sheehan, L.; Oexle, N.; Dubke, R.; Wan, H.T.; Corrigan, P.W. The Self-Stigma of Suicide Attempt Survivors. *Arch. Suicide Res.* **2020**, *24*, 34–47. [CrossRef]
21. Cavelti, M.; Kaess, M. Adolescent Suicide: An Individual Disaster, but a Systemic Failure. *Eur. Child. Adolesc. Psychiatry* **2021**, *30*, 987–990. [CrossRef]
22. Wasserman, D.; Carli, V.; Iosue, M.; Javed, A.; Herrman, H. Suicide Prevention in Childhood and Adolescence: A Narrative Review of Current Knowledge on Risk and Protective Factors and Effectiveness of Interventions. *Asia Pac. Psychiatry* **2021**, *13*, e12452. [CrossRef]
23. Zygo, M.; Pawłowska, B.; Potembska, E.; Dreher, P.; Kapka-Skrzypczak, L. Prevalence and Selected Risk Factors of Suicidal Ideation, Suicidal Tendencies and Suicide Attempts in Young People Aged 13–19 Years. *Ann. Agric. Environ. Med.* **2019**, *26*, 329–336. [CrossRef]
24. Deming, C.A.; Harris, J.A.; Castro-Ramirez, F.; Glenn, J.J.; Cha, C.B.; Millner, A.J.; Nock, M.K. Inconsistencies in Self-Reports of Suicidal Ideation and Attempts across Assessment Methods. *Psychol. Assess.* **2021**, *33*, 218–229. [CrossRef]
25. Coci, C.; Invernizzi, R.; Capone, L.; Casini, E.; Orlandi, M.; Galli, P.; Rossi, I.; Martinelli, O.; Borgatti, R.; Mensi, M.M.; et al. Psychological and Behavioral Characterization of Suicide Ideators and Suicide Attempters in Adolescence. *Front. Psychiatry* **2022**, *13*, 1009460. [CrossRef] [PubMed]
26. Klomek, A.B.; Orbach, I.; Sher, L.; Sommerfeld, E.; Diller, R.; Apter, A.; Shahar, G.; Zalsman, G. Quality of Depression Among Suicidal Inpatient Youth. *Arch. Suicide Res.* **2008**, *12*, 133–140. [CrossRef]
27. Grossberg, A.; Rice, T. Depression and Suicidal Behavior in Adolescents. *Med. Clin. North. Am.* **2023**, *107*, 169–182. [CrossRef]
28. Carballo, J.J.; Llorente, C.; Kehrmann, L.; Flamarique, I.; Zuddas, A.; Purper-Ouakil, D.; Hoekstra, P.J.; Coghill, D.; Schulze, U.M.E.; Dittmann, R.W.; et al. Psychosocial Risk Factors for Suicidality in Children and Adolescents. *Eur. Child. Adolesc. Psychiatry* **2020**, *29*, 759–776. [CrossRef]
29. Melhem, N.M.; Porta, G.; Oquendo, M.A.; Zelazny, J.; Keilp, J.G.; Iyengar, S.; Burke, A.; Birmaher, B.; Stanley, B.; Mann, J.J.; et al. Severity and Variability of Depression Symptoms Predicting Suicide Attempt in High-Risk Individuals. *JAMA Psychiatry* **2019**, *76*, 603–613. [CrossRef]
30. Orbach, I.; Milstein, I.; Har-Even, D.; Apter, A.; Tiano, S.; Elizur, A. A Multi-Attitude Suicide Tendency Scale for Adolescents. *Psychol. Assess.* **1991**, *3*, 398–404. [CrossRef]
31. Ferrara, M.; Terrinoni, A.; Williams, R. Non-Suicidal Self-Injury (Nssi) in Adolescent Inpatients: Assessing Personality Features and Attitude toward Death. *Child. Adolesc. Psychiatry Ment. Health* **2012**, *6*, 12. [CrossRef]

32. World Medical Association World Medical Association Declaration of Helsinki: Ethical Principles for Medical Research Involving Human Participants. *JAMA* **2025**, *333*, 71–74. [CrossRef]
33. Mensi, M.M. 20220612_DEP_SUICID_bdimast_MMM_01 2022.
34. Posner, K.; Brown, G.K.; Stanley, B.; Brent, D.A.; Yershova, K.V.; Oquendo, M.A.; Currier, G.W.; Melvin, G.A.; Greenhill, L.; Shen, S.; et al. The Columbia-Suicide Severity Rating Scale: Initial Validity and Internal Consistency Findings from Three Multisite Studies with Adolescents and Adults. *Am. J. Psychiatry* **2011**, *168*, 1266–1277. [CrossRef]
35. Hollingshead, A.B. *Four-Factor Index of Social Status*; Yale University: New Haven, CT, USA, 1975.
36. Wechsler, D. *Wechsler Intelligence Scale for Children-Fourth Edition (WISC-IV)*; Giunti Organizzazioni Speciali, Ed.: Firenze, Italy, 2003.
37. Wechsler, D. *Wechsler Adult Intelligence Scale-Fourth Edition (WAIS-IV)*; Giunti Organizzazioni Speciali, Ed.: Firenze, Italy, 2008.
38. Kaufman, J.; Birmaher, B.; Axelson, D.; Pereplitchikova, F.; Brent, D.; Ryan, N. *Schedule for Affective Disorders and Schizophrenia for School-Aged Children: Present and Lifetime Version (K-SADS-PL) DSM-5*; Child and Adolescent Research and Education: New Heaven, CT, USA, 2016.
39. Kaufman, J.; Birmaher, B.; Rao, U.; Ryan, N.; di Sogos, C.; Di Noia, S.P.; Fioriello, F.; Picchiotti, G. *K-SADS-PL DSM-5. Intervista Diagnostica per La Valutazione Dei Disturbi Psicopatologici in Bambini e Adolescenti. Schedule for Affective Disorders and Schizophrenia for School-Aged Children: Present and Lifetime Version (K-SADS-PL) DSM-5*; Erickson, Ed.: Trento, Italy, 2019.
40. American Psychiatric Association. *Diagnostic and Statistical Manual of Mental Disorders 5th Edition: DSM-5*, 5th ed.; American Psychiatric Association: Arlington, VA, USA, 2013.
41. Osman, A.; Barrios, F.X.; Grittmann, L.R.; Osman, J.R. The Multi-Attitude Suicide Tendency Scale: Psychometric Characteristics in an American Sample. *J. Clin. Psychol.* **1993**, *49*, 701–708. [CrossRef]
42. Osman, A.; Barrios, F.X.; Panak, W.F.; Osman, J.R.; Hoffman, J.; Hammer, R. Validation of the Multi-attitude Suicide Tendency Scale in Adolescent Samples. *J. Clin. Psychol.* **1994**, *50*, 847–855. [CrossRef] [PubMed]
43. Osman, A.; Gilpin, A.R.; Panak, W.F.; Kopper, B.A.; Barrios, F.X.; Gutierrez, P.M.; Chiros, C.E. The Multi-Attitude Suicide Tendency Scale: Further Validation with Adolescent Psychiatric Inpatients. *Suicide Life Threat. Behav.* **2000**, *30*, 377–385. [CrossRef] [PubMed]
44. Beck, A.T.; Beck, R.W. Screening Depressed Patients in Family Practice: A Rapid Technic. *Postgrad. Med.* **1972**, *52*, 81–85. [CrossRef] [PubMed]
45. JASP Team. *JASP*, Version 0.19.3; JASP Team: Amsterdam, The Netherlands, 2024.
46. R Core Team. *R: A Language and Environment for Statistical Computing*, Version 4.4.2; The R Core Team: Vienna, Austria, 2024.
47. Maggiolini, A.; Di Lorenzo, M.; Pisa, C. Atteggiamenti nei Confronti della Morte e del Suicidio in Adolescenza [Attitudes toward Facing Death and Suicide in Adolescence]. *Psichiatr. Psicoter.* **2012**, *31*, 268–284.
48. Bulat, L.R. Loneliness in the Context of Self-Harm Behaviors in Adolescence. In *Determinants of Loneliness*; IntechOpen: London, UK, 2024; ISBN 978-0-85466-550-1.
49. Wolfe, K.L.; Nakonezny, P.A.; Owen, V.J.; Rial, K.V.; Moorehead, A.P.; Kennard, B.D.; Emslie, G.J. Hopelessness as a Predictor of Suicide Ideation in Depressed Male and Female Adolescent Youth. *Suicide Life-Threat. Behav.* **2019**, *49*, 253–263. [CrossRef]
50. Ribeiro, J.D.; Huang, X.; Fox, K.R.; Franklin, J.C. Depression and Hopelessness as Risk Factors for Suicide Ideation, Attempts and Death: Meta-Analysis of Longitudinal Studies. *Br. J. Psychiatry* **2018**, *212*, 279–286. [CrossRef]
51. Penso, M.A.; Sena, D.P.A.D. A desesperança do jovem e o suicídio como solução. *Soc. Estado.* **2020**, *35*, 61–81. [CrossRef]
52. Wong, W.S. Attitudes toward Life and Death among Chinese Adolescents: The Chinese Version of the Multi-Attitude Suicide Tendency Scale. *Death Stud.* **2004**, *28*, 91–110. [CrossRef]
53. Riera-Serra, P.; Navarra-Ventura, G.; Castro, A.; Gili, M.; Salazar-Cedillo, A.; Ricci-Cabello, I.; Roldán-Espínola, L.; Coronado-Simsic, V.; García-Toro, M.; Gómez-Juanes, R.; et al. Clinical Predictors of Suicidal Ideation, Suicide Attempts and Suicide Death in Depressive Disorder: A Systematic Review and Meta-Analysis. *Eur. Arch. Psychiatry Clin. Neurosci.* **2024**, *274*, 1543–1563. [CrossRef]
54. Nobile, B.; Jaussent, I.; Kahn, J.P.; Leboyer, M.; Risch, N.; Olié, E.; Courtet, P. Risk Factors of Suicide Re-Attempt: A Two-Year Prospective Study. *J. Affect. Disord.* **2024**, *356*, 535–544. [CrossRef]
55. Millner, A.J.; Lee, M.D.; Hoyt, K.; Buckholtz, J.W.; Auerbach, R.P.; Nock, M.K. Are Suicide Attempters More Impulsive than Suicide Ideators? *General. Hosp. Psychiatry* **2020**, *63*, 103–110. [CrossRef] [PubMed]
56. Auerbach, R.P.; Stewart, J.G.; Johnson, S.L. Impulsivity and Suicidality in Adolescent Inpatients. *J. Abnorm. Child Psychol.* **2017**, *45*, 91. [CrossRef] [PubMed]
57. Rogantini, C.; Orlandi, M.; Vecchio, A.; Pratile, D.C.; Cabini, R.F.; Ballante, E.; De Giorgis, V.; Borgatti, R.; Mensi, M.M. Breakdown or Personality Disorder? Psychiatric Characterization and Developmental Pathways Towards Young Adulthood in Adolescents with Pathological Personality Structure. *Brain Sci.* **2024**, *14*, 1115. [CrossRef] [PubMed]

58. Karnick, A.T.; Fergerson, A.K.; Caulfield, N.M.; Buerke, M.; Albanese, B.J.; Schmidt, N.B.; Capron, D.W. Toward an Integrative Model of Transdiagnostic Risk Factors and Suicide: A Network Comparison of Psychiatric Outpatients. *J. Psychiatr. Res.* **2022**, *154*, 252–260. [CrossRef]
59. Solnek, B.L.; Seiter, T. How to Diagnose and Treat Depression. *Nurse Pract.* **2002**, *27*, 12–23. [CrossRef]
60. Masi, G.; Lenzi, F.; Fabiani, D.; Sudano, S.D.; D'Acunto, G.; Mucci, M. Suicidal ideation, suicidal attempts and non-suicidal self-injuries in referred adolescents. *Riv. Di Psichiatr.* **2020**, *55*, 168–174.
61. Klonsky, E.D.; May, A.M.; Glenn, C.R. The Relationship between Nonsuicidal Self-Injury and Attempted Suicide: Converging Evidence from Four Samples. *J. Abnorm. Psychol.* **2013**, *122*, 231–237. [CrossRef]
62. Miranda-Mendizabal, A.; Castellví, P.; Parés-Badell, O.; Alayo, I.; Almenara, J.; Alonso, I.; Blasco, M.J.; Cebrià, A.; Gabilondo, A.; Gili, M.; et al. Gender Differences in Suicidal Behavior in Adolescents and Young Adults: Systematic Review and Meta-Analysis of Longitudinal Studies. *Int. J. Public Health* **2019**, *64*, 265–283. [CrossRef]
63. Bosco, N.; Giaccherini, S.; Meringolo, P. A Gender Perspective about Young People's Seeking Help. *J. Prev. Interv. Community* **2020**, *48*, 132–146. [CrossRef]
64. Díez-Gómez, A.; Pérez-Albéniz, A.; Ortuño-Sierra, J.; Fonseca-Pedrero, E. SENTIA: An Adolescent Suicidal Behavior Assessment Scale. *Psicothema* **2020**, *32*, 382–389. [CrossRef]
65. Gipson, P.Y.; Agarwala, P.; Opperman, K.J.; Horwitz, A.; King, C.A. Columbia-Suicide Severity Rating Scale: Predictive Validity with Adolescent Psychiatric Emergency Patients. *Pediatr. Emerg. Care* **2015**, *31*, 88–94. [CrossRef] [PubMed]
66. Benchimol, E.I.; Smeeth, L.; Guttmann, A.; Harron, K.; Moher, D.; Petersen, I.; Sørensen, H.T.; von Elm, E.; Langan, S.M.; the RECORD Working Committee. The REporting of studies Conducted using Observational Routinely-collected health Data (RECORD) Statement. *PLoS Med.* **2015**, *12*, e1001885. Available online: https://www.equator-network.org/reporting-guidelines/record/ (accessed on 25 January 2025). [CrossRef] [PubMed]

Journal of
Clinical Medicine

MDPI

Article

Suicide Risk in People with Hearing Impairment in the Post-COVID-19 Period: The CaViDAuCo Study

Nerea Moreno-Herraiz [1], Iván Cavero-Redondo [1,*], Iris Otero-Luis [1], Carlos Pascual-Morena [2,3], María Dolores Gómez-Guijarro [1], Irene Martínez-García [1] and Alicia Saz-Lara [1]

1 Carvascare Research Group, University of Castilla-La Mancha, 16071 Cuenca, Spain; nerea.moreno@uclm.es (N.M.-H.); iris.otero@uclm.es (I.O.-L.); doloresgg18@gmail.com (M.D.G.-G.); irene.mgarcia@uclm.es (I.M.-G.); alicia.delsaz@uclm.es (A.S.-L.)

2 Health and Social Research Center, University of Castilla-La Mancha, 16071 Cuenca, Spain; carlos.pascual@uclm.es

3 Faculty of Nursing, University of Castilla-La Mancha, 02071 Albacete, Spain

* Correspondence: ivan.cavero@uclm.es

Abstract: Background/Objectives: During the COVID-19 pandemic, suicide risk increased in the general population and persisted in the post-pandemic period. People with hearing impairment faced communication barriers that negatively affected their mental health. However, there is no evidence on whether they have an increased suicide risk in the post-pandemic period. This study aimed to assess the association between mental disorders, quality of life, and suicide risk in individuals with hearing impairment in the post-COVID-19 period. **Methods**: A cross-sectional study was conducted with 103 participants with hearing impairment from the CaViDAuCo study. Adjusted and unadjusted differences in mental disorders (depression, anxiety, and stress) and quality of life (physical and mental) were analyzed using Student's t test and ANCOVA according to suicide risk. **Results**: Depression, anxiety, stress, and mental quality of life in people with hearing impairment were significantly associated with suicide risk (unadjusted, models 1 and 2, $p < 0.001$; Cohen's $d = 1.4$, 1.4, 1.3, and −1.0, respectively). Due to the cross-sectional design, no causal relationships can be established. **Conclusions**: In the post-pandemic period, participants with hearing impairment exhibited a significant association between suicide risk, mental disorders, and poor mental quality of life. Although causality cannot be established, and the results should be interpreted with caution due to the small sample size, these findings underscore the need to improve mental health accessibility and implement inclusive communication policies. Further research is needed to better understand these associations and design effective interventions that promote the mental health and quality of life of people with hearing impairment.

Keywords: COVID-19 pandemic; hearing impairment population; suicide risk; quality of life; mental disorders

1. Introduction

In December 2019, a sudden outbreak of severe infection associated with a new severe acute respiratory syndrome coronavirus (COVID-19) occurred in Wuhan, China, and rapidly spread worldwide, becoming a global pandemic [1,2]. Measures taken to prevent the spread of COVID-19 included house confinement, mobility restrictions, hand hygiene and hygienic measures, social distancing, and mandatory use of masks [3], but these measures caused psychological distress and had a major impact on the psychosocial well-being of the general population [4]. However, despite adopting these preventive measures, according to the Spanish National Institute of Statistics, deaths due to COVID-19 in 2020 totaled 33,312, and in 2021, they reached 29,300 [5].

These restrictions, particularly for people with hearing impairment (HI), have led to additional isolation and decreased accessibility in terms of social interaction, communication, and access to COVID-19-related information and resources, could contribute to poorer personal and emotional well-being [6,7]. Online activities and communications via video calls have increased, harming this population [4,8]. Face-covering mandatory hygiene masks have a major impact on communication, limiting facial expressions and preventing lip reading, not to mention being a major communication barrier if healthcare workers are wearing personal protective equipment (PPE) [6,8,9]. In addition, companions are restricted during healthcare, and it is highly important for people with HI to be accompanied by a family member or a sign language interpreter (SLI) to receive quality care and effective communication [8,10]. Finally, during the COVID-19 pandemic, continuous broadcasts of adequate and reliable information were inaccessible due to the lack of adaptations, such as the absence of SLIs and subtitles and the impossibility of accessing lip reading [8].

Concerning the COVID-19 pandemic itself, several previous studies have explored mental disorders and quality of life (QoL) in people with HI. The most frequently assessed mental disorders in this population were anxiety [11–16], depression [11,13–15,17], and stress [11,14,17]. According to these studies, people with HI suffered worse mental health than people without HI during the pandemic due to increased communication barriers, lack of access to information, and an increase in the number of mental disorders they already suffer from because HI is considered a risk factor for mental disorders [4,6,18].

Suicide, a worldwide public health problem, is associated with mental disorders according to the World Health Organization (WHO), and this connection is associated with an incidence of death by suicide every 40 s [19]. According to the Spanish National Institute of Statistics, there were 3941 deaths by suicide in Spain in 2020, an increase of 7.4% compared with 2019 [19]. However, the statistics only reflect deaths, not suicide attempts or suicidal ideation, which is estimated to be 20 times more frequent [20]. There are a number of possible mechanisms that explain how the suicide risk increases when people experience frustrated belongingness and an increased perceived burden due to repeated exposure to painful or fearful experiences [21]. These factors may be especially relevant for people with HI due to communication barriers, social isolation, limited access to information, and mental health resources [6,7], and they may exacerbate emotional distress, thereby increasing suicidal behaviors and ideation [6,7,21]. Another possible explanation is that people with HI are at greater risk of abuse due to persistent communication barriers, which limit their ability to seek help or report interpersonal violence [22,23]. Both physical and emotional abuse and neglect contribute to poor mental health among people with HI and may be associated with self-injurious thoughts and behaviors [23,24].

There is evidence that there was an increase in consultations for suicide attempts and suicidal ideation in the post-pandemic period [19], with a significant increase in the ratio of suicidal ideation to suicide attempts [20]. During the pandemic period, there were increases in symptoms of depression, anxiety, and insomnia in the general population and in people with HI in particular; these conditions have been observed alongside increased suicide risk [19], and suicidal ideation appeared to coincide with adjustment problems and loneliness. Although there is evidence of an increase in short-term mental disorders during the pandemic in people with HI, it is still necessary to investigate whether there have been any changes in the suicide risk of this population over the long-term.

Therefore, the aims of this study were as follows: (1) to assess the associations between mental disorders (depression, anxiety, and stress) and suicide risk in people with HI in the post-COVID-19 period; and (2) to assess the associations between quality of life—both physical and mental—and suicide risk in people with HI in the post-COVID-19 period.

2. Materials and Methods

2.1. Study Design, Participants, and Sample Size

The cross-sectional CaViDAuCo study was conducted in different centers and associations of people with HIs in Spain to analyze variables collected at a single point in time. Recruitment of participants was carried out at the University of Castilla-La Mancha, Cuenca, by the research staff (including physicians and nurses), who contacted a total of 57 centers and associations of people with HI in Spain, including ASPAS, APSORGU, APROSOJA, FASICAN, FESCAN, FEXAS, and FESORMANCHA, among others (Table S1). A convenience sampling method was used through an open call by email. Research staff sent both the questionnaires and informed consent forms by email. Participation was completely voluntary. The sample size was calculated a priori using Epidat 4.2 software based on an estimated large effect size (Cohen's $d = 1.0$) obtained from a previous study using the Overall Depression Severity and Impairment Scale [25]. This scale was selected exclusively for the purpose of estimating the sample size, as no prior studies assessing the association between mental disorders and suicide risk in populations with HIs were available at the time of study design. The Overall Depression Severity and Impairment Scale was chosen because of its conceptual similarity, as it assesses the severity of depression, which is a well-established predictor of suicidal behavior. This proxy approach allowed us to ensure a robust sample size to detect differences relevant to our primary hypothesis regarding the association between mental disorders and suicide risk. By converting the effect size to Cohen's d, we ensured a standardized and scale-independent estimate, which allows for valid extrapolation even when a different instrument was ultimately used in the study. However, we acknowledge that the use of a large effect size (Cohen's $d = 1.0$) in the sample size calculation may be optimistic and could inflate power estimates. Future studies should aim to use more conservative and empirically derived effect sizes as more data become available. Patients who met the inclusion and exclusion criteria were invited to participate in the study, and 103 participants were eventually enrolled between 1 March 2023 and 1 October 2023. This study followed the Strengthening the Reporting of Observational Studies in Epidemiology (STROBE) statement [26]. The eligibility criteria for individuals were as follows: (1) hearing impaired at birth or later; (2) over 18 years of age; and (3) used sign language, spoken language, or both. The exclusion criteria for individuals were as follows: (1) participated in another study; (2) provided no written informed consent; and (3) prior diagnosis of psychiatric pathology.

2.2. Ethical Considerations

The research protocol for this study was approved by the Clinical Research Ethics Committee of the Cuenca Health Area (REG: 2022/PI3322). Written informed consent to participate was obtained from all the subjects involved in the study.

2.3. Variables

The variables analyzed were collected via online self-administered questionnaires.

2.3.1. Main Variables

QoL (both physical and mental) was assessed using the SF12 health questionnaire. The subjects answered 12 questions about what they thought of their health and to what extent they were able to perform usual activities [27]. Once the answers were obtained, they were individually analyzed through the SF12 OrthoToolKit calculator [28], which calculates the physical and mental level scores for each subject (Table S2).

Depression, anxiety, and stress were assessed using the DASS-21 scale. The subjects responded to 21 questions on the scale, with four numerically ranked responses associated with the degree to which the statements had occurred during the past week. After the responses were obtained, item scores (subscales) for depression (items 3, 5, 10, 13, 16, 17, and 21), anxiety (items 2, 4, 7, 9, 15, 19, and 20), and stress (items 1, 6, 8, 11, 12, 14, and 18) were interpreted individually. For each subscale, the scores of the corresponding items are summed, and the result is then multiplied by two. The final total score was classified according to the following cut-off points to assess the degree of symptomatology: depression: normal (0–9), mild (10–13), moderate (14–20), severe (21–27), and extremely severe (28+); anxiety: normal (0–7), mild (8–9), moderate (10–14), severe (15–19), and extremely severe (20+); and stress: normal (0–14), mild (15–18), moderate (19–25), severe (26–33), and extremely severe (34+) [29] (Table S3).

Plutchik's Suicide Risk Scale. The subjects responded to the 15 questions of the scale only with affirmative or negative answers. The results were interpreted individually, with each affirmative response receiving 1 point and a negative response receiving 0 points, for a total possible score between 0 and 15 points. As the scale score increases, so does the suicide risk, establishing a cut-off point greater than or equal to 6 to consider the suicide risk to be significant [30] (Table S4).

2.3.2. Covariates

The self-reported covariates included in this study were age, sex, whether people were deaf from birth, hearing aids used, and the language used (sign language, spoken language, or both).

2.4. Statistical Analysis

Normal probability plots and the Kolmogorov–Smirnov test were used to verify the normality of the distribution of continuous variables. Descriptive data for the total sample are shown as the means and standard deviations (SDs) or proportions (%), as appropriate. The chi-square statistic was used to evaluate the prevalence of people at risk or not at risk of suicide according to the following categories: depression (mild, moderate, severe, or extremely severe), anxiety (mild, moderate, severe, or extremely severe), and stress (mild, moderate, severe, or extremely severe). In addition, the mean values and SDs were calculated for mental disorders (depression, anxiety and stress) and QoL (both physical and mental) according to suicide risk. Student's t test for independent samples and analysis of covariance (ANCOVA) were performed for the total sample between mental disorders and QoL and suicide risk. In addition, ANCOVA was performed adjusting for all variables, i.e., deaf at birth or later, hearing aids used and language used (sign language, spoken language, or both) as categorical covariates and age as a continuous covariate. Finally, we calculated Cohen's d for the effect size, considering the effect to be trivial (<0.2), small (0.2–0.5), medium (0.5–0.8), or large (>0.8) [31]. All analyses were performed for the overall population and by sex. All the statistical analyses were performed using IBM SPSS 28 (SPSS Inc., Chicago, IL, USA), and $p < 0.05$ was considered statistically significant.

3. Results

3.1. Characteristics of the Study Population (In the Post-COVID-19 Period)

The sample size previously calculated using Epidat software indicated that 37 participants would be needed to detect an estimated effect size (Cohen's d) of 1. Ultimately, the CaViDAuCo study included a total of 103 participants with HI aged between 19 and

74 years (mean age 35.4 ± 12.1 years). Among the total sample, 57 (55.3%) were women, and 46 (44.7%) were men. In addition, 64.1% were HIs from birth, and 45.6% used both sign language and spoken language. Table 1 shows the baseline characteristics of the included participants.

Table 1. Characteristics of the study participants.

Variable	Total (n = 103)	Men (n = 46)	Women (n = 57)
Age (years)	35.4 ± 12.1	34.7 ± 11.0	36.0 ± 12.9
Hearing impairment			
From birth	66 (64.1%)	34 (73.9%)	32 (56.1%)
Later	37 (35.9%)	12 (26.1%)	25 (43.9%)
Hearing aids			
Cochlear implants	27 (26.2%)	12 (26.1%)	15 (26.3%)
Hearing aids	42 (40.8%)	19 (41.3%)	23 (40.4%)
Both	13 (12.6%)	6 (13.0%)	7 (12.3%)
None	21 (20.4%)	9 (19.6%)	12 (21.1%)
Languages used			
Sign language	18 (17.5%)	9 (19.6%)	9 (15.8%)
Spoken language	38 (36.9%)	16 (34.8%)	22 (38.6%)
Both	47 (45.6%)	21 (45.7%)	26 (45.6%)
Mental disorders			
Depression	5.1 ± 4.7	4.8 ± 4.2	5.3 ± 5.0
Anxiety	3.6 ± 4.1	3.4 ± 3.6	3.8 ± 4.5
Stress	6.3 ± 4.8	5.9 ± 4.7	6.7 ± 4.8
Quality of life			
Physical QoL	52.2 ± 8.2	52.7 ± 7.8	51.8 ± 8.5
Mental QoL	45.7 ± 10.1	46.8 ± 9.6	44.9 ± 10.5

The data are shown as the mean ± standard deviation (SD) or number of subjects (percentage), n (%).

3.2. *Prevalence of Mental Disorders (Depression, Anxiety, and Stress) According to Suicide Risk*

Table 2 shows the prevalence of depression, anxiety, and stress according to categories (mild, moderate, severe, and extremely severe) in people with HI in the post-COVID-19 period according to suicide risk. Three years after the COVID-19 pandemic, the presence of mental disorders remained significantly associated with suicide risk. The prevalence of depression, anxiety, and stress was significantly higher among people at risk of suicide compared to those not at risk, both in the total population and in men and women. Specifically, depression, anxiety, and stress were more prevalent in the total population ($p < 0.001$), in men ($p = 0.002$, $p = 0.006$, and $p = 0.024$, respectively), and in women ($p < 0.001$, $p < 0.001$, and $p = 0.007$, respectively). Notably, men showed higher rates of extremely severe depression (33.3% vs. 15.4%) and extremely severe anxiety (44.4% vs. 15.4%) compared to women, as well as a higher prevalence of severe stress (33.3%). In contrast, women had higher rates of moderate depression (53.5% vs. 33.3%), severe anxiety (30.8% vs. 11.1%), and extremely severe stress (23.1%).

Table 2. Prevalence of mental disorders (depression, anxiety, and stress) according to suicide risk in the post-COVID-19 period.

	Total					Men					Women				
Variables	*n*	**Suicide Risk**	*n*	**No Suicide Risk**	*p*	*n*	**Suicide Risk**	*n*	**No Suicide Risk**	*p*	*n*	**Suicide Risk**	*n*	**No Suicide Risk**	*p*
Depression	22	81.8%	81	33.3%	<0.001	9	77.7%	37	27.0%	0.002	13	84.6%	44	38.6%	<0.001
Mild	1	4.5%	12	14.8%		0	0.0%	1	2.7%		1	7.7%	11	25.0%	
Moderate	10	45.5%	11	13.6%		3	33.3%	8	21.6%		7	53.5%	3	6.8%	
Severe	2	9.1%	3	3.7%		1	11.1%	1	2.7%		1	7.7%	2	4.5%	
Extremely severe	5	22.7%	1	1.2%		3	33.3%	0	0.0%		2	15.4%	1	2.3%	
Anxiety	22	72.7%	81	27.2%	<0.001	9	66.6%	37	21.6%	0.006	13	77.0%	44	31.8%	<0.001
Mild	3	13.6%	10	12.3%		1	11.1%	3	8.1%		2	15.4%	7	15.9%	
Moderate	2	9.1%	8	9.9%		0	0.0%	2	5.4%		2	15.4%	6	13.6%	
Severe	5	22.7%	2	2.5%		1	11.1%	2	5.4%		4	30.8%	0	0.0%	
Extremely severe	6	27.3%	2	2.5%		4	44.4%	1	2.7%		2	15.4%	1	2.3%	
Stress	22	59.0%	81	19.8%	<0.001	9	66.6%	37	21.6%	0.024	13	53.9%	44	18.2%	0.007
Mild	2	9.1%	8	9.9%		2	22.2%	4	10.8%		0	0.0%	4	9.1%	
Moderate	3	13.6%	4	4.9%		1	11.1%	2	5.4%		2	15.4%	2	4.5%	
Severe	5	22.7%	2	2.5%		3	33.3%	1	2.7%		2	15.4%	1	2.3%	
Extremely severe	3	13.6%	2	2.5%		0	0.0%	1	2.7%		3	23.1%	1	2.3%	

The data are shown as the number of subjects and percentage.

3.3. *Associations of Mental Disorders (Depression, Anxiety, and Stress) and Quality of Life (Physical and Mental) with Suicide Risk*

Table 3 shows the results of the mean differences in mental disorders and QoL according to suicide risk in the total population. In the post-pandemic period, people at suicide risk had higher values of depression, anxiety, and stress (9.6 ± 4.7, 7.5 ± 5.3, and 10.6 ± 4.7, respectively) than did people not at suicide risk (3.9 ± 3.8, 2.6 ± 3.0, and 5.2 ± 4.2, respectively) (for all variables, unadjusted model and models 1 and 2, $p < 0.001$). In addition, people at suicide risk had lower mental quality of life (38.6 ± 9.0) than people who were not at suicide risk (47.7 ± 9.5) (unadjusted model and models 1 and 2, $p < 0.001$).

Table 3. Unadjusted and adjusted differences in mental disorders (depression, anxiety, and stress) and quality of life (physical and mental) according to suicide risk in the post-COVID-19 period, analyzed using Student's *t* test and ANCOVA in the total population.

	Total					
Variable	**Suicide Risk (n = 22)**	**No Suicide Risk (n = 79)**	**Cohen's d (95% CIs)**	**Unadjusted Model**	**Model 1**	**Model 2**
Depression	9.6 ± 4.7	3.9 ± 3.8	1.4 (0.9, 1.9)	<0.001	<0.001	<0.001
Anxiety	7.5 ± 5.3	2.6 ± 3.0	1.4 (0.8, 1.9)	<0.001	<0.001	<0.001
Stress	10.6 ± 4.7	5.2 ± 4.2	1.3 (0.7, 1.8)	<0.001	<0.001	<0.001
Physical QoL	51.7 ± 10.1	52.3 ± 7.6	−0.1 (−0.5, 0.4)	0.763	0.576	0.613
Mental QoL	38.6 ± 9.0	47.7 ± 9.5	−1.0 (−1.5, −0.5)	<0.001	<0.001	<0.001

Model 1: adjusted for age and sex; Model 2: adjusted for age, sex, deafness at birth or later, hearing aids used, and language used.

Table 4 shows the results of the mean differences in mental disorders and QoL according to suicide risk in both men and women in the post-pandemic period. In men, those at suicide risk had higher values for depression, anxiety, and stress (10.1 ± 4.2, 7.7 ± 4.5, and 9.9 ± 3.9, respectively) than those who were not at suicide risk (3.5 ± 3.1, 2.4 ± 2.4, and 4.9 ± 4.5, respectively) (for depression and anxiety, unadjusted model and models 1 and 2, $p < 0.001$; for stress, unadjusted model, $p = 0.004$; model 1, $p = 0.006$; and model 2,

$p = 0.011$). Similarly, women at suicide risk had higher values of depression, anxiety, and stress (9.1 ± 5.2, 7.4 ± 5.9, and 11.0 ± 5.3, respectively) than did those who were not at suicide risk (4.1 ± 4.4, 2.7 ± 3.4, and 5.4 ± 3.9, respectively) (for depression, unadjusted model, $p < 0.001$; model 1, $p = 0.002$; and model 2, $p = 0.003$; for anxiety and stress, unadjusted model, models 1 and 2, $p < 0.001$). In addition, people at suicide risk had lower mental quality of life (36.1 ± 8.4) than people who were not at suicide risk (47.5 ± 9.7) (unadjusted model and model 1, $p < 0.001$; and model 2, $p = 0.001$).

Table 4. Unadjusted and adjusted differences in mental disorders (depression, anxiety, and stress) and quality of life (physical and mental) according to suicide risk in the post-COVID-19 period, analyzed using Student's *t* test and ANCOVA in men and women.

Variable	Suicide Risk (n = 22)	No Suicide Risk (n = 79)	Cohen's d (95% CIs)	Unadjusted Model	Model 1	Model 2
Men						
Depression	10.1 ± 4.2	3.5 ± 3.1	2.0 (1.4, 2.5)	<0.001	<0.001	<0.001
Anxiety	7.7 ± 4.5	2.4 ± 2.4	1.8 (1.3, 2.3)	<0.001	<0.001	<0.001
Stress	9.9 ± 3.9	4.9 ± 4.5	1.1 (0.6, 1.6)	0.004	0.006	0.011
Physical QoL	54.3 ± 6.1	52.3 ± 8.2	0.3 (−0.2, 0.7)	0.502	0.512	0.407
Mental QoL	42.3 ± 9.1	47.9 ± 9.5	−0.6 (−1.1, −0.1)	0.117	0.137	0.197
Women						
Depression	9.1 ± 5.2	4.1 ± 4.4	1.1 (0.6, 1.6)	<0.001	0.002	0.003
Anxiety	7.4 ± 5.9	2.7 ± 3.4	1.2 (0.7, 1.7)	<0.001	<0.001	<0.001
Stress	11.0 ± 5.3	5.4 ± 3.9	1.3 (0.8, 1.8)	<0.001	<0.001	<0.001
Physical QoL	49.9 ± 12.1	52.3 ± 7.2	−0.3 (−0.8, 0.2)	0.381	0.155	0.237
Mental QoL	36.1 ± 8.4	47.5 ± 9.7	−1.2 (−1.7, −0.7)	<0.001	<0.001	0.001

Model 1: adjusted for age; Model 2: adjusted for age, deafness at birth or later, hearing aids used, and language used.

4. Discussion

4.1. Main Findings

To our knowledge, this is the first study to evaluate the associations between mental disorders (such as depression, anxiety and stress) and QoL (both physical and mental) and suicide risk in a population with HI in the post-pandemic period. Our findings showed that in the post-pandemic period, depression (large effect), anxiety (large effect), stress (large effect) and mental QoL (trivial effect) could be positively associated with suicide risk, with higher scores than in individuals not at suicide risk in the population with HI. However, due to the lack of pre-pandemic data in people with HI, we cannot determine whether these risk levels have changed as a consequence of the pandemic.

Mental disorders and QoL during and during the post-COVID-19 period.

During the COVID-19 period, both the general population without HI [32–34] and those with HI experienced increased levels of mental disorders such as depression, anxiety and stress [10–12,14,16]. Similarly, physical and mental QoL declined in the general population [32], while people with HI reported even poorer QoL [35–37]. After 12 months, depression in the general population was observed, with a mild worsening trend and some individuals experiencing persistent or fluctuating psychological distress [38]. Psychological effects, such as anxiety, depression, and stress, may worsen over time and lead to long-term sequelae [38–40].

4.2. Mental Disorders in the Post-COVID-19 Period in the Population with Hearing Impairment

During the COVID-19 pandemic the mental health of people with HI has been affected, mental disorders have been observed such as depression, anxiety, and stress [6,11–13,15,17].

However, no prior evidence exists on the prevalence of these mental disorders in the post-pandemic period for this population. In the general population, a worsening mental disorders was observed during the pandemic period, and these have been identified as potential risk factors [41]. Suicide rates increased after the confinement period [42], and mental health issues and suicidal behaviors are expected to peak in the post-pandemic period [41], likely affecting specific groups such as people with HI. This population tends to have poorer mental health due to their disability [4,6,18,43] and may be at higher suicide risk than those without HI before the pandemic [43–47]. During the pandemic period, it has been observed that people with HI may be at higher suicide risk [48].

4.3. QoL in the Post-COVID-19 Period in the Population with Hearing Impairment

With respect to QoL, a decline in both physical and mental QoL was observed in the general population without HI during the lockdown period [32]. Following the lifting of restrictions, physical activity appeared to return to normal levels; however, a continued decline in mental activity was noted in the post-pandemic period [32]. While HI has been linked to lower QoL [43], studies have reported poorer QoL in people with HI during the pandemic period [35,37]. However, evidence of long-term changes in QoL following the end of restrictions, or in the absence of the pandemic, remains limited.

4.4. Barriers Faced by People with Hearing Impairment During the COVID-19 Period

The poorer mental health and mental QoL of people with HI may stem from a lack of coping skills and emotional awareness. Factors such as government measures, family loss, job disruptions, poverty, and psychological adversities during the pandemic may have contributed to this [49,50]. In addition, increased demand for mental health services has led to limitations, creating significant care gaps. Face-to-face care was often unavailable, shifting to remote interventions, which posed challenges for people with HI due to the lack of subtitles, SLI and the impossibility of lip reading [7,41,51]. Communication barriers were further exacerbated by PPE use and telecare [4,6,7], while masks also reduced perceived empathy, making communication even more difficult for people with HI [8,9].

Deficiencies in psychiatric emergency services, including suicide prevention [51], have been reported due to high demand and a shortage of mental health staff [52]. During the post-pandemic period, our findings showed that depression, anxiety, stress, and poor mental QoL in people with HI were observed alongside indicators of increased suicide risk. Therefore, it is crucial to improve online mental health resources and interventions for the overall population [41], particularly for individuals with HI, to ensure better accessibility through specialized applications and adaptations, such as written materials, images and videos, vibrations, colored lights, audio-to-text converters, and SLI [14,53–55].

In addition, most health professionals lack the necessary skills to communicate effectively with people with HI, causing stress and insecurity for both parties. It is essential that they understand the communication needs of people with HI and gain better insight into the deaf community [54,55]. For individuals with HI, support during healthcare is very important for optimal care and effective communication. However, during the pandemic, restrictions on accompanying persons, such as SLIs or family members, led to a lack of communication support for deaf individuals and for hard-of-hearing individuals [8,10].

During the COVID-19 period, irresponsible media coverage of suicide and repeated reports about the pandemic may have increased suicide risk and self-harm, especially among young people [41,51]. The prevalence of suicide is greater in individuals with previous suicide attempts, and self-harm ideations are more frequent than suicide attempts [20,42]. Many people avoid seeking mental health services due to stigma, often delaying care for 8–15 years [52]. In addition to mental disorders such as depression, anxiety, and stress, social isolation and loneliness could contribute to suicide risk, highlighting the need for support for those living alone [41]. Evidence suggests that people with HI experienced increased loneliness and isolation during the pandemic, with those living alone suffering more mental disorders than those living with others [14]. Additionally, poorer hearing ability has been linked to higher levels of loneliness [15].

Finally, studies [49,50] have shown that people with conditions that can contribute significantly to mental health are at increased risk of persistent psychological sequelae. HI is considered a risk factor for mental disorders [4,6,18]. For all the reasons mentioned above, mental disorders and poorer mental QoL in people with HI may persist in the post-pandemic period and could be associated with suicide risk, as suggested by our study.

In addition to the aforementioned psychosocial barriers, future research should also examine the impact of interpersonal factors such as abuse and neglect, which are often overlooked among people with HI due to persistent communication barriers. These experiences may exacerbate emotional distress and could be associated with increased suicide risk. Understanding these dynamics is crucial to developing more comprehensive suicide prevention strategies tailored to the specific vulnerabilities of this population and contributing positively to their mental health [22–24].

4.5. Limitations

This study has several limitations that should be considered. First, the sample size of people with HI was small (103 participants). Furthermore, since convenience sampling was used, there is a possibility of self-selection bias, which limits the representativeness of the sample and may influence the generalizability of the results. Second, although this was a study aimed at the population with HI, we must consider whether the questionnaires adapted for sign language were understandable and whether they were understood correctly, depending on the comprehension of this population. In addition, the questionnaires were self-reported online, which may influence the subjectivity of the participants. Third, due to the nature of the study design, a causal association cannot be established. Fourth, we did not assess the cause of HI, and this study may be biased toward people with HI at birth or later, so our results should be interpreted with caution. Fifth, the severity of each participant's disability was not assessed, only whether deafness was present at birth or acquired later and, if acquired, their age. Sixth, this study did not consider other covariates, such as other types of disability (visual, sensory, cognitive, etc.), ethnicity, comorbid medical diagnoses (such as diabetes, hypertension, etc.), and whether participants were taking medication. Seventh, although the sample size calculation was based on the Overall Depression Severity and Impairment Scale due to the lack of previous data in similar populations from the DASS-21, this scale was not used for data collection in our study. This could introduce slight discrepancies between the estimated and observed effect sizes, although the use of standardized metrics such as Cohen's d mitigates this limitation. Eighth, more superior suicide risk rating scales, such as the Columbia-Suicide Severity Rating Scale, the Beck Scale for Suicide Ideation, or the Suicide Behaviors Questionnaire—Revised, were not used; however, Plutchik's Suicide Risk Scale was used because in a population with HI, it can be flexibly adjusted or administered, as these participants may have difficulty expressing their emotions verbally due to limited access to spoken language. This scale allows for a more individualized approach than other more rigid scales. Ninth, the large effect sizes observed (e.g., Cohen's d >1.4) when comparing participants with and without suicide risk should be interpreted with caution. These values may reflect low within-group variability or small group sizes, especially given the limited number of participants at suicide risk (n = 22), rather than true population-level differences. This small sample may have increased the likelihood of statistical fluctuation and inflated effect size estimates.

Therefore, it is necessary to repeat the study with larger, more representative samples to confirm the magnitude of these associations. Furthermore, longitudinal studies with larger sample sizes and in different population types (in terms of age, gender, pathologies, etc.) are needed to further consolidate these findings.

5. Conclusions

In the post-pandemic period, people with HI continue to experience mental disorders, such as depression, anxiety, and stress, and have poor mental QoL. Given that mental disorders and poor mental QoL are risk factors for suicide, our findings indicate a significant association, rather than a causal relationship, between these factors and suicide risk in participants with HI. However, our results are based on a small sample size; therefore, they should be interpreted with caution and not generalized to the general population. It is essential to improve accessibility in mental health services by ensuring appropriate adaptations for people with HI, such as captioning, SLIs, images, and videos, among others. Additionally, raising awareness and implementing regional and national policies to improve communication tools can help address their specific needs and reduce the suicide risk. Further research is needed to better understand these associations and to design effective interventions that promote mental health and QoL in people with HI, helping reduce suicide risk.

Supplementary Materials: The following supporting information can be downloaded at: https://www.mdpi.com/article/10.3390/jcm14093130/s1, Table S1: Centres and associations for the hearing impaired in Spain included in the study; Table S2: SF-12 Health Questionnaire; Table S3: Depression, Anxiety and Stress Scale (DASS-21); Table S4: Plutchik's Suicide Risk Scale.

Author Contributions: Conceptualization: N.M.-H. and A.S.-L.; methodology: N.M.-H., A.S.-L. and I.C.-R.; software: I.C.-R. and C.P.-M.; validation: A.S.-L., I.O.-L., I.M.-G. and M.D.G.-G.; formal analysis: N.M.-H. and I.C.-R.; investigation: N.M.-H. and A.S.-L.; resources: N.M.-H., C.P.-M. and I.O.-L.; data curation: I.C.-R. and I.M.-G.; writing—original draft preparation: N.M.-H. and A.S.-L.; writing—review and editing: I.C.-R., C.P.-M. and I.O.-L.; visualization: I.M.-G. and M.D.G.-G.; supervision: A.S.-L. All authors have read and agreed to the published version of the manuscript.

Funding: This research was funded by ERDF funds and Carvascare Research Group from the Universidad de Castilla-La Mancha (2023-GRIN-34459). Nerea Moreno Herraiz is supported by a grant from Junta de Comunidades de Castilla-La Mancha (2023-PREJCCM-000062). Irene Martínez García has the support of a scholarship from science, innovation, and university (supported by a grant from science, innovation, and university) (FPU21/06866).

Institutional Review Board Statement: This study was conducted in accordance with the Declaration of Helsinki and was approved by the Clinical Research Ethics Committee of the Cuenca Health Area (REG: 2022/PI3322; 25 January 2023).

Informed Consent Statement: Written informed consent to participate was obtained from all the subjects involved in the study.

Data Availability Statement: The data are available in the manuscript or by contacting the corresponding author.

Conflicts of Interest: The authors declare no conflicts of interest. The funders had no role in the design of the study; in the collection, analyses, or interpretation of data; in the writing of the manuscript; or in the decision to publish the results.

Abbreviations

COVID-19	Coronavirus disease 2019
HI	Hearing impairment
PPE	Personal protective equipment
QoL	Quality of life
SLI	Sign language interpreter
WHO	World Health Organization

References

1. Zu, Z.Y.; Jiang, M.D.; Xu, P.P.; Chen, W.; Ni, Q.Q.; Lu, G.M.; Zhang, L.J. Coronavirus Disease 2019 (COVID-19): A Perspective from China. *Radiology* **2020**, *296*, E15–E25. [CrossRef] [PubMed]
2. Tu, Y.-F.; Chien, C.-S.; Yarmishyn, A.A.; Lin, Y.-Y.; Luo, Y.-H.; Lin, Y.-T.; Lai, W.-Y.; Yang, D.-M.; Chou, S.-J.; Yang, Y.-P.; et al. A review of SARS-CoV-2 and the Ongoing Clinical Trials. *Int. J. Mol. Sci.* **2020**, *21*, 2657. [CrossRef] [PubMed]
3. de Ministerio, S.; de Gobierno, E. Las 6 M Siempre En Mente. 17 February 2021. Available online: https://www.mscbs.gob.es/profesionales/saludPublica/ccayes/alertasActual/nCov/documentos/Infografia_6M.pdf (accessed on 23 October 2023).
4. Pineault, D. Impact of COVID-19 Pandemic on Mental Health and People with Hearing Problems. *Hear. J.* **2021**, *74*, 6. [CrossRef]
5. Instituto Nacional de Estadística (INE). Defunciones Por Causa de Muerte (lista reducida), Mes de Defunción Y Sexo. Años 2018–2022. Available online: https://www.ine.es/jaxi/Datos.htm?tpx=55863 (accessed on 23 October 2023).
6. Recio-Barbero, M.; Sáenz-Herrero, M.; Segarra, R. Deafness and mental health: Clinical challenges during the COVID-19 pandemic. *Psychol. Trauma.* **2020**, *12*, S212–S213. [CrossRef]
7. Trecca, E.M.C.; Gelardi, M.; Cassano, M. COVID-19 and hearing difficulties. *Am. J. Otolaryngol.* **2020**, *41*, 102496. [CrossRef]
8. Garg, S.; Deshmukh, C.P.; Singh, M.M.; Borle, A.; Wilson, B.S. Challenges of the Deaf and Hearing Impaired in the Masked World of COVID-19. *Indian J. Community Med.* **2021**, *46*, 11–14. [CrossRef]
9. Saunders, G.H.; Jackson, I.R.; Visram, A.S. Impacts of face coverings on communication: An indirect impact of COVID-19. *Int. J. Audiol.* **2021**, *60*, 495–506. [CrossRef]
10. Reed, N.S.; Assi, L.; Pedersen, E.; Alshabasy, Y.; Deemer, A.; Deal, J.A.; Willink, A.; Swenor, B.K. Accompaniment to healthcare visits: The impact of sensory impairment. *BMC Health Serv. Res.* **2020**, *20*, 990. [CrossRef] [PubMed]
11. Yang, Y.; Xiao, Y.; Liu, Y.; Li, Q.; Shan, C.; Chang, S.; Jen, P.H.-S. Mental Health and Psychological Impact on Students with or without Hearing Loss during the Recurrence of the COVID-19 Pandemic in China. *Int. J. Environ. Res. Public Health* **2021**, *18*, 1421. [CrossRef]
12. Ariapooran, S.; Khezeli, M. Symptoms of anxiety disorders in Iranian adolescents with hearing loss during the COVID-19 pandemic. *BMC Psychiatry* **2021**, *21*, 114. [CrossRef]
13. Necho, M.; Birkie, M.; Gelaye, H.; Beyene, A.; Belete, A.; Tsehay, M. Depression, anxiety symptoms, Insomnia, and coping during the COVID-19 pandemic period among individuals living with disabilities in Ethiopia, 2020. *PLoS ONE* **2020**, *15*, e0244530. [CrossRef] [PubMed]
14. Al Majali, S.A.; Alghazo, E.M. Mental health of individuals who are deaf during COVID-19: Depression, anxiety, aggression, and fear. *J. Community Psychol.* **2021**, *49*, 2134–2143. [CrossRef]
15. Littlejohn, J.; Venneri, A.; Marsden, A.; Plack, C.J. Self-reported hearing difficulties are associated with loneliness, depression and cognitive dysfunction during the COVID-19 pandemic. *Int. J. Audiol.* **2022**, *61*, 97–101. [CrossRef]
16. Dunn, C.C.; Stangl, E.; Oleson, J.; Smith, M.; Chipara, O.; Wu, Y.-H. The Influence of Forced Social Isolation on the Auditory Ecology and Psychosocial Functions of Listeners with Cochlear Implants During COVID-19 Mitigation Efforts. *Ear Hear.* **2021**, *42*, 20–28. [CrossRef]
17. Ariapooran, S.; Khezeli, M.; Batool, A. Post-Traumatic Stress Disorder (PTSD) and Depression in Iranian Adolescents with and Without Hearing Loss (HL) in Previous and During the Outbreak of the COVID-19. *Res. Sq.* **2021**. [CrossRef]
18. Peñacoba, C.; Garvi, D.; Gómez, L.; Álvarez, A. Psychological Well-Being, Emotional Intelligence, and Emotional Symptoms in Deaf Adults. *Am. Ann. Deaf.* **2020**, *165*, 436–452. [CrossRef]
19. Jerónimo, M.Á.; Piñar, S.; Samos, P.; González, A.M.; Bellsolà, M.; Sabaté, A.; León, J.; Aliart, X.; Martín, L.M.; Aceña, R.; et al. Intentos e ideas de suicidio durante la pandemia por COVID-19 en comparación con los años previos. *SJPMH* **2021**. [CrossRef]
20. Sànchez, J.G. Intento de suicidio antes y durante la pandemia de covid-19. Estudio comparativo desde el servicio de urgencias. *Semergen* **2023**, *49*, 101922. [CrossRef] [PubMed]
21. Van Orden, K.A.; Witte, T.K.; Cukrowicz, K.C.; Braithwaite, S.R.; Selby, E.A.; Joiner, T.E., Jr. The interpersonal theory of suicide. *Psychol. Rev.* **2010**, *117*, 575–600. [CrossRef]

22. Jagoe, C.; O'reilly, C.F.; James, L.E.; Khaled, E.; Alazzawi, H.; Enright, T. Interpersonal violence experienced by people with communication disabilities in Iraq: Sustainable Development Goals 16 and 5. *Int. J. Speech Lang. Pathol.* **2023**, *25*, 130–135. [CrossRef]
23. Olsson, S.; Dag, M.; Kullberg, C. Hard of Hearing Adults' Interpersonal Interactions and Relationships in Daily Life. *Disabilities* **2021**, *1*, 71–88. [CrossRef]
24. Chia, A.Y.; Hartanto, A.; Wan, T.S.; Teo, S.S.; Sim, L.; Kasturiratna, K.A.S. The Impact of Childhood Sexual, Physical and Emotional Abuse and Neglect on Suicidal Behavior and Non-Suicidal Self-Injury: A Systematic Review of Meta-analyses. *Psychiatr. Res. Commun.* **2025**, *5*, 100202. [CrossRef]
25. Gallagher, M.W.; Zvolensky, M.J.; Long, L.J.; Rogers, A.H.; Garey, L. The Impact of Covid-19 Experiences and Associated Stress on Anxiety, Depression, and Functional Impairment in American Adults. *Cognit. Ther. Res.* **2020**, *44*, 1043–1051. [CrossRef] [PubMed]
26. Von Elm, E.; Altman, D.G.; Egger, M.; Pocock, S.J.; Gøtzsche, P.C.; Vandenbroucke, J.P. The Strengthening the Reporting of Observational Studies in Epidemiology (STROBE) statement: Guidelines for reporting observational studies. *J. Clin. Epidemiol.* **2008**, *61*, 344–349. [CrossRef]
27. Gandek, B.; Ware, J.E.; Aaronson, N.K.; Apolone, G.; Bjorner, J.B.; Brazier, J.E.; Bullinger, M.; Kaasa, S.; Leplege, A.; Prieto, L.; et al. Cross-validation of item selection and scoring for the SF-12 Health Survey in nine countries: Results from the IQOLA Project. International Quality of Life Assessment. *J. Clin. Epidemiol.* **1998**, *51*, 1171–1178. [CrossRef]
28. SF-12 Score Calculator-OrthoToolKit. Available online: https://orthotoolkit.com/sf-12/ (accessed on 9 November 2023).
29. Lovibond, S.H.; Lovibond, P.F. *Manual for the Depression Anxiety Stress Scales*, 2nd ed.; Psychology Foundation of Australia: Sydney, Australia, 1995.
30. Plutchik, R.; Van Praag, H.; Conte, H.; Picard, S. Correlates of suicide and violent risk I: The suicide risk measure. *Compr. Psych.* **1989**, *30*, 296–302. [CrossRef]
31. Fritz, C.O.; Morris, P.E.; Richler, J.J. Effect size estimates: Current use, calculations, and interpretation. *J. Exp. Psychol. Gen.* **2012**, *141*, 2–18. [CrossRef]
32. Park, K.-H.; Kim, A.-R.; Yang, M.-A.; Lim, S.-J.; Park, J.-H. Impact of the COVID-19 pandemic on the lifestyle, mental health, and quality of life of adults in South Korea. *PLoS ONE* **2021**, *16*, e0247970. [CrossRef]
33. Pérez-Cano, H.J.; Moreno-Murguía, M.B.; Morales-López, O.; Crow-Buchanan, O.; English, J.A.; Lozano-Alcázar, J.; Somilleda-Ventura, S.A. Anxiety, depression, and stress in response to the coronavirus disease-19 pandemic. *Cirugia. Cir.* **2020**, *88*, 562–568. [CrossRef]
34. Salari, N.; Hosseinian-Far, A.; Jalali, R.; Vaisi-Raygani, A.; Rasoulpoor, S.; Mohammadi, M.; Rasoulpoor, S.; Khaledi-Paveh, B. Prevalence of stress, anxiety, depression among the general population during the COVID-19 pandemic: A systematic review and meta-analysis. *Glob. Health* **2020**, *16*, 57. [CrossRef]
35. Cavallaro, G.; Murri, A.; Nelson, E.; Gorrasi, R.; Quaranta, N. The Impact of the COVID-19 Lockdown on Quality of Life in Adult Cochlear Implant Users: A Survey Study. *Audiol. Res.* **2022**, *12*, 518–526. [CrossRef] [PubMed]
36. Ravens-Sieberer, U.; Kaman, A.; Erhart, M.; Devine, J.; Schlack, R.; Otto, C. Impact of the COVID-19 pandemic on quality of life and mental health in children and adolescents in Germany. *Eur. Child. Adolesc. Psychiatry* **2022**, *31*, 879–889. [CrossRef] [PubMed]
37. Khalaf, S.A.; Elhay, H.A.A.; Ghazy, H.K.; Goda, S.M. COVID-19 Pandemic Fear, Anxiety and Quality of Life among Adolescent Girls with Special Needs. *Tanta Sci. Nurs. J.* **2023**, *28*, 106–127. [CrossRef]
38. Lu, Z.-A.; Shi, L.; Que, J.-Y.; Zheng, Y.-B.; Wang, Q.-W.; Liu, W.-J.; Huang, Y.-T.; Shi, J.; Bao, Y.-P.; Lu, L. Long-term psychological profile of general population following COVID-19 outbreak: Symptom trajectories and evolution of psychopathological network. *Epidemiol. Psychiatr. Sci.* **2022**, *31*, e69. [CrossRef]
39. Gopal, A.; Sharma, A.J.; Subramanyam, M.A. Dynamics of psychological responses to COVID-19 in India: A longitudinal study. *PLoS ONE* **2020**, *15*, e0240650. [CrossRef] [PubMed]
40. Daly, M.; Sutin, A.R.; Robinson, E. Longitudinal changes in mental health and the COVID-19 pandemic: Evidence from the UK Household Longitudinal Study. *Psychol. Med.* **2022**, *52*, 2549–2558. [CrossRef]
41. Gunnell, D.; Appleby, L.; Arensman, E.; Hawton, K.; John, A.; Kapur, N.; Khan, M.; O'Connor, R.C.; Pirkis, J.; Caine, E.D. COVID-19 Suicide Prevention Research Collaboration. Suicide risk and prevention during the COVID-19 pandemic. *Lancet Psychiatry* **2020**, *7*, 468–471. [CrossRef]
42. Berardelli, I.; Sarubbi, S.; Rogante, E.; Cifrodelli, M.; Erbuto, D.; Innamorati, M.; Lester, D.; Pompili, M. The impact of the COVID-19 pandemic on suicide ideation and suicide attempts in a sample of psychiatric inpatients. *Psychiatry Res.* **2021**, *303*, 114072. [CrossRef]
43. Khurana, M.; Shoham, N.; Cooper, C.; Pitman, A.L. Association between sensory impairment and suicidal ideation and attempt: A cross-sectional analysis of nationally representative English household data. *BMJ Open* **2021**, *11*, e043179. [CrossRef]
44. Akram, B.; Batool, M. Suicidal Behavior Among the Youth with and Without Sensory Impairment: Prevalence and Comparison. *Omega* **2020**, *81*, 393–403. [CrossRef]

45. Fox, M.L.; James, T.G.; Barnett, S.L. Suicidal Behaviors and Help-Seeking Attitudes Among Deaf and Hard-of-Hearing College Students. *Suicide Life Threat. Behav.* **2020**, *50*, 387–396. [CrossRef] [PubMed]
46. Turner, O.; Windfuhr, K.; Kapur, N. Suicide in deaf populations: A literature review. *Ann. Gen. Psychiatry* **2007**, *6*, 26. [CrossRef] [PubMed]
47. Parker, M.; Duran, B.; Rhew, I.; Magarati, M.; Larimer, M.; Donovan, D. Risk and Protective Factors Associated with Moderate and Acute Suicidal Ideation among a National Sample of Tribal College and University Students 2015–2016. *J. Rural Health* **2021**, *37*, 545–553. [CrossRef]
48. Roy, N.; Amin, B.; Mamun, M.A.; Hossain, E.; Aktarujjaman; Sarker, B. Suicidal ideation among people with disabilities during the COVID-19 pandemic in Bangladesh: Prevalence and associated factors. *BJPsych Open* **2023**, *9*, e3. [CrossRef]
49. Ocampo-Eyzaguirre, D.; Correa-Reynaga, A.M. Situación emocional y resiliencia de estudiantes universitarios, pos-pandemia de la COVID-19. Norte de Potosí, Bolivia. *Soc. Tecnol.* **2022**, *6*, 17–32. [CrossRef]
50. Fernández González, D.; García Ramos, M.; Álvarez Héctor, G.; Morales Vento, E. Caracterización de la depresión en adultos mayores atendidos en consulta post-COVID-19. *Medimay* **2022**, *29*, 537–546. Available online: https://revcmhabana.sld.cu/index.php/rcmh/article/view/2260 (accessed on 15 December 2023).
51. Universidad Autónoma de Madrid (UAM). La OMS Publica Un Informe Sobre Las Consecuencias Que La Pandemia de La COVID-19 Ha Tenido En La Salud Mental Y En La Atención a Los Servicios de Salud Mental. 2022. Available online: https://www.uam.es/uam/investigacion/cultura-cientifica/noticias/covid-salud-mental (accessed on 1 January 2020).
52. Valencia Collazos, M. Trastornos mentales y problemas de salud mental. Día Mundial de la Salud Mental 2007. *Salud. Ment.* **2007**, *30*, 75–80. Available online: https://www.redalyc.org/articulo.oa?id=58230211 (accessed on 17 December 2023).
53. Naylor, G.; Burke, L.A.; Holman, J.A. Covid-19 Lockdown Affects Hearing Disability and Handicap in Diverse Ways: A Rapid Online Survey Study. *Ear Hear.* **2020**, *41*, 1442–1449. [CrossRef]
54. Corrales Pinto, M.; García Rodríguez, A.; Couto Calvo, M.V.; Díaz-Cueto Martínez, E. Obstáculos a derribar por el personal sanitario en la atención con discapacidad visual y auditiva. In *Conocimientos, Investigación y Prácticas en el Campo de la Salud*; Dykinson: Madrid, Spain, 2019; Volume 7, pp. 259–264.
55. Gutiérrez Domínguez, I.; García González, L. Comunicación del personal sanitario con pacientes con discapacidad auditiva. In *Revisión e Innovación en la Actuación de los Profesionales de la Salud*; Dykinson: Madrid, Spain, 2020; Volume 5, pp. 89–94.

Journal of
Clinical Medicine

MDPI

Article

Effect of the Narcissism Subscale "Threatened Self" on the Occurrence of Burnout Among Male Physicians

Antonia Tiziana Kreis [1,*], Roland von Känel [1], Sarah Andrea Holzgang [1], Aju Pazhenkottil [1,2,3], Jeffrey Walter Keller [1] and Mary Princip [1]

[1] Department of Consultation-Liaison Psychiatry and Psychosomatic Medicine, University Hospital Zurich, University of Zurich, 8091 Zurich, Switzerland
[2] Cardiac Imaging, Department of Nuclear Medicine, University Hospital Zurich, 8091 Zurich, Switzerland
[3] Department of Cardiology, University Hospital Zurich, 8091 Zurich, Switzerland
* Correspondence: antonia.kreis@uzh.ch; Tel.: +41-792625393

Abstract: Background/Objectives: Burnout is a highly prevalent issue among physicians. Recent research has indicated that personality traits, such as narcissism, may influence the development of burnout. This study investigates the relationship between the threatened self (TS) narcissism subscale and burnout in male physicians. **Methods:** We analyzed data from 60 male physicians in Switzerland, divided into burnout (n = 30) and control (n = 30) groups. Male physicians in Switzerland were recruited via hospitals, clinics, medical associations, professional journals, and direct email outreach. We assessed participants using the Maslach burnout inventory (MBI-HSS) and the Narcissism Inventory (NI-20). A generalized linear model (GLM) was used for the statistical analysis. **Results:** The results showed that lower TS scores were significantly associated with a reduced likelihood of burnout, suggesting that self-esteem instability and emotional vulnerability, characteristic of TS, may act as risk factors for burnout. Furthermore, we found that Effort–Reward Imbalance (ERI) was significantly associated with burnout. **Conclusions:** These findings highlight the importance of considering personality traits such as TS in burnout research and could be explored in further studies. In clinical practice, increasing therapists' awareness of TS may support more targeted interventions and help prevent the onset of burnout.

Keywords: narcissism; threatened self; burnout; physicians; job stress

1. Introduction

The increasing presence of the concept of burnout in societal discourses has led to a growing scientific interest in recent decades. Burnout is defined as a negative affective risk state for the development of mental and physical consequences and is characterized by three core symptoms, which are assessed with the Maslach burnout inventory (MBI) [1]: emotional exhaustion (EE), depersonalization (DP), and reduced personal accomplishment (PA) in terms of professional competencies [2]. Physicians are especially strongly affected by burnout, with an increasing trend in recent years [3,4]. Burnout negatively impacts both one's personal and professional well-being [5–11]. Among physicians, burnout is linked to compromised professionalism, a heightened risk of medical errors, diminished care quality [11], decreased patient satisfaction, and longer post-discharge recovery time in patients [12,13], as well as reduced career and work satisfaction [14,15]. Regarding the prevalence of burnout among Swiss physicians, a 2023 survey by the Association of Swiss Junior and Senior Hospital Doctors (VSAO) highlights a concerning decline in physician well-being. Indicators of poor health have worsened over the previous three

 https://doi.org/10.3390/jcm14103330

years: fatigue, emotional and physical exhaustion, and feelings of being overwhelmed have shown a marked increase among resident and senior physicians [16]. Further research shows an increasing prevalence of burnout among physicians in Switzerland [3], with younger physicians appearing to be particularly vulnerable [17].

While early research on burnout emphasized work-related factors, recent studies have increasingly recognized the role of personality characteristics in how individuals respond to different work situations, potentially increasing the risk of burnout [18,19]. A recent study identified a significant link between social comparison rumination and core components of burnout in students, particularly emotional exhaustion and cynicism. These findings underscore the potential role of maladaptive cognitive processes in the development of burnout. People with an overly idealized self-image may react strongly when others seem more successful or popular. This can lead to ongoing preoccupation and rumination about these social comparisons [20]. Among other personality traits, the impact of narcissism on burnout has been discussed. Before examining the role of narcissism in burnout, some general aspects of narcissism should be outlined, including the distinction between healthy and pathological forms, and with specific attention to the threatened self (TS), an important subdimension of narcissism.

Narcissism reflects an individual's ability to maintain a positive self-image through various cognitive, emotional, and behavioral regulatory processes [21]. This empowers the individual to seek validation, confirmation, and experiences of self-enhancement from the social environment [22]. Narcissism, as a regular aspect of personality, includes qualities such as high self-centeredness, a sense of superiority, a longing for admiration of others, and a tendency toward socially incompatible behaviors. A grandiose yet vulnerable self-concept explains the constant pursuit of external validation. The strong self-centeredness, coupled with a simultaneous lack of interest in others who are perceived as inferior, ultimately hinders the positive feedback that narcissistic personalities pursue [23]. The terms narcissism and narcissistic personality disorder have been used interchangeably for a long time. In recent times, the term narcissism has evolved to denote a personality variable in healthy individuals and should be distinguished from narcissistic personality disorder [24]. Differentiating precisely between healthy and pathological narcissism remains a challenge [25,26]. There are various approaches to describing and categorizing narcissism. Personality psychology distinguishes between grandiose and vulnerable manifestations of narcissistic traits. The transition from normative to pathological narcissism is marked by an increasing predominance of vulnerable characteristics [27].

The concept of the 'Threatened Self' (TS) was first introduced as a subdimension of narcissism in the original Narcissism Inventory (NI) developed by Deneke and Hilgenstock (1989) [28]. In its revised short form, the Narcissism Inventory-20 (NI-20), which is applied in the present study, narcissism is conceptualized along four dimensions, including the TS subscale [29]. These subscales are further described in detail in the following Methods section. TS reflects self-regulatory processes ranging from structural cohesion to narcissistic decompensation, indicating highly unstable self-esteem [28]. Despite its conceptual importance, research on the TS dimension is limited. In particular, the potential link between TS and burnout remains largely unexplored, highlighting a notable gap in the literature. TS represents an interesting aspect, particularly regarding underlying theories of the self. According to Claude Steele's (1988) [30] Self-Affirmation Theory, individuals are motivated to maintain a self-image that is coherent, morally adequate, and competent. When this self-image is threatened by failure, criticism, or social devaluation, for instance, it can trigger psychological defense mechanisms to protect the perceived integrity of the self [30]. This mechanism becomes particularly significant in the context of unstable self-esteem. Unstable self-esteem is considered a vulnerable predictor of maladaptive responses to self-threatening situations [31]. Individuals with unstable self-esteem are more prone to defensive reactions, such as externalizing blame or avoiding the source of threat. Coping with self-threat has also been investigated in the field of neuroscience; an fMRI study revealed that individuals with high self-esteem engage more strongly in self-enhancing strategies following a threat by more effectively inhibiting negative self-related information compared to those with low self-esteem [32]. Previous research has already identified a significant and positive association between narcissism and burnout and examined various aspects of this relationship [19,33–35]. There has been research on narcissism and burnout, exploring the subscales of adaptive and maladaptive narcissism [19] and research investigating grandiose narcissism, specifically admiration and rivalry in relation to burnout [36]. Schwarzkopf et al. (2016) examined the relationship between narcissistic personality traits and job burnout among 723 hospitalized patients with job-stress-related disorders, showing a significant correlation [34]. This study also examined the relationship between burnout and the four narcissism subscales of classic narcissistic self (CnS), idealistic self (IS), hypochondriac self (HS), and threatened self (TS), which are also employed in the present study. Rana et al. (2022) [35] examined the relationship between narcissism and burnout in a sample of surgeons in Germany, focusing on two dimensions of narcissism: "Admiration" and "Rivalry". High rivalry scores were linked to higher levels of burnout [35]. Other findings, comparing grandiose narcissism among surgeons, indicate that female participants exhibit significantly lower levels of narcissistic rivalry compared to their male colleagues [37]. This is an important finding pertaining to the present study, as our investigation was limited to male physicians. This decision has further reasons related to the study design, which are explained in more detail in the methodology section. Another recent study by Klerks et al. (2024) [38] examining the relationship between the dark triad (Machiavellianism, vulnerable and grandiose narcissism, and psychopathy) and burnout, mediated by perfectionistic self-presentation, found significant positive correlations between grandiose narcissism, academic burnout, and the Perfectionistic Self-Presentation Scale (PSPS). This study revealed that the relationship between grandiose narcissism and academic burnout was significantly mediated by the non-display of imperfections [38]. Burnout and narcissism among physicians have been explored to a limited extent, with the previously discussed study from 2022 specifically investigating this relationship in surgeons [35]. However, we further specify this research question by focusing directly on the TS narcissism subscale. While there has been existing research on narcissism and burnout among other study populations, as well as specifically on the TS subscale and burnout, the combination of these two components—the study population of physicians and TS—brings novelty to the field. Narcissism has been explored extensively; the TS subscale, which demonstrated the most significant associations with burnout compared to other dimensions in previous research [34], remains an area of untapped potential. Notably, there has been no prior investigation into the correlation between the TS subscale and physicians to our knowledge. In the present study, we examined the relationship between the TS narcissism subscale and burnout among physicians, exploring whether a high score of TS acts as a predictor for burnout.

Our hypothesis posits that TS serves as a positive predictor for the occurrence of burnout. The aim of this study is to gain a deeper understanding of this relationship, which may help identify a potential at-risk group and support its early recognition in the future. In addition, our findings may contribute to raising awareness of the influence of narcissistic personality traits on the development of burnout, highlighting possible clinical and therapeutic implications, and ultimately promoting a healthier workplace culture. By investigating TS as a potential predictor, this study addresses a notable gap in current research, as this subdimension of narcissism has rarely been examined in physician populations despite its theoretical relevance. As outlined above, TS plays a particularly important role in the psychological mechanisms underlying vulnerability to burnout, making it a compelling focus for further exploration.

2. Materials and Methods

2.1. Design

The following study is a secondary analysis of a previously conducted cross-sectional study that focused on the cardiovascular health of male physicians experiencing burnout [39]. We collected data between September 2019 and December 2021. Participation in this study was entirely voluntary, and we obtained informed consent from all participants. We recruited male physicians in Switzerland by contacting them through various channels, including hospitals, clinics, medical associations, professional publications, and direct email communication. Inclusion criteria were male physicians between 28 and 65 years of age, non-smokers for at least five years, and clinical burnout for the burnout group or absence of burnout for the control group based on the specified criteria. Exclusion criteria included any prior episode of clinical depression or burnout, current depression, cognitive impairment, a history of known heart disease, familial hypercholesterolemia, renal insufficiency, hypertension, diabetes, obesity, allergies to iodinated contrast media, contraindications to adenosine, beta-blockers, or isosorbide dinitrate, as well as a preference not to receive information regarding clinically relevant cardiac assessments. We included only male physicians based on the strict inclusion criteria of the parent study "Coronary microvascular function in male physicians with burnout and job stress". The parent study focused on working-age men (28–65 years) because the association between work stress and coronary heart disease has consistently been demonstrated in this group. In contrast, findings in women remain inconclusive, likely due to insufficient evidence and the fact that cardiovascular disease in women often manifests later in life, frequently beyond the typical working age [40]. Moreover, male physicians show a markedly higher rate of major adverse cardiovascular events than their female colleagues [41]. Finally, this decision aimed to minimize potential confounding factors, particularly hormonal influences on various blood biomarkers that were among the measures assessed. We included a total of 60 male participants in the study.

2.2. Ethics

This research project obtained approval from the local ethics committee of the State of Zurich, Switzerland (BASEC-Nr. 2018-01974). All participants provided written informed consent.

2.3. Participants

We included a total of 60 male participants in this study. These 60 participants were divided into two groups, consisting of 30 individuals each in the burnout and healthy control groups. We used the Maslach burnout inventory Human Services Survey (MBI-HSS; Mind Garden, Inc., Menlo Park, CA, USA) [42] and the Patient Health Questionnaire (PHQ-9; Pfizer Inc., New York, NY, USA) [43] to determine group assignments, conducting these surveys during the phone screening. To ensure a clear distinction between the two groups, we established cutoff values based on the review by Rotenstein et al. [44]. For the burnout group, the following cutoffs for the MBI-HSS were used: EE $\geq$ 27 and/or DP $\geq$ 10 (with a minimum EE of $\geq$20). For the healthy control group, the criteria were EE < 16 and DP < 7 [44]. We did not use the personal accomplishment (PA) subscale for group assignment, as previous research has shown that PA is relatively independent of the other two subscales [45–47]. In the case of the burnout group, a PHQ-9 score of $\leq$14, indicating at most moderate depressive symptoms, was required. For the healthy control group, a PHQ-9 score of ≤10, reflecting at most mild depressive symptoms, was necessary [48].

The total sample size was determined for the purpose of the parent study "Coronary microvascular function in male physicians with burnout and job stress" (Von Känel et al., 2023) [39], which involved extensive PET-based myocardial imaging. The decision was informed by previous institutional research conducted in patients with a sleep disorder [49], which indicated that a sample size of 23 participants per group was sufficient to detect a large effect (Cohen's d = 0.85) in adenosine-induced hyperemic myocardial blood flow, with 80% statistical power. To ensure adequate power and account for potential data loss, we aimed to enroll a total of 60 participants. Due to the complexity and resource-intensity of these procedures, a larger sample was not feasible.

2.4. Instruments

Participants completed the questionnaires NI20, ERI, and PSS-4 using printed forms on the day of the examination. For the MBI, all responses were taken from the examination day, except for one participant, for whom all MBI responses were missing and were therefore obtained from the initial phone screening.

Maslach burnout inventory (MBI): The MBI is a self-evaluation questionnaire used to assess the severity of burnout [1]. Our study used the 22-item German adaptation of the MBI-Human Services Survey [42]. Each of the 22 items is rated on a 7-point scale ranging from 0 ("never") to 6 ("daily"). These 22 items constitute the three dimensions of burnout: "Emotional exhaustion" (EE, nine items), "Depersonalization" (DP, five items), and "Personal achievement" (PA, eight items). The EE dimension examines feelings of being emotionally overwhelmed and exhausted because of work, while the DP dimension assesses a detached and impersonal response towards care recipients or patients. The PA dimension examines feelings of competence and successful accomplishments in one's work. Each of these dimensions can be evaluated independently. In this study, we identified a strong internal consistency for the EE dimension (Cronbach's $\alpha = 0.94$), as well as a good internal consistency for the DP dimensions (Cronbach's $\alpha = 0.89$) and PA (Cronbach's $\alpha = 0.81$).

Narcissism Inventory (NI-20): We used the 20-item short version of the self-reported Narcissism Inventory (NI-20) to measure narcissistic aspects [29]. The NI-20 items reflect a variety of narcissistic characteristics. As discussed by Deneke and Hilgenstock in 1989 [28], narcissistic self-regulation can be divided into four dimensions: threatened self (TS, seven items), classic narcissistic self (CnS, five items), idealistic self (IS, four items), and hypochondriac self (HS, four items). The TS dimension reflects self-organization ranging from cohesion to narcissistic decompensation, indicating unstable self-esteem. TS comprises 8 subscales, such as helpless self, loss of control over affects and impulses, derealization/depersonalization, basic potential of hope, worthless self, negative bodily self, social isolation, and withdrawal into feelings of harmony [29]. CnS corresponds to the traditional facet of narcissistic personality, emphasizing egocentrism or an inflated sense of one's abilities, reflecting aspects of narcissistic traits. The IS dimension addresses latent or overt anxiety about potential disappointment or emotional wounds in relationships, manifested through attempts to stabilize oneself by identifying with idealized models. HS, the fourth dimension, evaluates attention to one's own body and how it is perceived and utilized as an object, representing a hypochondriac anxiety-binding mode of self-regulation [29,50]. Participants assessed each item using a 5-point Likert scale, with options ranging from 1 (not applicable at all) to 5 (fully applicable). In our sample, the internal consistency of the dimension TS was Cronbach's $\alpha = 0.696$.

Perceived Stress Scale (PSS-4): We employed the 4-item German version of the PSS-4 to assess the extent to which individuals perceived situations as stressful during the past month [51]. This short version has demonstrated good internal consistency in a validation study [52]. Using a 5-point Likert scale, ranging from 0, representing "never", to 4, indicating "very often", questions were answered. A higher score on the PSS-4 signifies a higher level of perceived stress. In our sample, the total score showed an excellent internal consistency, with Cronbach's $\alpha = 0.86$.

Effort–Reward Imbalance (ERI): We evaluated job-related stress using the German short form of the Effort–Reward Imbalance questionnaire (ERI; University of Düsseldorf, Düsseldorf, Germany). The questionnaire includes three items assessing the effort put into work, seven about the rewards obtained at work, and six items measuring overcommitment [53]. Each item is rated on a 4-point Likert scale, ranging from 1, indicating 'strongly disagree', to 4, indicating 'strongly agree'. We calculated the effort–reward ratio while considering a correction factor to address the differing number of effort and reward items. A higher ratio signifies higher job stress. In our sample, the internal consistency for the effort scale showed a Cronbach's α of 0.76 and 0.77 for the reward scale. This German-language version also demonstrated satisfactory psychometric properties in a validation study, supporting its continued use in research and practice [54]. In two studies conducted among physicians in Switzerland, the ERI questionnaire was applied, and the validity for use in this context was demonstrated [55,56].

2.5. Statistical Analysis

The present analysis represents a secondary analysis derived from the parent study "Coronary microvascular function in male physicians with burnout and job stress". We performed statistical analyses using R statistical software version 4.4.1 [57]. A p-value below 0.05 was considered statistically significant.

Although the sample size has been predetermined, a crude post hoc sample size calculation based on the number of predictors was performed for verification purposes, using the formula $n = 20 + (10 \times \text{predictors})$, which resulted in a required sample size of 60. The statistical power of our final model was assessed using the pwr package (version 1.3-0).

Group comparisons to compare demographic data were either unpaired t-tests or Chi-squared tests where appropriate.

A linear regression analysis was conducted. Due to a single highly influential outlier in the calculations, the analysis was performed twice: once with the outlier and once without. Model quality metrics, i.e., R squared values, were calculated using 10-fold cross-validation.

Furthermore, we used a logistic regression with the outcome burnout and the independent variable TS of the 20-item Narcissism Inventory. We tested the impact of TS on the occurrence of burnout, calculating odds ratios to quantify the strength of the association. In our model, we controlled for PSS-4, ERI, and age. As a model quality metric, we calculated the average area under the receiver operating characteristic curve (ROC AUC), sensitivity, and specificity using 10-fold cross-validation. No explicit threshold optimization was applied; thus, the predefined cut-off was left at 0.5. Finally, we calculated the classification accuracy of the model on the original data set.

3. Results

The demographic characteristics of the burnout group and the control group exhibited notable similarities, except for age and job satisfaction (Table 1) [58,59]. Both groups demonstrated comparable features in terms of body mass index, marital status, job status, weekly working hours, provision of night shifts, and employment status. However, physicians in the burnout group were younger ($p = 0.012$) and reported significantly lower job satisfaction ($p < 0.001$). The medical specialties were distributed as follows: approximately one-third were internists, slightly less than one-fifth were surgeons, and one-tenth were psychiatrists. There was no significant difference observed between the two groups regarding medical specialties. The two groups exhibited significant differences in the total MBI score ($p < 0.001$) the scores of the three MBI subscales (EE ($p < 0.001$), DP ($p < 0.001$), and PA ($p < 0.001$)), as expected, due to the deliberate formation of extreme groups based on burnout severity. Furthermore, the groups differed significantly in the TS narcissism subscale ($p < 0.001$), PSS-4 ($p < 0.001$), and ERI ($p = 0.002$), including all the ERI subscales (Effort subscale ($p < 0.001$), Reward subscale ($p = 0.001$), and Overcommitment subscale ($p < 0.001$) (Table 2). With an R^2 exceeding 0.6, the model's power was calculated to be 100%, as the explained variance was substantially higher than initially expected.

In the correlation matrix (Figure 1), several relationships were observed among the variables, with the strongest correlation found between MBI and TS. In the linear regression analyses, with the outlier included (Table 3) and excluded (Table 4), burnout was significantly associated with TS and age. However, in the model excluding the outlier, a significant association with Effort–Reward Imbalance (ERI) was also found. Moreover, the results indicated that a lower age was associated with higher burnout scores. Using a 10-fold cross validation, our model explains, on average, about 57% of the variance in the validation data set. Excluding the outliner, this average explained variance increases to 63%.

Using a logistic regression, Table 5 shows how a lower score on the TS narcissism subscale is significantly associated with a reduced likelihood of experiencing burnout. Controlling for PSS-4 and age, we found no significant associations, except for ERI. Like the TS, a lower ERI score is significantly associated with a reduced risk of experiencing burnout. Using 10-fold cross-validation, the model demonstrated excellent discrimination with an ROC AUC of 0.944. Sensitivity was 82%, and specificity was 80%. Applying the model to the original data set resulted in a classification accuracy of 81.4%.

Table 1. Sample characteristics.

Characteristic		Total Sample, n = 60		Burnout, n = 30				Control, n = 30					
		n (%)	Mean (SD)	n (%)	Mean (SD)	Median	IQR	n (%)	Mean (SD)	Median	IQR	z-Value	p-Value
Age (years)			49.85 (9.59)		46.77 (10.56)	45	18.25		52.93 (7.48)	52	12	−2.29	0.012
Body mass index (m^2/kg)			24.99 (2.96)		25.63 (3.09)	25.25	3.29		24.35 (2.72)	23.92	2.90	1.75	0.094
Marital status	Married	44 (73%)		21 (70%)				23 (77%)					0.359
	Other	16 (27%)		9 (30%)				7 (23%)					
Job status	full time	48 (80%)		25 (83%)				23 (77%)					0.527
	part time	12 (20%)		5 (17%)				7 (23%)					
Working hours per week			56.03 (10.40)		57.35 (8.99)	60.00	13.75		54.72 (11.66)	55.00	14.375		0.332
Night work		35 (58%)		18 (60%)				17 (57%)					1.000
Employment	Self-employed	20 (33%)		10 (33%)				10 (33%)					
	hospital	38 (63%)		19 (63%)				19 (63%)					
	Self-employed and hospital	2 (3.3%)		1 (3.3%)				1 (3.3%)					

Table 1. *Cont.*

Characteristic		Total Sample, n = 60		Burnout, n = 30				Control, n = 30					
		n (%)	Mean (SD)	n (%)	Mean (SD)	Median	IQR	n (%)	Mean (SD)	Median	IQR	z-Value	p-Value
Job satisfaction	Very dissatisfied	1 (1.7%)		1 (3.3%)				0 (0%)					<0.001
	dissatisfied	1 (1.7%)		1 (3.3%)				0 (0%)					
	Partly satisfied, partly dissatisfied	14 (23%)		14 (47%)				0 (0%)					
	satisfied	21 (35%)		11 (37%)				10 (33%)					
	Very satisfied	23 (38%)		3 (10%)				20 (67%)					
Medical specialty	Psychiatry	6 (10%)		2 (6.7%)				4 (13.3%)					0.181
	Cardiology	3 (5%)		1 (3.3%)				2 (6.7%)					
	Internal medicine	20 (33%)		12 (40%)				8 (27%)					
	Oncology	4 (6.7%)		0 (0%)				4 (13%)					
	Surgery	11 (18.3%)		4 (13.3%)				7 (23.3%)					
	Neurology	3 (5%)		2 (6.7%)				1 (3.3%)					
	Other	13 (22%)		9 (30%)				4 (13.3%)					

Table 2. Descriptive statistics of Maslach burnout inventory, Narcissism Inventory TS (NI-2O), Effort–Reward Imbalance (ERI), and Perceived Stress Scale (PSS-4).

Variables		Total Sample, n = 60	Burnout, n = 30			Control, n = 30				
		Mean (SD)	Mean (SD)	Median	IQR	Mean (SD)	Median	IQR	z-Value	p-Value
Maslach Burnout Inventory (MBI)	Total score	1.68 (1.11)	2.68 (0.57)	2.62	0.91	0.68 (0.33)	0.71	0.50	6.65	<0.001
	Emotional Exhaustion	19.53 (12.78)	31.13 (5.84)	30.50	8.75	7.93 (4.43)	7.00	6.75	6.66	<0.001
	Depersonalization	8.05 (7.26)	13.77 (6.08)	12.00	8.75	2.33 (1.67)	2.00	2.00	6.45	<0.001
	Personal accomplishment	8.68 (5.58)	12.43 (4.61)	12.00	6.75	4.93 (3.6)	5.00	5.00	5.45	<0.001
Narcissism Inventory (NI20)	Threatened Self	1.55 (0.54)	1.87 (0.56)	1.71	0.71	1.25 (0.30)	1.14	0.29		<0.001
Perceived Stress Scale Sum Score (PSS-4)		4.66 (3.10)	6.45 (2.73)	7.00	4.00	2.93 (2.39)	3.00	2.75		<0.001
Effort–Reward Imbalance Questionnaire (ERI)	Effort–Reward Ratio	1.33 (1.22)	1.84 (1.54)	1.46	0.74	0.84 (0.41)	0.76	0.50	3.477	0.002
	Effort Subscale	6.36 (2.22)	7.69 (1.37)	8.00	2.00	5.01 (2.13)	5.00	2.00		<0.001
	Reward Subscale	13.53 (3.80)	11.97 (3.89)	12.00	6.00	15.03 (3.09)	15.00	4.00		0.001
	Overcommitment Subscale	8.48 (3.78)	10.68 (2.88)	11.00	4.25	6.43 (3.37)	7.00	4.00		<0.001

Table 3. Linear regression with outlier.

Coefficients:	Estimate	Std. Error	z-Value	p	CI Lower	CI Upper
(Intercept)	1.32	0.64	2.08	0.04 *	0.045	2.60
Narcissism Subscale "Threatened self"	1.10	0.21	5.14	<0.001 ***	0.669	1.52

Table 3. *Cont.*

Coefficients:	Estimate	Std. Error	z-Value	p	CI Lower	CI Upper
PSS-4 Sum score	0.04	0.038	1.09	0.28	−0.035	0.117
Effort–Reward Ratio	0.05	0.08	0.68	0.50	−0.106	0.216
Age	−0.35	0.10	−3.47	0.001 **	−0.055	−0.015

CI Lower = lower bound of the 95% confidence interval, CI Upper = upper bound of the 95% confidence interval, * = $p = 0.01$, ** = $p = 0.001$, *** = $p = 0$

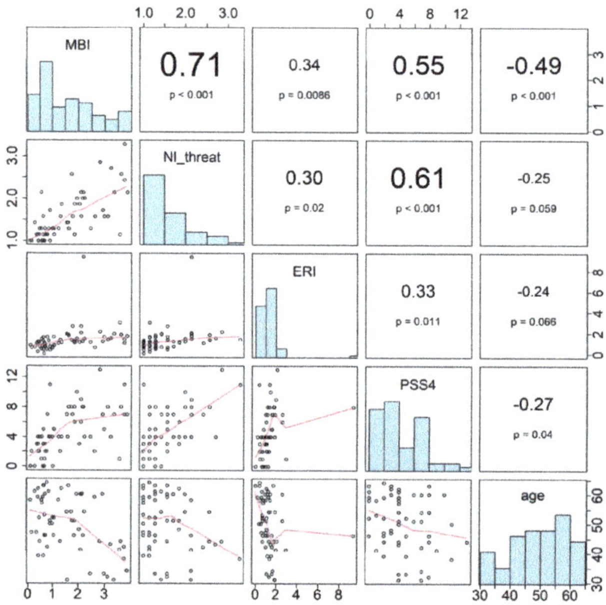

Figure 1. Pearson correlation of Maslach burnout inventory (MBI), Narcissism Inventory TS (NI-threat), Effort–Reward Imbalance (ERI), Perceived Stress Scale (PSS4), and age.

Table 4. Linear regression without outlier.

Coefficients:	Estimate	Std. Error	z-Value	p	CI Lower	CI Upper
(Intercept)	0.71	0.66	1.07	0.288	−0.615	2.03
Narcissism Subscale "Threatened self"	1.06	0.20	5.16	<0.001 ***	0.646	1.47
PSS-4 Sum score	0.03	0.04	0.68	0.498	−0.049	0.099
Effort–Reward Ratio	0.42	0.17	2.49	0.016 *	0.081	0.756
Age	−0.028	0.01	−2.84	0.006 **	−0.049	−0.008

CI Lower = lower bound of the 95% confidence interval, CI Upper = upper bound of the 95% confidence interval, * = $p = 0.01$, ** = $p = 0.001$, *** = $p = 0$

Table 5. Generalized linear model for analyzing the threatened self narcissism subscale as a predictor of burnout.

Coefficients:	Estimate	Odds Ratio	Std. Error	z-Value	p	CI Lower	CI Upper
(Intercept)	7.36	-	3.26	2.26	0.024 *	0.819	13.900
Narcissism Subscale "Threatened self"	−2.62	0.07	1.24	−2.12	0.034 *	−5.110	−0.140
PSS-4 Sum score	−0.33	0.72	0.18	−1.82	0.068	−0.685	0.032

Table 5. *Cont.*

Coefficients:	Estimate	Odds Ratio	Std. Error	z-Value	p	CI Lower	CI Upper
Effort–Reward Ratio	−2.30	0.10	0.96	−2.39	0.017 *	−4.220	−0.374
Age	0.02	1.02	0.05	0.34	0.733	−0.080	0.113

* = p = 0.01.

4. Discussion

In this study, we explored the relationship between the TS narcissism subscale and burnout among a group of male physicians with burnout and a control group. Our findings indicate a significant association, suggesting that a lower score on the TS narcissism subscale is associated with a reduced likelihood of experiencing burnout. Therefore, we conclude that narcissism may function as a predictor for burnout. Our findings are consistent with previous research, which showed a significant association between burnout and narcissism [19,33,34]. Narcissism has already been assessed and investigated in various ways, using different methods and across different study populations [19,33–35]. The understanding and assessment of narcissism in terms of narcissistic personality disorder, pathological narcissism, and normal narcissism have been complex. There is an effort to address the challenge of reconciling inconsistent definitions of narcissism within the fields of clinical psychology, psychiatry, and social/personality psychology to capture this diverse concept within a comprehensive construct [21].

The TS narcissism dimension comprises eight subscales: helpless self, loss of control over affects and impulses, derealization/depersonalization, basic potential of hope, worthless self, negative bodily self, social isolation, and withdrawal into feelings of harmony [29]. When considering these subscales, most of the subscales entail inherently taxing and exhausting states. We can further argue that since emotional exhaustion represents a crucial dimension of burnout, such exhausting states pose a significant risk for burnout. The attributes of TS are virtually archaic, basal feelings that intuitively suggest a risk for psychological decompensation. Conversely, we know from a psychological perspective that a strong sense of self-worth, social integration, and feelings of security have a protective effect on stress experience and burnout [60,61]. The very contrasting emotional states such as "helpless self", "worthless self", or "social isolation" are characteristic of TS [29]. Unlike other narcissistic traits, such as the classic narcissistic self, which involves overestimating one's abilities or seeking constant validation [29], the traits of TS pose a consistent risk for burnout due to a fundamental disruption of the self. While grandiosity fantasies may significantly impact one's experiences and social relationships, the self is not affected as profoundly as with TS.

Focusing on the professional role of physicians, within the healthcare sector, physicians often encounter patients who exhibit neediness, hopelessness, and strong emotional burdens [62,63]. However, these patients are not threatened by a narcissistic self but rather by an illness. The symptoms of TS are reflected in affected physicians from an external source, potentially amplifying their own struggles with narcissistic structures of the threatened self, such as hopelessness or social isolation. Consequently, this situation may activate or exacerbate existing narcissistic issues and feelings of inadequacy.

Another finding of this study pertains to the relationship between ERI and burnout. Previous research shows inconsistency regarding the influence of ERI on burnout. While a significant positive impact of ERI on burnout has been demonstrated [64,65], a longitudinal cohort study found that ERI was not longitudinally associated with any of the burnout dimensions when controlling for confounders [66]. In the present study, after controlling for PSS-4 and age, it was demonstrated that a lower ERI score is significantly associated with a reduced risk of experiencing burnout. The inconclusive results across studies suggest the need for further research to explore the relationship between these components. We included participants who had to explicitly state that they had had job stress over 6 months at least, so an association would be highly expected.

Furthermore, we observed a linear association between a younger age and higher levels of burnout. This finding is consistent with the previous literature and may be attributed to lower professional experience and a resulting higher vulnerability to being overwhelmed.

In this study, the burnout group averaged 57.35 working hours per week. In contrast, non-physicians in Switzerland work an average of 41.7 h per week, with a legally regulated maximum working time of 45 h per week [67]. These additional working hours reduce opportunities for social balance and increase the risk of social isolation.

Furthermore, despite great and important efforts in recent decades to change societal stigmas, the display of weakness is traditionally viewed as a non-masculine trait [68,69]. This perception may be heightened when traits like strength, security, and the role of a harbinger of hope are projected onto physicians as a professional group. A 2020 study explored how gendered ways of thinking relate to the perception of role models in medical education. The findings revealed that male students rarely identified female doctors as role models, and male role models were generally perceived as more admirable than their female counterparts. These results highlight the ongoing influence of gendered perceptions that subtly shape the professional ideals and attitudes of medical students [70]. This can be linked to TS insofar as the mentioned masculine traits conflict with the features of TS, potentially accentuating them and thereby increasing the risk of burnout. However, this interpretation remains speculative, and further research needs to explore how men, grappling with weakened or threatened self-perceptions, possibly clash with their ideals of masculinity and the physician's role, thereby engendering an emotionally taxing conflict, which in turn potentially heightens the risk for burnout.

Preventive measures to reduce burnout often target individual-focused interventions such as counseling, supervision, or relaxation exercises, as well as work-related interventions such as altering workflow or work organization [71]. Screening for at-risk individuals is not a practical preventive measure for narcissism. Instead, the focus can be on raising awareness among therapists working with people who are already suffering burnout, particularly in addressing aspects of the threatened self and potentially providing therapy, especially in the patient group of male physicians with burnout. TS exhibits fewer aspects of external behavior than of internal experiences, making it important to address this internal experience therapeutically. Thus, this awareness can potentially act as relapse prevention through increased diagnosis.

Our study has several noteworthy limitations. First, the sample size was relatively small (n = 60), which may reduce the statistical power and limit the generalizability of the findings. Additionally, it was divided into two predetermined extreme groups based on the severity of burnout, thereby hindering us from analyzing continuous scores of the MBI. With the ethics committee's approval, we had to slightly relax the criteria to attain the recruitment target of 60 participants, potentially introducing methodological limitations. While we only selected male physicians for our study based on the stringent inclusion criteria of the parent study, "*Coronary microvascular function in male physicians with burnout and job stress*", this approach aimed to minimize confounding variables, such as hormonal influences. Moreover, while we exclusively examined physicians working in Switzerland, our study population encompassed different medical specialties, enabling a broader and more generalized representation of physicians. Furthermore, since participation in our study was voluntary and contingent upon participants' interest, we cannot disregard the possibility of both a self-selection bias and a self-reporting bias. The cross-sectional design of our study does not permit a causal conclusion regarding the association between the TS narcissism subscale and burnout. However, it can be argued that a personality variable represents a long-term condition, thus suggesting that a causal relationship can be assumed. Therefore, it is legitimate to use a predictive statistical model, such as the generalized linear model in our case. Due to the small sample size, we were not able to conduct a more detailed analysis of the eight subdimensions of the TS subscale. Such an analysis could have provided valuable insights into which specific aspects of TS have the strongest influence on burnout. Furthermore, there are several potential influencing factors, such as a history of trauma, that may impact the observed associations. These should be explored in future research. Additionally, the study was conducted during the COVID-19 pandemic. The impact of COVID-19 on the mental health of healthcare workers remains a subject of inconsistent findings in the literature. While some studies suggest that clinically relevant symptoms of anxiety and depression occurred at comparable rates before and during the pandemic [72,73], others report a marked increase in psychological distress among healthcare professionals [74]. Regarding the present study, it can be noted that this was a period when physicians faced exceptional challenges, which might have diminished their capacity to engage in this study and potentially affected their mental well-being.

5. Conclusions

In this study, we investigated the effect of the TS narcissism subscale on the occurrence of burnout. Our findings suggest that the increased display of the TS narcissism subscale acts as a positive predictor for experiencing burnout. However, studies with larger samples are needed to expand upon our findings. In particular, the inclusion of female physicians is warranted to examine whether the association between narcissism and burnout differs by gender. Longitudinal designs may further help to clarify causal relationships and reveal how narcissistic traits influence the development of burnout over time. Additionally, future research could explore early identification strategies and evaluate targeted therapeutic interventions for healthcare professionals exhibiting elevated levels of narcissistic traits, with the aim of preventing or mitigating burnout.

Author Contributions: Conceptualization, R.v.K., M.P., S.A.H. and A.P.; methodology, A.T.K.; validation, A.T.K.; formal analysis, A.T.K. and J.W.K.; investigation, M.P., R.v.K., S.A.H. and A.P.; data curation, M.P., R.v.K., S.A.H., A.P. and A.T.K.; writing—original draft preparation, A.T.K.; writing—review and editing, A.T.K., M.P., R.v.K., S.A.H., A.P. and J.W.K.; visualization, A.T.K. and J.W.K.; supervision, R.v.K.; project administration, M.P. and S.A.H.; funding acquisition, R.v.K. All authors have read and agreed to the published version of the manuscript.

Funding: This research was funded by an institutional grant from the University of Zurich to the clinical director Roland Von Känel.

Institutional Review Board Statement: The study was conducted according to the guidelines of the Declaration of Helsinki, and approved by the Ethics Committee of Zurich (BASEC-Nr. 2018-01974, 17 December 2018).

Informed Consent Statement: Written informed consent was obtained from all participants involved in the study.

Data Availability Statement: The data sets used and analyzed during the current study are available from the corresponding author upon reasonable request. Data cannot be publicly disclosed due to privacy and ethical restrictions.

Conflicts of Interest: The authors declare no conflicts of interest. The funders had no role in the design of the study; in the collection, analyses, or interpretation of data; in the writing of the manuscript; or in the decision to publish the results.

Abbreviations

The following abbreviations are used in this manuscript:

CnS	Classic narcissistic self
DP	Depersonalization
EE	Emotional exhaustion
ERI	Effort–Reward Imbalance
HS	Hypochondriac self
IS	Idealistic self
MBI	Maslach Burnout Inventory
NI-20	Narcissism Inventory
PA	Personal accomplishment
PHQ-9	Patient Health Questionnaire
PSS4	Perceived Stress Scale
TS	Threatened self

References

1. Maslach, C.; Jackson, S.E.; Leiter, M.P. Maslach Burnout Inventory: Third edition. In *Evaluating Stress: A Book of Resourzces*; Scarecrow Education: Lanham, MD, USA, 1997; pp. 191–218.
2. Maslach, C.; Jackson, S. The Measurement of Experienced Burnout. *J. Organ. Behav.* **1981**, *2*, 99–113. [CrossRef]
3. Arigoni, F.; Bovier, P.A.; Sappino, A.P. Trend of burnout among Swiss doctors. *Swiss Med. Wkly.* **2010**, *140*, w13070. [CrossRef] [PubMed]
4. Shanafelt, T.D.; Hasan, O.; Dyrbye, L.N.; Sinsky, C.; Satele, D.; Sloan, J.; West, C.P. Changes in Burnout and Satisfaction With Work-Life Balance in Physicians and the General US Working Population Between 2011 and 2014. *Mayo Clin. Proc.* **2015**, *90*, 1600–1613. [CrossRef]
5. Shanafelt, T.D.; Noseworthy, J.H. Executive Leadership and Physician Well-being: Nine Organizational Strategies to Promote Engagement and Reduce Burnout. *Mayo Clin. Proc.* **2017**, *92*, 129–146. [CrossRef] [PubMed]
6. Govardhan, L.M.; Pinelli, V.; Schnatz, P.F. Burnout, depression and job satisfaction in obstetrics and gynecology residents. *Conn. Med.* **2012**, *76*, 389–395. [PubMed]
7. Pereira-Lima, K.; Loureiro, S.R. Burnout, anxiety, depression, and social skills in medical residents. *Psychol. Health Med.* **2015**, *20*, 353–362. [CrossRef] [PubMed]
8. Rath, K.S.; Huffman, L.B.; Phillips, G.S.; Carpenter, K.M.; Fowler, J.M. Burnout and associated factors among members of the Society of Gynecologic Oncology. *Am. J. Obstet. Gynecol.* **2015**, *213*, 824.e1–824.e9. [CrossRef]
9. Talih, F.; Warakian, R.; Ajaltouni, J.; Shehab, A.A.; Tamim, H. Correlates of Depression and Burnout Among Residents in a Lebanese Academic Medical Center: A Cross-Sectional Study. *Acad. Psychiatry* **2016**, *40*, 38–45. [CrossRef]
10. Pompili, M.; Innamorati, M.; Narciso, V.; Kotzalidis, G.D.; Dominici, G.; Talamo, A.; Girardi, P.; Lester, D.; Tatarelli, R. Burnout, hopelessness and suicide risk in medical doctors. *Clin. Ter.* **2010**, *161*, 511–514.
11. Shanafelt, T.D.; Balch, C.M.; Bechamps, G.; Russell, T.; Dyrbye, L.; Satele, D.; Collicott, P.; Novotny, P.J.; Sloan, J.; Freischlag, J. Burnout and medical errors among American surgeons. *Ann. Surg.* **2010**, *251*, 995–1000. [CrossRef]
12. Anagnostopoulos, F.; Liolios, E.; Persefonis, G.; Slater, J.; Kafetsios, K.; Niakas, D. Physician burnout and patient satisfaction with consultation in primary health care settings: Evidence of relationships from a one-with-many design. *J. Clin. Psychol. Med. Settings* **2012**, *19*, 401–410. [CrossRef] [PubMed]
13. Halbesleben, J.R.; Rathert, C. Linking physician burnout and patient outcomes: Exploring the dyadic relationship between physicians and patients. *Health Care Manag. Rev.* **2008**, *33*, 29–39. [CrossRef] [PubMed]
14. Goldberg, R.; Boss, R.W.; Chan, L.; Goldberg, J.; Mallon, W.K.; Moradzadeh, D.; Goodman, E.A.; McConkie, M.L. Burnout and its correlates in emergency physicians: Four years' experience with a wellness booth. *Acad. Emerg. Med.* **1996**, *3*, 1156–1164. [CrossRef]
15. Sharma, A.; Sharp, D.M.; Walker, L.G.; Monson, J.R. Stress and burnout in colorectal and vascular surgical consultants working in the UK National Health Service. *Psychooncology* **2008**, *17*, 570–576. [CrossRef]
16. Gut, A.; Fröhli, D. *Arbeitssituation der Assistenz- und Oberärztinnen und -ärzte Management Summary zur Mitgliederbefragung 2023 im Auftrag des Verbands Schweizerischer Assistenz- und Oberärztinnen und -ärzte (vsao)*; Verband Schweizerischer Assistenz- und Oberärztinnen und -ärzte (vsao): Bern, Switzerland, 2023.
17. Lindemann, F.; Rozsnyai, Z.; Zumbrunn, B.; Laukenmann, J.; Kronenberg, R.; Streit, S. Assessing the mental wellbeing of next generation general practitioners: A cross-sectional survey. *BJGP Open* **2019**, *3*, bjgpopen19X101671. [CrossRef] [PubMed]

18. Alarcon, G.; Eschleman, K.J.; Bowling, N.A. Relationships between personality variables and burnout: A meta-analysis. *Work. Stress* **2009**, *23*, 244–263. [CrossRef]
19. von Känel, R.; Herr, R.M.; AEM, V.A.N.V.; Schmidt, B. Association of adaptive and maladaptive narcissism with personal burnout: Findings from a cross-sectional study. *Ind. Health* **2017**, *55*, 233–242. [CrossRef] [PubMed]
20. Flett, G.L.; Nepon, T.; Hewitt, P.L.; Su, C.; Yacyshyn, C.; Moore, K.; Lahijanian, A. The Social Comparison Rumination Scale: Development, Psychometric Properties, and Associations With Perfectionism, Narcissism, Burnout, and Distress. *J. Psychoeduc. Assess.* **2024**, *42*, 685–704. [CrossRef] [PubMed]
21. Pincus, A.L.; Lukowitsky, M.R. Pathological narcissism and narcissistic personality disorder. *Annu. Rev. Clin. Psychol.* **2010**, *6*, 421–446. [CrossRef]
22. Pincus, A.L.; Ansell, E.B.; Pimentel, C.A.; Cain, N.M.; Wright, A.G.C.; Levy, K.N. Initial construction and validation of the Pathological Narcissism Inventory. *Psychol. Assess.* **2009**, *21*, 365–379. [CrossRef] [PubMed]
23. Morf, C.C.; Rhodewalt, F. Unraveling the paradoxes of narcissism: A dynamic self-regulatory processing model. *Psychol. Inq.* **2001**, *12*, 177–196. [CrossRef]
24. Ritter, K.; Lammers, C.-H. Narzissmus—Persönlichkeitsvariable und persönlichkeitsstörung = Narcissism—Variable of personality and personality disorder. *PPmP Psychother. Psychosom. Med. Psychol.* **2007**, *57*, 53–60. [CrossRef]
25. Emmons, R.A. Factor analysis and construct validity of the Narcissistic Personality Inventory. *J. Personal. Assess.* **1984**, *48*, 291–300. [CrossRef] [PubMed]
26. Emmons, R.A. Narcissism: Theory and measurement. *J. Personal. Soc. Psychol.* **1987**, *52*, 11–17. [CrossRef] [PubMed]
27. Wilfer, T.; Spitzer, C.; Lammers, C.H. Narcissism-Normal, pathological, grandiose, vulnerable? *Nervenarzt* **2024**, *95*, 1052–1062. [CrossRef]
28. Deneke, F.-W.; Hilgenstock, B. *Das Narzissmusinventar*; Huber: Atlanta, GA, USA, 1989.
29. Daig, I.; Burkert, S.; Fischer, H.F.; Kienast, T.; Klapp, B.F.; Fliege, H. Development and factorial validation of a short version of the narcissism inventory (NI-20). *Psychopathology* **2010**, *43*, 150–158. [CrossRef]
30. Steele, C.M. The Psychology of Self-Affirmation: Sustaining the Integrity of the Self. In *Advances in Experimental Social Psychology*; Berkowitz, L., Ed.; Academic Press: Cambridge, MA, USA, 1988; Volume 21, pp. 261–302.
31. Kernis, M.H. Measuring self-esteem in context: The importance of stability of self-esteem in psychological functioning. *J. Personal.* **2005**, *73*, 1569–1605. [CrossRef] [PubMed]
32. Hoefler, A.; Athenstaedt, U.; Corcoran, K.; Ebner, F.; Ischebeck, A. Coping with Self-Threat and the Evaluation of Self-Related Traits: An fMRI Study. *PLoS ONE* **2015**, *10*, e0136027. [CrossRef]
33. Barnett, M.D.; Flores, J. Narcissus, exhausted: Self-compassion mediates the relationship between narcissism and school burnout. *Personal. Individ. Differ.* **2016**, *97*, 102–108. [CrossRef]
34. Schwarzkopf, K.; Straus, D.; Porschke, H.; Znoj, H.; Conrad, N.; Schmidt-Trucksäss, A.; von Känel, R. Empirical evidence for a relationship between narcissistic personality traits and job burnout. *Burn. Res.* **2016**, *3*, 25–33. [CrossRef]
35. Rana, M.; Riedel, E.; Czens, F.; Petersohn, H.; Moellmann, H.L.; Schorn, L. When Do Narcissists Burn Out? The Bright and Dark Side of Narcissism in Surgeons. *Int. J. Environ. Res. Public Health* **2022**, *19*, 15123. [CrossRef] [PubMed]
36. Shanafelt, T.D.; Raymond, M.; Kosty, M.; Satele, D.; Horn, L.; Pippen, J.; Chu, Q.; Chew, H.; Clark, W.B.; Hanley, A.E.; et al. Satisfaction with work-life balance and the career and retirement plans of US oncologists. *J. Clin. Oncol.* **2014**, *32*, 1127–1135. [CrossRef] [PubMed]
37. Moellmann, H.L.; Rana, M.; Daseking, M.; Petersohn, H. Exploring grandiose narcissism among surgeons: A comparative analysis. *Sci. Rep.* **2024**, *14*, 11665. [CrossRef] [PubMed]
38. Klerks, M.; Dumitrescu, R.; De Caluwé, E. The relationship between the Dark Triad and academic burnout mediated by perfectionistic self-presentation. *Acta Psychol.* **2024**, *250*, 104499. [CrossRef] [PubMed]
39. von Känel, R.; Princip, M.; Holzgang, S.A.; Garefa, C.; Rossi, A.; Benz, D.C.; Giannopoulos, A.A.; Kaufmann, P.A.; Buechel, R.R.; Zuccarella-Hackl, C.; et al. Coronary microvascular function in male physicians with burnout and job stress: An observational study. *BMC Med.* **2023**, *21*, 477. [CrossRef] [PubMed]
40. Sara, J.D.; Prasad, M.; Eleid, M.F.; Zhang, M.; Widmer, R.J.; Lerman, A. Association Between Work-Related Stress and Coronary Heart Disease: A Review of Prospective Studies Through the Job Strain, Effort-Reward Balance, and Organizational Justice Models. *J. Am. Heart Assoc.* **2018**, *7*, e008073. [CrossRef]
41. Ko, D.T.; Chu, A.; Austin, P.C.; Johnston, S.; Nallamothu, B.K.; Roifman, I.; Tusevljak, N.; Udell, J.A.; Frank, E. Comparison of Cardiovascular Risk Factors and Outcomes Among Practicing Physicians vs the General Population in Ontario, Canada. *JAMA Netw. Open* **2019**, *2*, e1915983. [CrossRef]
42. Büssing, A.; Perrar, K.-M. Die Messung von Burnout Untersuchung einer deutschen Fassung des Maslach Burnout Inventory (MBI-D) = Measuring burnout: A study of a German version of the Maslach Burnout Inventory (MBI-D). *Diagnostica* **1992**, *38*, 328–353.

43. Gräfe, K.; Zipfel, S.; Herzog, W.; Löwe, B. Screening psychischer Störungen mit dem "Gesundheitsfragebogen für Patienten (PHQ-D)". *Diagnostica* **2004**, *50*, 171–181. [CrossRef]
44. Rotenstein, L.S.; Torre, M.; Ramos, M.A.; Rosales, R.C.; Guille, C.; Sen, S.; Mata, D.A. Prevalence of Burnout Among Physicians: A Systematic Review. *JAMA* **2018**, *320*, 1131–1150. [CrossRef]
45. Lee, R.T.; Ashforth, B.E. A meta-analytic examination of the correlates of the three dimensions of job burnout. *J. Appl. Psychol.* **1996**, *81*, 123–133. [CrossRef] [PubMed]
46. Leiter, M.P. Burnout as a developmental process: Consideration of models. In *Professional Burnout: Recent Developments in Theory and Research*; Schaufeli, W.B., Maslach, C., Marek, T., Eds.; Series in Applied Psychology: Social Issues and Questions; Taylor & Francis: Philadelphia, PA, USA, 1993; pp. 237–250.
47. Cordes, C.L.; Dougherty, T.W. A Review and an Integration of Research on Job Burnout. *Acad. Manag. Rev.* **1993**, *18*, 621–656. [CrossRef]
48. Kroenke, K.; Spitzer, R.L.; Williams, J.B. The PHQ-9: Validity of a brief depression severity measure. *J. Gen. Intern. Med.* **2001**, *16*, 606–613. [CrossRef] [PubMed]
49. Schwarz, E.I.; Schlatzer, C.; Stehli, J.; Kaufmann, P.A.; Bloch, K.E.; Stradling, J.R.; Kohler, M. Effect of CPAP Withdrawal on myocardial perfusion in OSA: A randomized controlled trial. *Respirology* **2016**, *21*, 1126–1133. [CrossRef]
50. Walter, M.; Dammann, G.; Küchenhoff, J.; Frommer, J.; Schoeneich, F.; Danzer, G.; Klapp, B.F. Psychosocial situation of living donors: Moods, complaints, and self-image before and after liver transplantation. *Med. Sci. Monit.* **2005**, *11*, Cr503–Cr509. [PubMed]
51. Cohen, S.; Kamarck, T.; Mermelstein, R. A global measure of perceived stress. *J. Health Soc. Behav.* **1983**, *24*, 385–396. [CrossRef] [PubMed]
52. Klein, E.M.; Brähler, E.; Dreier, M.; Reinecke, L.; Müller, K.W.; Schmutzer, G.; Wölfling, K.; Beutel, M.E. The German version of the Perceived Stress Scale—Psychometric characteristics in a representative German community sample. *BMC Psychiatry* **2016**, *16*, 159. [CrossRef] [PubMed]
53. Siegrist, J.; Wege, N.; Pühlhofer, F.; Wahrendorf, M. A short generic measure of work stress in the era of globalization: Effort-reward imbalance. *Int. Arch. Occup. Environ. Health* **2009**, *82*, 1005–1013. [CrossRef]
54. Rödel, A.; Siegrist, J.; Hessel, A.; Brähler, E. Fragebogen zur Messung beruflicher Gratifikationskrisen. *Z. Für Differ. Und Diagn. Psychol.* **2004**, *25*, 227–238. [CrossRef]
55. Hämmig, O.; Brauchli, R.; Bauer, G.F. Effort-reward and work-life imbalance, general stress and burnout among employees of a large public hospital in Switzerland. *Swiss Med. Wkly.* **2012**, *142*, w13577. [CrossRef] [PubMed]
56. Buddeberg-Fischer, B.; Klaghofer, R.; Abel, T.; Buddeberg, C. Junior physicians' workplace experiences in clinical fields in German-speaking Switzerland. *Swiss Med. Wkly.* **2005**, *135*, 19–26. [CrossRef] [PubMed]
57. R Core Team. *R: A Language and Environment for Statistical Computing*; R Foundation for Statistical Computing: Vienna, Austria, 2022.
58. Holzgang, S.A.; Pazhenkottil, A.P.; Princip, M.; Auschra, B.; Euler, S.; von Känel, R. Burnout among Male Physicians: A Controlled Study on Pathological Personality Traits and Facets. *Psych* **2023**, *5*, 1–13. [CrossRef]
59. Holzgang, S.A.; Princip, M.; Pazhenkottil, A.P.; Auschra, B.; von Känel, R. Underutilization of effective coping styles in male physicians with burnout. *PLoS ONE* **2023**, *18*, e0291380. [CrossRef]
60. Kilic, R.; Nasello, J.A.; Melchior, V.; Triffaux, J.M. Academic burnout among medical students: Respective importance of risk and protective factors. *Public Health* **2021**, *198*, 187–195. [CrossRef] [PubMed]
61. Weilenmann, S.; Schnyder, U.; Keller, N.; Corda, C.; Spiller, T.R.; Brugger, F.; Parkinson, B.; von Känel, R.; Pfaltz, M.C. Self-worth and bonding emotions are related to well-being in health-care providers: A cross-sectional study. *BMC Med. Educ.* **2021**, *21*, 290. [CrossRef] [PubMed]
62. Puig Llobet, M.; Sánchez Ortega, M.; Lluch-Canut, M.; Moreno-Arroyo, M.; Hidalgo Blanco, M.; Roldán-Merino, J. Positive Mental Health and Self-Care in Patients with Chronic Physical Health Problems: Implications for Evidence-based Practice. *Worldviews Evid. Based Nurs.* **2020**, *17*, 293–300. [CrossRef] [PubMed]
63. Fröhlich-Rüfenacht, S.; Rousselot, A.; Künzler, A. Psychosoziale Aspekte chronischer Erkrankungen und deren Einfluss auf die Behandlung. *Swiss Med. Forum Schweiz. Med. Forum* **2013**, *13*. Available online: https://www.chronischkrank.ch/wp-content/uploads/2016/09/smf-01425pdf (accessed on 23 February 2024). [CrossRef]
64. Raju, A.; Nithiya, D.R.; Tipandjan, A. Relationship between burnout, effort-reward imbalance, and insomnia among Informational Technology professionals. *J. Educ. Health Promot.* **2022**, *11*, 296. [CrossRef] [PubMed]
65. Alvarado, L.E.; Bretones, F.D.; Rodríguez, J.A. The Effort-Reward Model and Its Effect on Burnout Among Nurses in Ecuador. *Front. Psychol.* **2021**, *12*, 760570. [CrossRef]
66. Shoman, Y.; Ranjbar, S.; Strippoli, M.P.; von Känel, R.; Preisig, M.; Guseva Canu, I. Relationship Between Effort-Reward Imbalance, Over-Commitment and Occupational Burnout in the General Population: A Prospective Cohort Study. *Int. J. Public Health* **2023**, *68*, 1606160. [CrossRef]

67. Alle Schweizer Bundesbehörden. Tatsächliche Arbeitsstunden. Tatsächliches Arbeitsvolumen, Entwicklung der Arbeitszeit. Available online: https://www.bfs.admin.ch/bfs/de/home/statistiken/arbeit-erwerb/erwerbstaetigkeit-arbeitszeit/arbeitszeit/tatsaechliche-arbeitsstunden.html (accessed on 23 February 2024).
68. Seidler, Z.E.; Dawes, A.J.; Rice, S.M.; Oliffe, J.L.; Dhillon, H.M. The role of masculinity in men's help-seeking for depression: A systematic review. *Clin. Psychol. Rev.* **2016**, *49*, 106–118. [CrossRef] [PubMed]
69. Fleming, P.J.; Lee, J.G.; Dworkin, S.L. "Real men don't": Constructions of masculinity and inadvertent harm in public health interventions. *Am. J. Public Health* **2014**, *104*, 1029–1035. [CrossRef] [PubMed]
70. Lindberg, O. Gender and role models in the education of medical doctors: A qualitative exploration of gendered ways of thinking. *Int. J. Med. Educ.* **2020**, *11*, 31–36. [CrossRef]
71. Walter, U.; Krugmann, C.S.; Plaumann, M. Preventing burnout? A systematic review of effectiveness of individual and combined approaches. *Bundesgesundheitsblatt Gesundheitsforschung Gesundheitsschutz* **2012**, *55*, 172–182. [CrossRef]
72. Weilenmann, S.; Ernst, J.; Petry, H.; Pfaltz, M.C.; Sazpinar, O.; Gehrke, S.; Paolercio, F.; von Känel, R.; Spiller, T.R. Health Care Workers' Mental Health During the First Weeks of the SARS-CoV-2 Pandemic in Switzerland-A Cross-Sectional Study. *Front. Psychiatry* **2021**, *12*, 594340. [CrossRef] [PubMed]
73. Wozniak, H.; Benzakour, L.; Moullec, G.; Buetti, N.; Nguyen, A.; Corbaz, S.; Roos, P.; Vieux, L.; Suard, J.C.; Weissbrodt, R.; et al. Mental health outcomes of ICU and non-ICU healthcare workers during the COVID-19 outbreak: A cross-sectional study. *Ann. Intensive Care* **2021**, *11*, 106. [CrossRef]
74. Sebo, P.; Favrod-Coune, T.; Mahler, L.; Moussa, A.; Cohidon, C.; Broers, B. A cross-sectional study of the health status of Swiss primary care physicians. *Sci. Rep.* **2021**, *11*, 23459. [CrossRef]

Journal of
Clinical Medicine

Article

Context, Timing and Individualized Care: A Realist Evaluation of Safety Planning for Individuals Living with Suicide-Related Thoughts and Behaviours, Their Families and Friends and Service Providers

Elisa Hollenberg [1,†], Hwayeon Danielle Shin [1,2,†], Nadine Reid [1,2], Vicky Stergiopoulos [1,2,3], Laurent Lestage [4], Gina Nicoll [1], Alyna Walji [1] and Juveria Zaheer [1,2,3,*]

1 Centre for Addiction and Mental Health, 1001 Queen Street West, Toronto, ON M6J 1H4, Canada; elisa.hollenberg@camh.ca (E.H.); danielle.shin@camh.ca (H.D.S.); nadine.reid@camh.ca (N.R.); vicky.stergiopoulos@camh.ca (V.S.); regina.nicoll@camh.ca (G.N.); alyna.walji@camh.ca (A.W.)

2 Institute of Health Policy, Management and Evaluation, University of Toronto, 155 College Street, 4th Floor, Toronto, ON M5T 3M6, Canada

3 Department of Psychiatry, Temerty Faculty of Medicine, University of Toronto, 250 College Street, 8th Floor, Toronto, ON M5T 1R8, Canada

4 Département de Psychiatrie et D'addictologie, Université de Montréal, Pavillon Roger-Gaudry 2900, Boulevard Édouard-Montpetit, Montréal, QC H3T 1J4, Canada; laurent.lestage@umontreal.ca

* Correspondence: juveria.zaheer@camh.ca; Tel.: +1-416-535-8501 (ext. 34201)

† These authors contributed equally to this work.

Abstract: Background/Objectives: This research aimed to identify and investigate how context facilitates or hinders safety planning interventions (SPIs) intended to manage suicidal ideation (SI) and behaviour (SB) from the perspective of service users, friends, family members, service providers and other key informants. Additionally, this research aimed to identify underlying mechanisms influencing the effective and acceptable management of SI and SB across these groups. **Methods**: A realist evaluation framework (i.e., Context + Mechanism = Outcome; CMO) was used to inform the qualitative study design, which explores whether SPIs are perceived as effective (i.e., outcome) and examines the underlying mechanism(s) and specific contexts involved. A total of 28 service users, 11 family members or friends and 15 key informants, including service providers and other stakeholders, participated in semi-structured interviews. A total of 18 frontline service providers also participated in three focus groups. These interviews and focus groups were analyzed to develop a shared model capturing the mechanisms and contexts influencing effective SPI implementation. Data was collected between September 2019 and December 2021. **Results**: The model consists of three pillars: (1) understanding the importance of context, timing and relationships in safety planning, (2) identifying perceived barriers and facilitators to safety planning as described by service users, family members and service providers, (3) bridging the gap between evidence and experience in implementing safety planning interventions. **Conclusions**: While SPIs are evidence-based interventions, contextual factors and perceived barriers and facilitators can impact implementation and outcomes in mental health care settings. Understanding these factors can help to explain differences in outcomes within and across patient populations and care settings, and addressing perceived challenges can improve implementation and experiences for service users, family members and service providers.

Keywords: suicide prevention; realist evaluation; complex interventions

1. Introduction

Suicide is a major health concern internationally, and it has been reported that 700,000 people die by suicide every year [1,2]. In Canada, the estimated economic cost per death, resulting from reduced productivity, increased health service utilization, disability and premature death, exceeds CAN 1,000,000 [3]. Experiencing suicidal thoughts or behaviours is painful and distressing and requires treatment and support; these experiences are associated with high rates of comorbidity, marginalization, premature mortality and poor access to mental health care [4]. Safety planning interventions (SPIs) are considered one of the best available brief interventions in suicide prevention and are well supported by existing evidence [5–7]. SPIs are a collaborative process between health care professionals and service users working together to develop a plan to manage suicidal ideation (SI) and behaviour (SB). The main elements of the safety plan as originally developed include identifying the following: (1) warning signs, (2) internal coping strategies, (3) socialization strategies for distraction and support, (4) social contacts for assistance in resolving suicidal crises, (5) professional and agency contacts to help resolve suicidal crises, (6) means restriction [8]. SPIs have been shown to decrease suicidal behaviour by up to 45% [9].

Two systematic reviews [6,7] and one meta-analysis [5] illustrate the positive effects of SPIs in reducing suicidal ideation (SI) or suicidal behaviour (SB) based on outcomes that evaluate the intervention as a whole. However, limited qualitative research explores why and how SPIs work and the perceived feasibility, effectiveness and acceptability of their component elements [6,10]. Qualitative studies have been heterogeneous, examining SPIs in different contexts (e.g., perceptions of SPI at discharge from the emergency department (ED) with brief follow-up contact phone calls [11–13], SPI prior to discharge from inpatient units [14–16], in therapeutic groups [17], using online apps [18], in specialized programs for veterans [19–21], in community outpatient services [22] or in peer support programs [23]). These studies have focused on a range of demographic groups including veterans on their own [13,19] or with providers and/or family members [17,20,23]; health care providers for veterans [12,16]; youth and their family members [15]; the general population presenting at the ED [11] or discharged [14] from general hospitals; youth, adults, family members and clinicians for SPI app users [18]; and staff in a program for people of refugee and asylum-seeker backgrounds [22].

There are several evidence-based suicide prevention interventions beyond SPI, including pharmacological treatments. In emergency departments, medications such as antidepressants are considered an important part of suicide prevention care due to their therapeutic effects, while taking care to limit access to potentially harmful substances [24]. If a patient diagnosed with a psychiatric illness is already taking medication and is responding well to it, the emergency department may initiate prescriptions, with plans for close follow-up care after discharge [24]. However, the evidence supporting the effectiveness of some psychiatric medications for suicide prevention remains inconclusive. For example, lithium has historically been recommended for managing depressive symptoms and reducing suicide risk, but recent studies have presented conflicting findings regarding its effectiveness [25]. While there is an ongoing debate about this, for treatment-resistant depression—when patients fail to respond to two antidepressants—an Italian expert panel reached a strong consensus on the use of lithium [26]. However, in Canada, its use has declined over the past decade [27] and also remains limited in the United States, possibly due to concerns about renal toxicity and the aggressive marketing of alternative medications [28].

While mental health diagnoses are commonly understood as risk factors for suicide, it is critical to acknowledge that suicide can also occur among individuals without a formal diagnosis. In a retrospective analysis of 174,001 suicide decedents from 37 U.S.

states between 2003 and 2017, 58.2% had no known mental illness [29]. This broadens the scope of prevention efforts and challenges assumptions that tie suicide risk exclusively to diagnosable mental illness. In this context, the present paper contributes to the literature by moving beyond the question of what works in suicide prevention. Focusing on SPI, the paper asks under what circumstances interventions are effective, recognizing the importance of tailoring strategies to the varied realities of those at risk.

Research Aim and Questions

This study aimed to better understand experiences of safety planning in health care settings across Ontario, Canada. A realist evaluation framework was used to identify and investigate how context facilitates or hinders SPIs intended to manage SI and SB from the perspective of service users, friends, families, service providers and other supports. We interviewed participants from a variety of settings to better understand the specific contextual factors related to emergency care and beyond for implementing SPIs.

Specific research questions included the following:

(1) What are the experiences of individuals (context) who have experienced SI and/or SB regarding safety planning interventions that may interact, influence, modify, facilitate or hinder the intervention and its outcome?
(2) What are the components of safety planning interventions (mechanism-resource—key elements of the SPI itself and/or its implementation) that are perceived to be helpful or unhelpful for individuals (mechanism-reasoning—the human response to SPIs) who have experienced SI and/or SB?
(3) What are the perspectives of families, friends, caregivers and service providers who have supported someone who has experienced SI and/or SB, in relation to the context, mechanisms and outcomes of safety planning interventions?

2. Materials and Methods

2.1. Realist Evaluation Approach

A realist evaluation design [30] addressed the research aims above. One major assumption of this methodology is that interventions work differently in different contexts for different people, which aligns well with suicide, SI and SB being understood as complex phenomena with psychological, biological, social and cultural underpinnings. Prevention strategies that work for one individual may not work for or work differently for another. Suicide-specific interventions, including SPIs, are assumed to be complex interventions, involving multiple interacting components, feedback mechanisms and alternative and simultaneous causal strands [31].

Realist evaluation uses the CMO (i.e., Context + Mechanism = Outcome) framework [30]. The resulting CMO configurations articulate whether SPI works or does not work (i.e., outcome) in the presence of the underlying mechanism(s) taking place in particular contexts (Table 1). This manuscript was prepared using the RAMESES II reporting standards for realist evaluations (Supplemental File S1, Table S1) [32] and the COREQ checklist for qualitative research reporting (Supplemental File S2, Table S2) [33].

Table 1. Realist CMO definition of terms.

Domain	Definition
Context (C)	Contexts are all factors that are not part of the intervention itself, and features of conditions in which interventions are introduced that are relevant to mechanisms' operation [30]. Contexts interact, influence, modify, facilitate or hinder the intervention and its outcome (e.g., effectiveness) [30].
Mechanism (M)	Mechanisms are the combination of the intended and unintended resources offered by an intervention, as well as the reactions and/or responses (e.g., cognitive, emotional, motivational reasoning, physical) to those resources that make an intervention work [34]. Mechanisms can be further classified as (1) the resources provided by the program (M-resource) or (2) the human response to receiving those resources (M-reasoning) [34].
Outcome (O)	Outcomes are the results of an intervention with multiple underlying mechanisms, which can lead to different effects on individuals in various situations, resulting in the possibility of multiple outcomes [30].
	"CMO configuring is a heuristic used to generate causative explanations about outcomes in the observed data. A CMO configuration may be about the whole [intervention] or only certain aspects" [35] (p. 3).

2.2. Sampling and Recruitment

2.2.1. Service Users, Friends, Family Members and Other Supports

Convenience sampling for approximately 20 service users and 10–20 friends, family members and other supports was employed by posting informational study flyers on research boards at the Centre for Addiction and Mental Health (CAMH) and at the Canadian Mental Health Association (CMHA) in Toronto, Ontario, Canada. CAMH is Canada's largest mental health teaching hospital and home to the only standalone psychiatric ED in Ontario. CMHA is a mental health community care setting. The study team contacted service providers in these settings and notified them about the study, inviting them to refer interested individuals. In such instances, service providers provided potential participants with a copy of the study flyer and study information sheet containing the study contact information. Potential participants could independently contact the study team or, if they wished, their verbal consent would be obtained by their service provider, to later be contacted by the study team for further information and enrollment. The study was also posted on the CAMH research registry and CAMH 'Research Connect' webpage that hosts a database of CAMH studies, with a link to the study poster. Other recruitment strategies for this group included social media posts on 'X'.

To be eligible to participate, service users needed to be older than 18 years, have had at least one occurrence of SI or SB in their lifetime and live in Ontario. Service users were ineligible if they could not speak English fluently, were acutely ill or hospitalized, had significant visual, auditory or cognitive impairments or lived outside of Ontario. Friends or family members, including individuals bereaved by suicide, were eligible if they were currently or had previously supported a service user who had experienced SI or SB. Participants in this subgroup were ineligible if they could not speak English fluently.

2.2.2. Key Informants and Service Providers

Key informants at CAMH and CMHA were purposively identified for an approximate sample of 10 participants by the study team for interviews according to known areas of expertise and experience and then contacted by the principal investigator (PI) by e-mail with a personalized request to participate, the electronic study poster attached and a connection to the study coordinator.

To recruit an approximate sample of 20 to 30 service providers for focus groups, convenience sampling was used by posting a series of study flyers in CAMH staff rooms as permitted, such that service providers could self-refer. Further, the PI was provided with a list of physicians and allied health staff by CAMH and CMHA programs and sent a personalized request by e-mail for programs to participate; an electronic version of the study poster was included in which interested participants were directed to contact the study coordinator.

To be eligible to participate in a focus group (service providers) or interview (key informants), participants had a role as a leader, physician or allied health worker experienced in working in a health care setting providing care for people who are experiencing SI and/or SB.

Ethics approval was granted by the Research Ethics Board (REB) at CAMH in Toronto, Ontario, Canada, on 1 August 2019 (REB#041-2019).

2.3. Data Collection

Informed consent was obtained from all participants. Semi-structured interviews were conducted with key informants, service users, friends and family members to explore experiences with SI and/or SB or in providing or organizing care and experiences with suicide interventions such as safety planning. Interviews were conducted remotely due to COVID-19 pandemic restrictions with service users and friends or family members [by J.Z.] between November 2020 and December 2021 by videoconference or phone. Data was collected from key informants (interviews) and service providers (focus groups) [by N.R., J.Z. and E.H.] in person between September 2019 and March 2020 and remotely between February 2021 and August 2021. Only participants and researchers were present during interviews and focus groups. Participants were asked about their previous experiences with safety planning in any context in Ontario, Canada, what was most helpful, least helpful, most challenging and why, for their individual help-seeking and care, caregiving or service delivery experiences. They were subsequently shown a copy of the CAMH Emergency Department SPI template adapted from Stanley and Brown [8] (see Appendix A) and asked for their thoughts and about anything that could be added or modified to make it more helpful. The interview guide was developed and reviewed in collaboration with a team member with lived experience [G.N.].

Interviews with service users, friends and family members lasted between 30 and 90 min. At the end of each interview, participants' demographic characteristics were captured with a demographic survey administered by the interviewer. Interviews with key informants and focus groups with service providers were between 60 and 90 min long. Demographics were captured after these sessions with an online survey. Based on these survey results, the researchers built on the convenience sampling approach to balance the number of participants by broad gender categories (men, women) as recruitment progressed. Field notes were made following interviews and focus groups. All interviews were audio-recorded, transcribed verbatim and de-identified. Transcripts were available for participant review and revision upon request, although none were asked for. Data collection was followed by regular team discussion of developing patterns. Sampling continued until there was a consensus that there were multiple examples of similar participant experiences in relation to the research questions, adequate variation in the viewpoints expressed, rich descriptions of such experiences, with no new information or topics emerging, indicating saturation in themes at the level of sampling [36,37].

To ensure the safety of participants, several strategies were used. A three-question screening tool for suicide risk was administered at the beginning and end of each interview with service user participants. In the case of an increase in risk identified by this tool, a range of resources were readily available to both the researcher and participants including but not limited to counselling, connection to crisis lines and emergency support.

2.4. Data Analysis

All interview data were coded, analyzed thematically [38] and then configured using the CMO framework, aligned with the realist approach using NVivo 12 software (QSR International, Burlington, MA, USA). Analysis began with the reading and re-reading of service user transcripts by the authors E.H. and J.Z. and key informant transcripts by E.H., J.Z. and N.R. During this process, open codes were generated by each author and compared to build an initial coding strategy. Six transcripts were then coded independently, any interpretation discrepancies were resolved via discussion and new codes were generated before finalizing the coding strategy. The remaining service user and key informant interviews were coded by E.H. During the coding of the remaining transcripts, any emergent codes and sub-codes were identified and discussed between E.H. and J.Z. until a consensus was reached.

A subset of three friend and family member interviews were then read and coded by E.H. and J.Z. to determine the applicability of the final service user coding strategy. It was determined that the service user coding strategy could be applied directly, with the addition of some agreed-upon emergent codes specific to the friend and family member experience. The service user NVivo 12 coding tree was duplicated and further developed with the additional codes, and then the family member and friend transcripts were coded by E.H.

During the initial and subsequent interview coding, memos were made by E.H. and J.Z. to note insights and connections across content and codes. Coded data and memos were searched for repeated patterns of meanings to re-organize codes and compile a report with broader themes, summaries and analysis specifically for the safety planning intervention. Consensus was reached regarding thematic saturation based on the presence of recurring themes with no new ones, no additional information or relationships identified [39], with an understanding that all themes were not discussed in equal proportions by all types of participants (e.g., service users, service providers, key informants or family members). Rather, triangulation was used to add the voices of other participant groups for themes that were saturated in one group when they were discussed by participants in other groups in ways that confirmed, contrasted with or complemented views for the theme that was developed for the first group.

The steps mentioned above were completed by authors, E.H., N.R. and J.Z. as indicated, who have extensive experience in qualitative research. The overall process was supervised by J.Z., a clinician scientist who has clinical and research expertise in suicide intervention and realist evaluation. For the realist evaluation level of analysis, E.H., H.D.S. and J.Z. read and re-read the thematically coded material and memos, and re-read transcripts when necessary, to organize the identified themes into CMO configurations. To do so, coded material under each initial theme was analyzed descriptively to indicate how aspects of context, mechanism-resource, mechanism-reasoning or outcomes were represented in the data. The newly described CMO coded material was then examined by the authors to understand the extent of coded material with similar or contrasting CMO factors. Alternative CMO explanations were explored, and considerations were made as to whether new themes were necessary. Revised overarching themes and sub-themes were then developed with new CMO definitions to include data with exemplary quotes representing both similar and different viewpoints. A model with three pillars was developed to further group themes conceptually. Other authors (G.N. and N.R.) reviewed and provided feedback for these themes and the model, which were finalized through group discussion.

Demographic characteristics were analyzed descriptively. A reflexivity statement [40] for the authors is contained in Appendix B.

3. Results

In total, 28 service users, 11 friends and family members and 15 key informants participated in an interview, for a total of 54 interviews (1 interview was with 2 family members). Three service user participants completed a second interview due to having more to share than was possible during one interview, an option discussed during the consent process. Eighteen service providers participated in three focus groups. Seven people consented but did not complete the study interview.

Half of the service users identified as women (n = 14; 50%), ranging from 20 to 59 years of age, and half identified as racialized (n = 14, 50%). All but one participant reported having at least one mental health diagnosis. A total of 82% of participants reported having two or more mental health diagnoses, demonstrating a high level of comorbidity among the population. Most friends and family members identified as women (n = 7; 64%), ranging from 26 to 78 years of age, and most of them identified as white (n = 9, 82%). No friends and family members were connected in any way to the service users interviewed. All of the friends and family members reported that the individual they supported had at least one mental health diagnosis and almost half had a substance use disorder. Please see Tables 2–6 for detailed demographic breakdowns.

Table 2. Service user demographic characteristics.

Characteristics	*n* (%)
n	28 (100)
Average Age (years, range)	32.9 (20–59)
Gender	
Woman [1]	14 (50)
Man [1]	10 (36)
Non-binary	4 (14)
Race	
Racialized [2]	14 (50)
White	14 (50)
Marital Status	
Married/partnered	7 (25)
Single/divorced	20 (71)
Education	
Completed college/university	19 (68)
Less than college/university	9 (32)
Employment	
Employed	
Full-time	8 (29)
Part-time	6 (21)
Unemployed	13 (46)

Table 2. *Cont.*

Characteristics	n (%)
Source of Income [3]	
Average number of income sources (range)	1.2 (0–3)
Employment	13 (46)
Social support [4]	12 (43)
Family support/savings	8 (29)
Student loan	4 (14)
Living with	
Alone	12 (43)
Family	7 (29)
Spouse/partner	4 (14)
Friend/roommate	3 (11)
No answer	2 (7)

[1] Includes cis and trans women/men. [2] Includes East Asian, South Asian, Black-Caribbean, Black-North American, Latin American, Middle Eastern and two or more racial/ethnic groups. [3] Categories are not mutually exclusive. [4] Includes Ontario Disability Support Program (ODSP), Employment Insurance (EI), Canadian Emergency Response Benefit (CERB) and long-term disability.

Table 3. Mental health characteristics of service users.

Characteristics	n (%)
n	28 (100)
Previous Emergency Department (ED) Visit	
Yes	19 (70)
Previous Hospitalization	
Yes	15 (54)
Average number of hospitalizations (range)	3.1 (2–6)
Current Diagnoses	
Average number of diagnoses (range)	2.9 (0–6)
Depression and related [1]	23 (82)
Anxiety disorders [2] and Obsessive-compulsive disorder (OCD)	17 (61)
Post-traumatic stress disorder (PTSD) and related [3]	15 (54)
Borderline Personality Disorder	10 (36)
Bipolar Disorder	5 (18)
Substance Use Disorder	3 (11)
Attention-deficit/hyperactivity disorder (ADHD)	3 (11)
Other [4]	4 (14)
Comorbidity	
Yes	23 (82)
Treatment team	
Primary care provider	16 (62)
Psychiatrist	11 (42)

Table 3. *Cont.*

Characteristics	n (%)
Specialist physician	3 (12)
Allied Health	
Therapist	11 (44)
Social worker	3 (12)
Case worker	3 (12)
Allied health linked with psychiatry [5]	4 (15)
Peer support	2 (8)

[1] Includes depression, chronic depression, Major Depressive Disorder, Major Depressive Episode and Adjustment Disorder. [2] Includes Generalized Anxiety Disorder, Social Anxiety Disorder and Panic Disorder. [3] Includes PTSD, Complex post-traumatic stress disorder (CPTSD), Dissociation Disorder and Dissociative Identity Disorder. [4] Includes Schizophrenia, Autism Spectrum Disorder and Unspecified Eating Disorder. [5] Includes aftercare, online programs and care at psychiatric hospitals.

Table 4. Friend and family demographic characteristics.

Characteristics	n (%)
n	11 (100)
Average Age (years, range)	50.6 (26–78)
Gender	
Woman [1]	7 (64)
Man	2 (18)
Not listed	10 (1)
Race	
Racialized [2]	2 (18)
White	9 (82)
Marital Status	
Married/partnered	7 (64)
Single/divorced	4 (36)
Has Children	
Yes	6 (55)
Average number ofchildren (range)	2.7 (2–3)
Education	
Completed college/university	7 (36)
Less than college/university	4 (36)
Employment	
Employed	
Full-time	27 (3)
Part-time	2 (18)
Self-employed	2 (18)
Unemployed	2 (18)
Retired	2 (18)

Table 4. *Cont.*

Characteristics	*n* (%)
Source of Income [3]	
Average number of income sources (range)	1.2 (0–2)
Employment	6 (55)
Social support [4]	2 (18)
Family support/savings	6 (55)
Living with	
Alone	2 (18)
Spouse/family	8 (73)
Friend/roommate	1 (9)

[1] Includes cis and trans women/men. [2] Includes Black-African and two or more racial or ethnic groups. [3] Categories are not mutually exclusive. [4] Categories are not mutually exclusive.

Table 5. Description of friend and family mental health characteristics.

Characteristics	*n* (%)
n	11 (100)
Previous Hospitalization	
Yes	11 (100)
Average number of hospitalizations (range)	5.3 (1–20)
Current Diagnoses	
Average number of diagnoses (range)	1.9 (1–4)
Depression	5 (45)
Anxiety	1 (9)
PTSD	1 (9)
Borderline Personality Disorder	3 (27)
Substance Use Disorder	6 (55)
Other [1]	4 (36)

[1] Includes Somatic Symptom Disorder, an eating disorder, a reading disorder and psychosis.

Table 6. Key informant and service provider demographic characteristics.

Characteristics	*n* (%)
n	33 (100)
Gender	
Woman	25 (76)
Man	8 (24)
Role [1]	
Frontline clinician [2]	18 (55)
Physician	9 (27)
Administration/leadership	11 (33)

Table 6. *Cont.*

Characteristics	*n* (%)
Ethnicity	
White	19 (58)
Racialized	13 (39)
Prefer not to answer	1 (3)

[1] Categories are not mutually exclusive. [2] Includes nurses, social workers, occupational therapists, case managers and program managers.

3.1. Themes and CMO Configurations

This section presents the qualitative results in a model with three pillars: (1) understanding the importance of context, timing and relationships in safety planning; (2) identifying perceived barriers and facilitators to safety planning as described by service users, family members and service providers; (3) bridging the gap between evidence and experience in implementing safety planning interventions. Each pillar contains content that is further described using realist evaluation CMO concepts: context, mechanism (mechanism-resource or mechanism-reasoning) and outcome. The analysis demonstrates the influence of context and mechanisms on SPI processes.

3.1.1. Model Part 1: The Importance of Context, Timing and Relationships

Timing

Creating a safety plan when experiencing acute SI or SB may be challenging.

When individuals experiencing SI or SB first arrive at an emergency department, they are often in an acute crisis state, and thinking beyond their current difficulties can be challenging (context). The timing of introducing safety planning (mechanism-resource), as well as the state of the service user's condition (context), matters. One service user expressed difficulty engaging in safety planning because they were overwhelmed and did not have the emotional capacity (mechanism-reasoning).

> *I will say that when I had come into the ER...they had given me a piece of paper (...) and they were like, can you fill this out? And it was about suicidal thoughts, and I was like, completely overwhelmed, and it was like, what are your coping skills? Or what keeps you safe? And when you're in a headspace where you're not wanting to do that, you're like, why the hell are you giving this to me?*
>
> (SU004)

Service providers similarly noted the difficulty for individuals in crisis to create a safety plan:

> *When people are in crisis, their brains don't work well. And to be able to kind of identify those things, the person might just say, I don't know! I don't know! I don't know!*
>
> (KI1015)

Several participants specifically discussed difficulty answering a 'reasons for living' question if they were experiencing intense distress.

> *The one that I've never liked is step number 2 there, remind myself of my reasons for living (...) when you're in the middle of a crisis, it's not always the most practical to then say to yourself, remind myself of my reasons for living. (...) If you weren't constantly thinking back and forth about suicide or things that are crappy, then you could probably just move on. Right?*
>
> (SU010)

To create a thoughtful and meaningful safety plan, other conditions are required. One participant suggested that safety planning would be more effective when a person is feeling better (context).

I don't know if I would be in the mindset to write things down when I was, like, at my worst. Maybe if you can get them to a point where they're a little more cheerful, you know, finding a reason to be good and healthy.

(SU013)

Relationships

Safety planning as a conversation, not a checklist.

Relationships are important when developing safety plans. If safety planning is part of a broader conversation (context), it can be helpful and meaningful (resource-reasoning). However, if safety planning is reduced to just another checklist (mechanism-resource) to satisfy organizational requirements, it may lose effectiveness (outcome). One service provider stated,

It can be something that's meaningful, powerful, relevant, and it can be something that is just a matter of ticking some boxes and making sure they have the thing.

(KI1015)

Another noted that a mandatory formal template might risk being reduced to a checklist:

I worry always with checklists and so on about the seductive quality. So, instead of doing the template as part of a larger conversation, getting to know the patient, we simply ask very quickly, you know, what are your warning signs, right?

(KI1009)

One service provider indicated that creating a safety plan in longer-term therapeutic relationships (context) allows more time to explore underlying reasons and core issues leading to SI (mechanism-resource) and opens a deeper conversation about how to manage difficult feelings and situations (outcome).

I would say anyone who we're acutely worried about safety leaves with a safety plan of sorts, whether it's like, one of those forms all written out, or whether it's like, 'here's what number to call or who to reach out to'. Safety planning, I would say, is an active part of any session with somebody who is acutely suicidal, for sure (. . . .) And we have the luxury of therapy appointments with longitudinal care, where we can dig into this stuff that's causing the suicidality. I feel like spending more time there gives you way more bang for your buck, and people leave not suicidal because you've actually addressed the core issues that are leading to suicidal thoughts.

(FG3, P2)

A participant described how creating a safety plan (outcome) with a professional (mechanism-resource) between crises (context) was helpful to review what worked and what did not, and to adapt the safety plan as needed, over time (outcome).

I've done it several times with different professionals. I find that useful because they can suggest things to add, or maybe when they've seen me in a crisis state, they're like, oh, remember we tried this and it worked? I was just so out of it that I didn't remember we did that.

(SU025)

Other Relationships for Developing Safety Plans.

Several respondents discussed developing their safety plan in a group therapy context (mechanism-resource) which was helpful, because the group's input generated more ideas (outcome).

We did it together at the trauma therapy program. Yeah, because, like, a lot of the other women in the group had ideas that would have never occurred to me on my own. Ah, I found it helpful.

(SU001)

Other participants had created safety plans with friends (context), sharing ideas and ways to keep safe (mechanism-reasoning) and taking more time (context) than would be possible with a health care professional.

(. . .) just in terms of time and patience, because health care providers, obviously, are kind of on a fixed schedule. So, they have 15 min to do safety planning with you, and maybe you need longer than that, whereas with my friends, I've had situations where if we need to go to the other person's house and get slushies at 7–11 and take 45 min to even start to safety plan, that's okay because we have time for each other.

(SU007)

Participants also suggested safety planning templates online (mechanism-resource) to complete (outcome) independently (context) in their own time (context), with existing examples of safety plans they could draw upon for ideas (mechanism-resource).

I think it's nice to have ones that you can fill out on your own, like, maybe if I was at that place where I still didn't trust providers or if I wasn't in therapy at a certain time, it'd be great to be able to go to a website and have blank templates, or maybe even see examples.

(SU025)

The data showed variation in the context, timing and relationships in which safety planning can occur, particularly when an individual is feeling less distressed between crises. This process can help with insight and the recall of previous solutions, generate more ideas for keeping safe and provide more time for completion.

3.1.2. Model Part 2: Perceived Facilitators and Barriers to Safety Planning

Individual Differences in Safety Planning

Use of safety plans during an acute phase of illness or a crisis.

Individual differences may affect the implementation of safety plans. Some participants anticipated challenges implementing plans when in an acute phase of illness or a crisis, whereas others found safety plans the most helpful at exactly these times.

The barrier of experiencing an acute crisis (context) for not only creating but using (outcome) the safety plan was mentioned by various respondents. One respondent said that they did not think individuals experiencing intense suicide-related thoughts would use a safety plan when in crisis.

Um, yeah, I think it's important. But it's—the only sort of complicating thing is if you are in a really severe crisis, and you're really, really dedicated to ending your life, I think you wouldn't necessarily follow that.

(SU028)

Another participant felt they would not personally use a safety plan in an acute phase:

I don't know how other people have dealt with using these, but when I'm in crisis again, I look at that and I'm like, I don't care. And you can make the plan, but the likelihood of somebody using it is, at least for myself, is very slim. They're like, you can use this if you're suicidal, and I'm like, no!

(SU004)

Another described the difficulty of reaching out for help or emerging from their despair, meaning that even if they knew what resources were available, they might not use them.

I found that sometimes you don't want to get better, like you don't want to see the positives, you don't want to see the light, and kind of get yourself out of it, you just want to kind of mope in that feeling, not that it's any fault of your own, but you're kind of stuck there and you want to hurt yourself sometimes, and you are thinking about that. And you kind of don't want the help or to reach out.

(SU011)

A family member similarly expressed concern that an individual may not use a safety plan if they are experiencing acute distress.

Well, if you say it and then write things down (. . .) if you have some contact numbers, it might do some good. But if a person is really wanting to end it—they really want to take their life, you know.

(F006)

Alternatively, other participants described safety plans as protective when experiencing suicidal thoughts:

I think it is helpful for me. I mean, I have a bit of a mental checklist, I'm like, okay, if I start feeling terrible again, go to the ER, like just knowing that's a possibility.

(SU024)

I think it's like maybe something to fall back on when your own thoughts are dangerous.

(SU017)

One described their safety plan as something available to them when and if they needed it:

I love the idea of a contingency plan, so when you're, like, down, that sounds like a great idea. I think people, as in nature, we live in waves. So, it's bound to happen, you know, you feel great, and then tomorrow, maybe not, because that's how it works. You know, we can't be happy all the time, like you wouldn't like it if it was all darkness—you wouldn't like it if it was light all the time, right? You gotta know darkness to distinguish the light, right? Everything comes and goes. Like a wave.

(SU013)

Diagnosis, sense of self, control and coping.

Service providers differentiated between those who would benefit (outcome) from safety planning (mechanism-resource) and those who may not, based on their diagnosis (context) or the degree to which SI is a part of an individual's sense of self, control and coping (context).

One service provider spoke of the great value of safety planning with patients who 'don't usually want to die' but are impulsive and so are scared of their suicidal thoughts.

(. . .) there's patients who actually really don't want to die, but deal with this impulsive suicidality that comes on, and things go really dark on them really quickly. This would be more for Borderline Personality (. . .) and they're actually scared by their own suicidality, and those patients actually are the best ones for safety planning, because they really want to safety plan.

(KI1010)

For individuals with ambivalence towards living or dying, more in-depth work is needed to understand these emotions than safety planning alone. The same service provider stated,

> *There's other people who are more ambivalent (. . .) they won't commit to using a safety plan because there's still this part of them that actually wants to die. And it's not purely impulsive, it's more, it's thought out and they're really considering it (. . ..) and so safety planning alone is not going to be effective. You need to go deeper and really try to work at the part that wants to die and try to help them understand it in a deeper way.*
>
> (KI1010)

For people who experience chronic suicidal thoughts, they are part of their identity (mechanism-reasoning), and safety planning needs to be approached differently:

> *For her, it's part of her identity, and part of who she is, and it's a control issue to maintain her ownership of her suicidality. And she does not want that fixed, and she does not want that examined and she does not like that kind of planning. So, when I do safety planning with her, in quotes, it's like what are you doing this week? Are you going to therapy next week?*
>
> (KI1014)

Another service provider discussed challenges they have experienced in safety planning with individuals with chronic suicidal ideation:

> *For a large number of folks with chronic suicidality, the response is so automatic that having this safety plan, they don't access it. So, it's something that they're actually doing (. . .) for the clinician (. . .) and not for themselves, ultimately.*
>
> (FG3, P3)

Family and Social Networks

Positive support from family and social networks.

The social network (context) of individuals living with suicide-related thoughts and behaviours (e.g., families and friends who are involved in providing longer-term care) is often engaged through safety planning (mechanism-resource) to provide support or implement key aspects of the safety plan (outcome).

Several respondents listed family members or friends as key contacts on their safety plans. These contacts can remind individuals with SI and SB to notice warning signs and practice coping skills, provide direct emotional support and encourage them to seek help when needed.

> *(. . .) it's like a plan of, like, tangible actions to take if you feel that you're in a mental health crisis, and maybe suicidal, or liable to self-harm. So, in my case, a lot of it is around, sort of, the people who are my supports. So, when I'm in that moment, I always try to call somebody, like my sister or my mom, or my partner. And I don't want to be alone. So, I'll—if my roommates aren't home, I would ask to go over to somebody's house.*
>
> (SU028)

Sometimes, service users made specific plans in advance, with their friends, for how they might provide support. One participant explained how a plan was shared and then implemented with their inner circle:

> *I circulated it to my inner circle, my friends, so that they would know what to do, how to help me, because I think everybody's unique and you know, when I'm in a particular zone, maybe I just need them to listen rather than go, oh, you know, it's not that bad, you know, it could be much worse or something.*

(SU018)

A service provider similarly suggested that the safety plan be shared with family and friends to involve them in how best to respond:

> *We do the wellness planning, and talk about involving loved ones in either in the planning or share the plan with them. I'll often say, you know, this is a chance for you to talk to your family, parents, partner, how do you want them to respond.*
>
> (KI1015)

Lack of family or social networks.

When individuals are faced with worsening suicidal thoughts/behaviours, social support (mechanism-resource) can help individuals to put their safety plan into practice (outcome) for social distraction (mechanism-resource) or direct support (mechanism-resource) during a suicidal crisis. However, when individuals lack a trusted social network (context), these mechanisms become unavailable:

> *I was asked at [hospital #1] to do a safety plan... They would ask about people that I could contact when I'm feeling down or feeling at risk, but I don't feel like I have someone that I truly trust to be in that role. So, I never found that my safety plan is sufficient.*
>
> (SU005)
>
> *I think it's a useful tool, just because it reminds you of people that you have there for you, and things that help, that are immediately accessible. But I also acknowledge that at some points in my life, it was harder because I did not have people to put on there.*
>
> (SU008)

In addition, the 'reaching out' aspect of a safety plan (mechanism-reasoning) might be challenging for individuals who experience difficulties with social interactions (context):

> *It's been hard for me to follow the plans that have just been like, call someone, or speak to someone, because of—oh, oh, part of the general anxiety.*
>
> (SU017)

Lack of support for friends and family members to help implement a safety plan.

Individuals who support someone with suicide-related thoughts or behaviours to implement a safety plan (mechanism-resource) may encounter difficulties (outcome) if they do not have adequate information, resources, time, the capacity or do not feel safe enough (context) to help implement the plan.

Friends and family members find it helpful to be involved in the safety planning process, especially if they are invited to be part of the process at the beginning. However, they acknowledge that there can be challenges to implementing a safety plan. Several friends and family members expressed, for example, that they cannot be present 24/7 to ensure safety.

> *I couldn't be there 24/7 and my siblings tried to be and were probably mad at me because I wasn't. But you can't be there if—you can't watch someone 24 h a day.*
>
> (F004)

Some friends and family members reported wanting to help, but ultimately felt uncomfortable or even unsafe (context) being involved in care.

> *Because once it [the situation with their family member] reached physical violence, she [a therapist] was just like, you need out right now... So, for me, it's like I can do it, I can do it. I think that was my downfall, is because I believed that I could do it so much that I ended up causing myself more trauma. I really felt like I could do it all. Until it reached the point where I couldn't, and then I crashed.*

(F009)

A few friends and family members provided examples of times when having access to a safety plan on its own was not enough for them to fully understand the situation (context), when the person they supported was discharged to their care. In one case, the plan on its own (mechanism-resource) was not enough to fully understand the situation (context), since the service user had not disclosed their suicide-related thoughts or behaviours. An individual may not wish to disclose such thoughts, due to stigma or shame, to protect the friend or family member in question or any other variety of reasons.

> *[She] gave us the papers but she had blocked off things. What she blocked off was the beginning of it where it says, I came to [hospital] after a serious attempt on my life. She cut that off... and gave us the photocopy copy of her safety plan.... We never got the picture. We never connected the dots. And that's where I have such regret because even with that information, this happened. I read her safety plan. And I thought [the family member] was doing really well. Even with having that safety plan in place, I was naive, and I was feeling like [the family member] was doing well. And I was so wrong. I was so wrong.*
>
> (F008)

Another family member similarly expressed that they did not know the level of severity of the situation. She echoed a need for family members to have more complete information about the situation of the person they support.

> *I think it would have been helpful for her and me, you know. That's something you do with the patient and whomever they're living with, their caregiver. And we could discuss it. You know, I think, going back to (...) I knew at the end she was trying to protect me, and she wasn't telling me everything. But if there was a forum where she could be open, it was encouraged with a doctor, any kind of support person, where the three of us, or you know, talk about that together, I think that would be... because then you can talk to one another more easily.*
>
> (F001)

Some service providers concurred that family members were not often involved in safety planning and suggested that barriers like the time required, obtaining consent and confidentiality made collaboration more difficult:

> *I can't even think, like, maybe a few examples in our day treatment service, where we've actually pulled family into the suicide risk assessment, right? Maybe not the assessment so much as like the safety planning. [I: I imagine one of the barriers is time?] Time and then, I think like, consent and willingness. [I: Confidentiality?] Confidentiality, yeah.*
>
> (KI1004)

Others considered the involvement of family members an important area of program development:

> *There's also potential to grow, in terms of having more safety plan[ing] and involving family members.*
>
> (FG1, P2)

In other program contexts, the involvement of family members was more common, and these barriers were not as apparent:

> *We're approaching it with them almost like, your safety plan is like first aid for suicidal thoughts, when these thoughts hit you go into action with doing these steps. And the families come onboard and they learn the safety plan, and I get them to put it on their phone and they print out copies and really visualizing them using it.*

(KI1010)

In adolescent care contexts, the involvement of family members was considered a key aspect of safety planning:

We create a safety plan often with these high-risk kids, with the collaboration with their parents. (. . ..) [In] family meetings (. . .) I always tell youth that safety is not a secret. So It's not something I'm going to keep secret from your family, whether you like it or not. So suicide is always something we talk frankly about in family meetings and with parents.

(KI1008)

In summary, although friends and family members were generally in support of safety plans, they realized that depending on their personal context, access to information, ability to provide support and the context of the individual, safety plans may not be possible to implement as intended.

3.1.3. Model Part 3: Bridging the Gap Between Evidence and Experience in Implementation

Creating Personalized Tailored Safety Plans in a Preferred Format Helps with Use

It is helpful to create a personalized safety plan for content and format such that it is more effective for the individual (mechanism-reasoning), with it also being easy to access (context) such that they are more likely to use it (outcome).

One participant spoke of the importance of creating a safety plan with elements that are already part of their everyday life (mechanism-reasoning) such that their plan is simply a reminder (outcome) to access the supports that they would normally use (context).

(. . .) I've made mine very much real life. Like it's things that are in my house, my friends' numbers are on there, like we've worked out, sort of, when I'll call them for support what they might do . . . they're things that I would already would naturally be doing, they're just sort of written down on a paper. So, I see it more as a reminder than something that, like, I'm forced to do or have to do.

(SU025)

The format could also be individualized. Some structured their safety plan as a personalized visual 'mind-map' or flowchart. These participants planned multiple options (mechanism-reasoning) in case some pathways did not provide the support needed (outcome).

I tend to think of safety planning almost as a mind map, where it's like if this happens then do this, and if this happens, then you go this way. (. . .) So, it's like a flowchart . . . I think that it can adapt to how my circumstances might change, and it makes it easier to follow because when I'm in a lot of distress, I really need it clearly laid out, like this is my next step. . . I always make sure that I have multiple options so there's never one end choice, because sometimes things don't work. . .So, I try to structure it in a way where I'm never going to get to a point where, like, okay, this was my last option, because that's gonna be unsafe for me.

(SU007)

The location of where the plan (mechanism-resource) was accessed (context) was also important, to ensure it could be easily found (outcome) during a crisis. One individual stated that storing their safety plan in a meaningful consistent location helped with its use.

(. . .) it's a quick reference, because when I'm like that emotional, I'm not really logical anymore, it's hard for me to remember things, but I know where my paper is. Or for me,

it's in my art books, and I know what page to flip to, and then it's something I know and I'm familiar with, so that's kind of comforting, like, yeah, I've done this before, I start here, and then I try this.

(SU025)

Others liked an idea introduced by the interviewer of creating a safety plan on an app (mechanism-resource) where they could find it easily (outcome), although they had not accessed one in this way before.

I think an app is really helpful and [hospital] actually had an app that I used for similar things. And like, mood tracking and tracking triggers and that was really helpful.

(SU008)

Others preferred pen and paper (context) in relation to format:

Maybe I'm still a little, I'm more pen and paper than most people, I think.

(SU024)

I'm sort of a visual person. So, if I had a plan written somewhere, and I could visualize the plan.

(SU015)

Rating Systems Contribute to the Implementation of Safety Plans

Various participants discussed incorporating a self-rating system (mechanism-resource) into their safety plans, to identify 'warning signs' of an increase in emotional distress (context), such that they could implement steps to keep themselves safe, prior to encountering a crisis situation (outcomes). The rating system could be conducted independently or in collaboration with others. One participant stated,

There's different levels [in the safety plan]. So, like, up until about a 9.5 out of 10, I can help myself. And if it gets to a 9.6, that's when I need to call on the professionals.

(SU025)

Other participants built a rating system that was then shared with a friend, family member or health care provider whom they saw regularly. As part of the plan, agreed-upon steps could be taken if an individual's rating reached a certain level. One participant explained how they used this rating system with a friend:

I definitely have, my safety plan, in terms of when I know I'm getting to a point of mental distress, I feel like I have that conversation with my best friend, where I give him a barometer of what I'm feeling. So, like, 0 being like, my batteries are out, I'm zero, I'm no life, I'm going to commit suicide, and 8 being the happiest I've ever been on earth. So, every so often, you know, I face challenges just like everybody else, my friend will ask me, hey, where are you on your scale? And like, I'll say straight up, like, I feel like I'm a 2 today, and then my best friend knows to jump into action.

(SU002)

An example of the use of an informal rating system used with a trusted health professional who has been seen over the long term was discussed by another participant:

Late last week, I definitely went through a hard time. And I called his office, he called me back, he's like, I can just tell in your voice, and he's like, what's your rating? And he trusts me that that rating is very accurate. And so it helps to have that, where we have an established rating system, but I bring it up when I feel I need to (. . .) you just have a code of, like, no, this is serious now.

(SU025)

Service providers also endorsed the value of incorporating rating systems into safety plans, especially for individuals with ongoing or chronic experiences of suicidal thoughts and behaviours that can occasionally become acute. The respondent calls this an 'acute-upon-chronic' situation and may use advance directives, as described below:

> *I think it's sometimes difficult with the chronically suicidal folks. I have a lot of patients that constantly think about ending their lives, or constantly don't want to be alive. I differentiate the risk when I look at their behaviours and what has changed. So, some of my patients, we have a safety plan and are very clear that if you tell me a certain thing, I'm going to send you to the Emerge, regardless of what else comes after that. So, if you tell me you're, for example, at acute risk or you've done a certain thing, there's no questions asked, you're going to the Emerge. And it may just be for a night, but that just means that in that moment, you're not safe. So, I have agreements with some patients around how I know whether they're safe or unsafe.*
>
> (KI1008)

The same provider described how colours can be effective rating systems for some individuals:

> *She has colours that work for her. She's like, if I'm in the red zone, I will try to kill myself. She came in, she said I'm in the red zone, and I was like, great, well, I guess you're going to the Emerge. (. . .) this is a kid who's made eight suicide attempts.*
>
> (KI1008)

The above steps of implementing a rating system (mechanism-resource) in a safety plan helps with determining the next steps for the kind of support needed (outcome), at a point prior to an individual being so severely distressed that they might not be able to or wish to access support (context). That is, the 'warning signs' are identified through comparing them to an individualized baseline score on the safety plan such that the individual can access support as needed. In these examples, the rating system is most often established between crises, when an individual and their support person(s) are able to collaboratively discuss a shared rating scale.

4. Discussion

Our research findings resulted in the construction of a model with three pillars of important considerations for implementing safety plans. The relevance of context and mechanisms (realist evaluation concepts) to SPI outcomes were discussed for the themes within each pillar. We will discuss the findings in relation to the current literature to understand their broader relevance. We will also compare the findings to the Stanley and Brown SPI model [8] upon which many SPIs are based and evaluated [6], to understand the differences or similarities between lived experience and the expected functioning of widely known SPI mechanisms.

First, the results revealed that while safety planning is perceived as a potentially effective intervention, context, timing and relationships are important in creating safety plans. For example, the timing of introducing safety planning during an acute crisis (context) can present challenges. Additionally, identifying aspects like 'reasons for living' (mechanism) at a time of emotional distress may cause individuals to feel disregarded and they may struggle to focus upon or find authentic answers.

Challenges for individuals to engage in creating a safety plan when they are having difficulty thinking at a time of acute crisis (context) were also identified in other qualitative studies [11,16,22]. Individuals in a UK study presenting at the ED with self-harm or SI expressed difficulty engaging in safety planning due to feeling overwhelmed and that they often could not remember what was discussed once they returned home [11]. Providers further observed that readiness to engage in plan creation was often challenged by difficulty for individuals in seeing alternatives to suicide at times of acute crisis [16,22]. The issue of when to complete the safety plan is referred to in the Stanley and Brown [8] model by having the SPI occur after a risk assessment that seeks to learn what led to the current crisis, builds rapport and identifies warning signs that can be included in a safety plan. Building a trusting relationship (mechanism) is an important first step to safety planning in this model. Although building a relationship may not completely moderate the difficulty of filling out a safety plan at a time of acute crisis, it may help with the process.

The value of creating a safety plan relationally, through therapeutic conversations (mechanism) rather than viewing safety plans as a checklist, was the second important factor discussed by health providers and service users in the current study and has been widely noted elsewhere. In another study, veterans suggested that the safety plan template itself does not need modification, but to improve plan development, active listening and skillful prompting by a health care provider are required [19]. In a recent qualitative systematic review and meta-synthesis of experiences of SPIs, it was found that the quality of the therapeutic interaction was more important than the resulting plan itself [10]. Adequate time and training are considered necessary to support person-centered, collaborative discussions and to prevent the SPI process from being reduced to 'risk mitigation' [10] or a 'checklist'. Importantly, in relation to the existing evidence-base for SPIs, collaborative co-creation is a core principle of interventions evaluated to have positive effects [6]. The Stanley and Brown model specifies that 20 to 45 min is the expected time required for this collaborative discussion [8].

In contrast to safety planning at the time of intense SI or SB, we found that embedding the process within existing therapeutic relationships between acute phases of illness (context) is experienced positively. This approach can invite discussion of contributing factors (context) to SI and may improve relevance over more time-constrained processes with health care providers. Other qualitative studies similarly report that ongoing SPI practices (mechanism) are positively perceived due to problem-solving discussions that are helpful to update existing plans [10,11,14,16,22]. The mechanism of continuing SPI practices in outpatient settings beyond initial plan creation is included in the Stanley and Brown model [8]. Other relational mechanisms through which safety plans can be created that are positively perceived within the current study and in the emerging literature include outpatient therapy groups or peer support [17,23].

In addition to the themes of timing, context and relationships described above, this study also describes facilitators and barriers to safety plan implementation as the second pillar of its model. For this pillar, individual-level differences (context) play an important role. Some participants strongly doubted they would be able, or were not able, to implement safety plans when in crisis (context), whereas others would consult the plan at exactly that time (mechanism-reasoning). Service users from a number of other studies similarly described much more difficulty and less motivation in implementing safety planning tools or strategies when experiencing intense distress, despair, depression or when in a 'red zone' or crisis [10,18–20].

Due to the prevalence of this finding, it has been suggested that cognitive and problem-solving abilities and self-regulatory behavioural coping strategies that are key to the overall SPI mechanism may not be as accessible in times of crisis [10,18]. Consequently, relying on other SPI mechanisms such as means-restrictions or family support is emphasized in some of the literature [10]. Notably, such cognitive barriers to implementing a safety plan while in crisis are anticipated in the original SPI design by Stanley and Brown [8]. The intervention suggests that after initial plan development but before implementation, clinicians troubleshoot potential barriers, prioritizing the strategies most likely or least likely to be used. Despite this mechanism, based on this study and others, using safety plans at a time of crisis remains difficult for some individuals. In the Recommendations Section to follow, adding a safety rating system or linking warning signs to strategies in SPIs are two mechanisms suggested to enhance SPIs. Such steps may help to prevent situations from escalating to a crisis when safety plans are not as useful for some people, and also to reduce cognitive load with specific advance directives should a crisis occur.

Another facilitator or barrier to SPIs was noted by service providers in relation to individual differences (context) that affect SPI implementation based on working with persons who struggle with SI but do not want to end their lives, others who are ambivalent or those for whom SI is related to core coping mechanisms. Notably, different individual characteristics and diagnoses were identified in other qualitative studies than in the current study as facilitators or barriers to SPI implementation [11,16]. Due to the disparity in perception, more research is needed to understand the importance of individual differences for SPI implementation. Furthermore, clinical supervision is suggested to address fixed beliefs by providers about the value of SPI for individuals with certain diagnoses, fears about possible negative effects of safety planning (e.g., evoking trauma) and other factors [11,14,22]. The Stanley and Brown SPI model includes an explanation that the use of the SPI may need to be adapted depending on the population, but it does not deeply examine the impact of individual differences. Many social and environmental factors place individuals at a disproportionate risk of SI and/or SB. One example is the link between childhood maltreatment and self-injurious thoughts and behaviours [41,42]; therefore, trauma-informed approaches to SPI may be relevant for tailoring interventions for this group. The findings of the current study and others substantiate the importance of individual differences as a barrier or facilitator to the functioning of SPI mechanisms.

In the second pillar exploring barriers and facilitators to SPIs, positive support from family and social networks was another key facilitator of safety plan implementation. Friends and family were often named as contacts in safety plans, acting as a critical mechanism (e.g., recognizing and responding to warning signs with social support and distraction or reminders about coping skills and other strategies). Sharing safety plans with social networks in advance (mechanism) was also discussed as highly valued to develop shared understandings of how best to respond. The effectiveness of this mechanism was strongly echoed by participants in other qualitative studies who sought support from friends or family when warning signs arose, for social distraction, to help ensure safety, to provide assistance in contacting mental health resources and for overall plan implementation [10,19–21].

While social network involvement is a key mechanism of SPIs, barriers to implementing this factor due to sparse networks (context) are not discussed in the Stanley and Brown SPI model [8]. The current qualitative study and others clearly demonstrate that some individuals have very few trusted family members, friends or social supports they can include in a safety plan [10,14,16,18,19,22,23]. A suggested intervention (mechanism-resource) from the literature to address this difficulty is to support service users to build new relationships or revitalize old ones [19]; once the individual's social context is shifted, the social support mechanism in safety planning can be more easily accessed.

At times, family members or friends felt unable to implement a plan due to a lack of information, resources, time, capacity or feeling safe enough to do so (context). This finding was echoed by recommendations by family members in another study that more information and mental health psychoeducation would help to make their involvement more useful [20]. The inclusion of friends or family members in SPI processes was variable in the current study, depending on the organizational context, but was seen as a valuable area for program improvement. Overall, friend or family member involvement in SPI processes (e.g., initial safety plan creation, at review appointments or receiving support from providers) is not part of the Stanley and Brown SPI model [8]. However, such mechanisms are widely recognized to enhance safety planning across the literature [10,15,19–21]. Some studies even suggest constructing separate safety plans for service users and family members [15] or modifying a service user plan to incorporate instructions for family members [20] since there are different needs and roles.

4.1. Recommendations

This study identified ways to improve implementation in its third pillar, 'bridging the gap between evidence and experience in implementation'. The findings reflect that the extent to which the plan is personalized (mechanism) impacts the willingness to use the plan (outcome). Some methods to personalize include ensuring the safety plan is reviewed and up to date, formatted according to an individual's preference (e.g., flowchart or list) (mechanism), accessible and/or portable according to individual preference (e.g., printed card, sheet of paper or electronic) (mechanism). Formatting plans flexibly with photographs, images or drawings to bridge language barriers [22], using targeted language and layouts for youth and children [15] and modified or supplemental templates for family members [15,20] are further proposed in the literature to personalize plans and optimize use.

Another key recommendation for safety planning is a rating system (mechanism) established in comparison to a personalized 'baseline' within a safety plan to identify 'warning signs' of an increase in emotional distress such that steps can be taken prior to encountering a crisis situation. Such rating systems can be used independently or with family members, friends or professionals. A similar innovation was suggested in another study with adolescents engaged to provide input for an SPI design for their demographic [15]. Like in the current study, rating scales were suggested for the rapid communication of internal states to chosen support individuals using numbers to track moods which could result in pre-determined types of support or reminders of coping skills (strategies) to prevent escalation [15].

Notably, the idea of linking 'warning signs' to strategies more generally (without the added mechanism of rating scales) was also suggested in the current study by participants who structured safety plans as a flowchart with 'if this happens/then do this' scenarios. Similar suggestions are made in other qualitative studies to improve safety plans by pairing anticipated scenarios with actions that could be used in a crisis [21] or linking warning signs and strategies in a safety plan app to provide reminders during a suicidal crisis [19,43]. Service providers also discussed the importance of making such linkages [16]. Rating scales and linking warning signs and strategies are not included in the Stanley and Brown SPI [8] and represent two innovations to prevent situations from escalating to crises and, if they do, to reduce cognitive load at that point when safety plans have been found more difficult to implement for some individuals.

A summary of the above recommendations that emerged directly from the findings in pillar three, and additional suggestions woven throughout the discussion based on comparison of the findings from other pillars with the literature, are summarized in Appendix C. Below is a table derived from this appendix with an actionable summary for clinicians and administrators (Table 7).

Table 7. Recommendations for clinicians and administrators with regard to SPIs.

SPI Mechanisms	Recommendation
Introducing Safety Plans (Timing)	Complete risk assessment prior to safety planning to hear what led to the current crisis, to build rapport and to identify warning signs that can be included in a safety plan (first step in the Stanley and Brown [8] SPI). Consider the importance of timing and context when co-creating safety plans. Possibly delay, or complete risk assessment as above and establish a trusting relationship first, if in acute crisis.
Safety Plan Creation	Co-create a safety plan relationally and collaboratively rather than completing it as a 'checklist' to fulfill instrumental or 'risk mitigation' goals required by the organization. Time for safety plan completion (20–45 min recommended in the Stanley and Brown [8] SPI). SPI training in all aspects of the Stanley and Brown SPI model [8]. Active listening and skillful prompting by clinician; attend to quality of the therapeutic relationship. During safety plan creation, before finalizing the plan, troubleshoot barriers to implementation during a crisis by prioritizing the strategies most likely and least likely to be used during this time (mechanism in the Stanley and Brown [8] SPI).
Ongoing Safety Planning	Continue SPI practices within an ongoing professional therapeutic relationship in the outpatient context (recommended by the Stanley and Brown [8] SPI). Review what has worked and not worked during times of crisis; discuss things to add based on reflection (e.g., new warning signs, strategies, contacts); update plan accordingly.
Troubleshooting Implementation Issues Some service users doubt they will use safety plans in a time of crisis or have experience in not using them at this time.	During safety plan creation, before finalizing the plan, troubleshoot barriers to implementation during a crisis by prioritizing the strategies most likely and least likely to be used during a crisis situation (mechanism in the Stanley and Brown [8] SPI). Ensure means-restrictions and chosen family and/or friend supports are in place as a result of prior safety planning to accommodate inability to use safety plans during crisis situations. Add safety scales with linked strategies and/or link warning signs and strategies within SPIs. Update as needed through ongoing SPI practices. Share rating scales with chosen family members and/or friends, to ensure shared language to communicate distress and pre-determined strategies when crisis situations occur. These approaches may reduce cognitive load during a crisis and facilitate implementation of safety plan strategies that may not be normally possible due to difficulties with problem-solving and behavioural self-regulation at this time.
Adapting SPIs for Individual Differences Individual differences related to diagnosis, sense of self, control and coping may either facilitate or prevent engagement with, or use of, safety plans.	Maintain awareness of variation in responses to SPIs. Introduce safety planning to individuals who may find it helpful. Adapt SPIs to focus on the short-term or introduce other adaptations for individuals who may see SI or SB as part of their identity, sense of control or coping. As appropriate for individuals with longstanding SI and/or SB, facilitate therapeutic processes to explore root causes. Trauma-informed approaches to care and clinical supervision.

Table 7. *Cont.*

SPI Mechanisms	Recommendation
Family and Social Network Involvement	List the chosen social supports on the safety plan for social distraction or to contact during a suicidal crisis. Share the safety plan with chosen members of the social network. When trusted family members or social networks are lacking, support service users to build new relationships or revitalize old ones [19]; once the individual's social context is shifted, the social support mechanisms in safety planning can be more easily accessed. To increase safety and effectiveness, involve chosen family members and/or friends in SPI processes with adequate information about the service user's situation and warning signs, offer mental health psychoeducation sessions, construct separate safety plans tailored to support person needs and/or add professional contacts for family and friend support.
Formatting SPIs	The extent to which the plan is personalized and accessible impacts the willingness and ability to use the plan. Ensure the safety plan is up to date, including content formatted according to an individual's preference (e.g., flowchart or list, language, visual cues), accessible and/or portable according to individual preference (e.g., printed wallet card, sheet of paper or electronic).

4.2. Future Directions for Research

As noted earlier, more research is needed to understand how individual differences (context) affect safety planning and what corresponding adaptations to SPIs may be needed. The CAMH Suicide Prevention Cohort Study (CAMH-SPCS), which was work that grew out of the current study, will recruit 500 individuals with SI and SB who present to the CAMH ED to better understand their trajectories and needs. A qualitative component will interview a subset across different age, gender, ethnicity and diagnosis categories and will interview one friend or family member per participant separately to understand their perspectives of evidence-based interventions, including safety planning. This study will add to the existing understanding of how safety planning can apply to different types of individuals.

Furthermore, evidence-based interventions for suicide prevention, such as SPIs, are not consistently implemented or provided to all patients who might need them [44]. More efforts are needed to implement SPIs in the right context and with the right mechanisms for each person to ensure the anticipated outcomes of SPIs can be realized. To contribute to this work, a current implementation research study will further explore barriers and facilitators in delivering SPIs from emergency department clinicians' perspectives for alternative (app) and paper-based modalities and collaboratively design strategies to address these barriers [45]. Such efforts will provide further valuable insights into how SPIs can be optimized, adapted and effectively implemented while maintaining their intended outcomes.

4.3. Strengths and Limitations

The use of the realist evaluation design is a strength of this study since it examines contextual factors and mechanisms that facilitate or hinder the outcomes of safety planning interventions. This methodology has not yet been applied to SPIs. The study compares its findings to prior qualitative studies, contributing to credibility and transferability, two aspects of trustworthiness in qualitative research [46]. A further strength is the triangulation of perspectives about SPIs from a relatively large and heterogeneous sample of service user participants with those of friends, family members and service users, which further contributes to credibility and transferability. There was rigorous coding and analysis of transcribed interviews, reflexive practice through memo writing and peer review of coding and manuscript writing, which contributes to dependability and confirmability [46].

A key limitation is that although many participants shared views on safety planning, the specific type of safety planning model experienced was not explored in the primary study to know whether all of the steps were completed (e.g., Stanley and Brown SPI [8]). Thus, the safety planning interventions experienced across participants may have differed. In addition, the research goals did not include examining implementation differences across different care contexts such as emergency care, inpatient units or community follow-up. Regardless, the findings reflect very similar experiences for participants in this study as in other qualitative studies with known intervention types and care settings, which contributes to credibility and transferability. Future directions for research, moreover, include examining implementation issues in the emergency department, specifically.

A further limitation is that the study did not purposively or theoretically sample for language spoken, geographical or socio-demographic diversity and only recruited English-speaking individuals. Furthermore, while the demographic characteristics indicated diversity for gender identity, race and socio-economic factors, the findings were not analyzed to explore whether certain groups may have unique needs and preferences. While the sampling and analysis approach may limit transferability [46], this limitation was moderated by comparisons in the discussion with prior qualitative research across various demographic groups in various geographic regions that demonstrated similarities across multiple findings.

5. Conclusions

In this paper, qualitative interviews were used to better understand the lived experiences of individuals who have experienced SI and/or SB with SPIs. Friends, family members and health care providers were also interviewed about their views. A realist evaluation analysis distilled which contexts and mechanisms influenced SPI implementation. A resulting model was developed with three pillars: (1) understanding the importance of context, timing and relationships in safety planning; (2) understanding perceived barriers and facilitators to safety planning; (3) bridging the gap between evidence and experience in implementation. Taken together, and compared to the current literature and the Stanley and Brown SPI [8], the results demonstrate the value of certain SPI mechanisms and draw attention to others for which taking context into consideration, or adding interventions, would enhance SPI outcomes.

Supplementary Materials: The following supporting information can be downloaded at https://www.mdpi.com/article/10.3390/jcm14124047/s1, Supplemental File S1, Table S1: RAMESES II reporting standards for realist evaluations: checklist; Supplemental File S2, Table S2: Consolidated criteria for reporting qualitative studies (COREQ): 32-item checklist.

Author Contributions: Conceptualization, E.H., H.D.S., N.R., V.S. and J.Z.; Data curation, E.H. and J.Z.; Formal analysis, E.H., H.D.S., N.R., A.W. and J.Z.; Funding acquisition, V.S. and J.Z.; Investigation, J.Z.; Methodology, E.H., H.D.S., N.R., V.S., G.N. and J.Z.; Project administration, E.H. and J.Z.; Supervision, J.Z.; Validation, E.H., H.D.S. and J.Z.; Visualization, E.H. and J.Z.; Writing—original draft, E.H., H.D.S. and J.Z.; Writing—review and editing, E.H., H.D.S., N.R., V.S., L.L., G.N., A.W. and J.Z. All authors have read and agreed to the published version of the manuscript.

Funding: This research was funded by a Canadian Institutes of Health Research (CIHR) foundation grant (201409FDN-332964-FDN-CEAH-150099) awarded to V. Stergiopoulos.

Institutional Review Board Statement: This study was conducted according to the guidelines of the Declaration of Helsinki and approved by the Research Ethics Board of the Centre for Addiction and Mental Health (REB#041-2019, 1 August 2019).

Informed Consent Statement: Informed consent was obtained from all subjects involved in this study.

Data Availability Statement: The data presented in this study are available on request from the corresponding author. The data are not publicly available due to privacy and ethical restrictions.

Conflicts of Interest: The authors declare no conflicts of interest.

Abbreviations

The following abbreviations are used in this manuscript:

ADHD	Attention-deficity/hyperactivity disorder
CAD	Canadian Dollar
CAMH	Centre for Addiction and Mental Health
CERB	Canadian Emergency Response Benefit
CMHA	Canadian Mental Health Association
CMO	Context + Mechanism = Outcome
CPSTD	Complex post-traumatic stress disorder
EI	Employment Insurance
ED	Emergency Department
OCD	Obsessive-compulsive disorder
ODSP	Ontario Disability Support Program
PTSD	Post-traumatic stress disorder
SI	Suicidal Ideation
SB	Suicidal Behaviours
SPIs	Safety Planning Interventions

Appendix A

Centre for Addiction and Mental Health (CAMH) Safety Plan Template

The following safety plan template is adapted from Stanley and Brown's 2012 paper entitled 'Safety Planning Intervention: A Brief Intervention to Mitigate Risk for Suicide' [8] and the CAMH Suicide Prevention and Assessment Handbook (2011).

Table A1. Centre for Addiction and Mental Health (CAMH) safety plan template.

Safety Plan
Step 1: Warning signs that I may not be safe
1.
2.
3.
Step 2: Remind myself of my reasons for living
1.
2.
3.

Table A1. *Cont.*

Safety Plan
Step 3: Coping strategies that I use to distract myself or feel better
1. 2. 3.
Step 4: Social situations and people that can help distract me
1. 2. 3.
Step 5: People who I can ask for help
1. 2. 3.
Step 6: Professionals or agencies I can contact during a crisis
1. 2. 3.
Step 6: Professionals or agencies I can contact during a crisis
1. 2. 3. 4. 5.
Step 7: Making my environment safe
1. 2. 3.

Appendix B

Author Reflexivity Statement

The qualitative and realist evaluation methodologies used in this study both adopt an interpretive epistemological stance, proposing that human knowledge is socially constructed. The realist methodology additionally adopts an ontological position that there is a separate 'reality' apart from human observation, but that this 'reality' can be perceived only partially, due to how it is filtered through language, culture and other factors [40]. Due to these philosophical perspectives, both research methodologies suggest that the positioning of the researchers be made transparent, in what is known as 'reflexivity'. Reflexivity asks the researchers to examine and then share how the research context (e.g., culture, health care system, local policies or service frameworks) and the researchers' backgrounds and perspectives may influence study design, implementation, analysis, writing and other research processes.

Due to these principles, it is important to acknowledge that a number of the research team members have worked as psychiatrists (L.L., V.S., J.Z.) or in research roles (H.D.S.) in CAMH's Gerald Sheff and Shanitha Kachan Emergency Department (ED), Canada's largest mental health teaching hospital and only standalone psychiatric ED in Canada. This ED receives over 15,000 visits annually, and approximately 1/3 of these visits have identified suicidal ideation (SI) or suicide-related behaviours (SB) at triage. In the CAMH ED, there is a standard SPI template adapted from Stanley and Brown [8]. Upon discharge from the ED, individuals leave with a paper-based, personalized safety plan. Several authors, therefore, were familiar with how SPIs were implemented and experienced in this context prior to the study.

One objective of the study was to understand the lived experiences of SPIs from various perspectives (service users, friends, family and service providers) and what components were helpful or not helpful in the ED context but also in other Ontario, Canada, health care and community contexts, as reflected by its broad recruitment strategy. Therefore, perceptions of the SPI process at the CAMH ED needed to be considered by some authors when collecting or analyzing the current study data. In addition to acknowledging prior experience with SPIs, the researchers' broader backgrounds are important to acknowledge for their possible influence. Overall, the researchers brought clinical practice experience, lived experience and research experience to this study. They all have longstanding relationships within the health context in Ontario. The researchers disclosed their roles and positionality in the informed consent document and at the beginning of interviews or focus groups.

E.H. (MSW, she/her) is a research coordinator with qualitative research expertise in the area of SI and SB, a registered social worker, and has previously worked as a community mental health provider for the friends and family members of people with SI and SB, as well as being a family member herself. H.D.S. (RN, PhD, she/her) is a registered nurse with experience in emergency and mental health nursing with extensive experience in qualitative research, collaborative research and implementation research in the mental health context including suicide prevention. N.R. (PhD, she/her) is a researcher and evaluator with expertise in realist evaluation and qualitative research methods centred in equity and engagement. V.S. (MD, she/her) is a psychiatrist and health services researcher who often works with patients who have experienced SI and SB. L.L. (MD, he/him) is an emergency department psychiatrist who often works with patients who have experienced SI and SB. G.N. (she/her) is a research assistant with lived experience of mental illness and suicide and has expertise in research and peer support. A.W. (MSW, she/her) is a research analyst with qualitative research experience in mental health and addictions and a registered social worker who frequently works with people who experience SI and SB. J.Z. (MD, she/her) is an emergency department psychiatrist and researcher with qualitative research expertise. She often works with patients who have experienced SI and SB.

During the study, different views and perspectives were acknowledged and shared among research team members. This process resulted in increased reflexivity and conversations about how best to interpret the data. Consequently, one of the goals of reflexivity to broaden the conversation and to include alternate perspectives was accomplished [40].

Appendix C

Summary of Findings and Recommendations

Table A2. Summary of findings and recommendations.

Theme	Context	Mechanism	Outcome	Recommendation
Pillar 1: Importance of Timing, Context and Relationships				
Timing				
Creating a safety plan or identifying reasons for living when experiencing acute SI or SB may be challenging.	Acute crisis.	Introducing safety planning. Creating a safety plan. Discussing reasons for living.	Overwhelmed. Feeling disregarded or unheard. Struggles to focus upon or find authentic answers to safety planning questions.	Complete risk assessment prior to safety planning to hear about what led to the current crisis, to build rapport, and to identify warning signs that can be included in a safety plan (first step in the Stanley and Brown SPI). Build a trusting relationship as a first step to co-creating a safety plan. Consider the importance of timing of the intervention and context of the service user, when co-creating safety plans.
Relationships				
Co-create a safety plan relationally and collaboratively rather than completing it as a 'checklist' to fulfill instrumental or 'risk mitigation' goals required by the organization.	Time for safety plan completion (20–45 min recommended in the Stanley and Brown SPI). Availability of a clinician with SPI training in all aspects of the Stanley and Brown SPI model (including aspects of the SPI that are not included in the safety planning template alone, but can be found in the original intervention protocol).	Clinician and service user co-create the safety plan collaboratively. Active listening by clinician. Skillful prompting by clinician. Attend to quality of the therapeutic relationship (which is considered more important than the resulting safety plan by service users). During safety plan creation, before finalizing the plan, troubleshoot barriers to implementation during a crisis by prioritizing the strategies most likely and least likely to be used during this time (mechanism in the Stanley and Brown SPI).	Safety plan that is personalized and reflects authentic input from the service user that the individual can take with them.	See content in the adjacent context and mechanism columns for this theme.

Table A2. *Cont.*

Theme	Context	Mechanism	Outcome	Recommendation
Embed safety plan within existing therapeutic relationships.	Access to therapeutic relationship in the outpatient context. Skilled clinicians who can discuss the underlying causes of SI or SB.	Continue SPI practices within an ongoing professional therapeutic relationship in the outpatient context (recommended by the Stanley and Brown SPI when possible). Review what has worked and not worked during times of crisis; discuss things to add based on reflection (e.g., new warning signs, strategies, contacts); update plan accordingly. Engage in therapeutic discussions about the underlying causes of SI or SB.	Revised and updated safety plan. Barriers to implementation may be discussed through review. The underlying causes of SI or SB may be discussed in some contexts to help with reflection and healing.	See content in the adjacent context and mechanism columns for this theme.
Other relationships for creating safety plans.	Therapeutic group settings with a focus on SPI. Access to supportive peers who are knowledgeable about, and able to assist with safety plan creation. Access to online templates or apps for safety planning; trusted professional support may not be available.	Therapeutic groups may provide education and structure a process for safety planning with peers and clinician-facilitators. Peers may engage in informal collaborative safety planning outside of the clinical context. Service users may access online SPI tools independently, outside of the clinical context.	Safety plans are created through group processes, resulting in peer-support and generating more ideas. Safety plans are created with peer-support and possibly more time than is available in clinical contexts. Safety plans are created independently, which may be useful in ties when trusted professional support is not available.	Explore alternative relational mechanisms to create safety plans, such as therapeutic groups; peer support; and online safety planning resources that can be used independently at times when trusted professional support is not available.
Pillar 2: Perceived Facilitators and Barriers to Safety Planning				
Individual Differences in Safety Planning				
Use of safety plans during an acute phase of illness or a crisis				

Table A2. *Cont.*

Theme	Context	Mechanism	Outcome	Recommendation
Some service users doubt they will use safety plans in a time of crisis or have experience in not using them at this time.	Acute crisis. 'Red zone.' Intense depression. Lack of motivation. Despair.	Cognitive and problem-solving abilities and self-regulatory strategies to implement safety plan mechanisms are not accessible to the service user.	Safety plan not used.	During safety plan creation, before finalizing the plan, troubleshoot barriers to implementation during a crisis during by prioritizing strategies most likely and least likely to be used during a crisis situation (mechanism in the Stanley and Brown SPI). Ensure means-restrictions and family support are in place as a result of prior safety planning to accommodate inability to use safety plans during crisis situations. Add safety scales with linked strategies and/or link warning signs and strategies within SPIs. Share rating scales with support networks (including available friends, family and clinicians) to ensure there is a shared language for service users to communicate distress and pre-determined strategies to enact when crisis situations occur.
		Diagnosis, sense of self, control and coping		
Individual differences related to diagnosis, sense of self, control and coping may either facilitate or prevent engagement with, or use of safety plans.	Individuals who struggle with SI but do not want to end their lives may find SPI helpful. Individuals who are ambivalent or for whom SI is related to identity or core coping mechanisms may not engage in SPI or find SPI helpful. Access to outpatient context for SPI practice. Skilled clinicians able to facilitate therapeutic processes to explore the root causes of SI or SB.	Introduce safety planning to individuals who may find it helpful. Adapt SPI to focus on the short-term or introduce other adaptations for individuals who may see SI or SB as part of their identity, sense of control or coping. Work with individuals with chronic SI to explore the root causes of SI or SB.	Adapted safety plan interventions to needs of specific individuals. Increased awareness and understanding of self and root causes of SI and SB for individuals who engage in therapy.	Develop or maintain awareness of variation in responses to SPIs depending on the context of the individual. Clinical supervision to help with clinician 'fixed' beliefs about the ability of individuals with particular diagnoses to engage in safety planning and to provide support around fears about possible negative effects of safety planning (e.g., evoking trauma).

Table A2. *Cont.*

Theme	Context	Mechanism	Outcome	Recommendation
Family and social networks				
Positive support from family and social networks				
Positive support from family and social networks is a key facilitator to safety plan implementation.	Positive relationships with a number of friends, family members and social networks that can be listed for social distraction or SI or SB crisis support on a safety plan.	List social supports on the safety plan for social distraction or to contact during a suicidal crisis, as appropriate. Share safety plan with members of the social network.	Service users will contact the friends, family members or members of their social network listed on their safety plan for support when needed. Members of the social network may recognize and respond to warming signs, provide social distraction or support during a suicidal crisis.	See content in the adjacent mechanism column for this theme.
Lack of family or social networks				
Individuals with sparse social networks cannot draw upon key SPI mechanisms involving social distraction or direct support for SI or SB.	Some individuals do not have any trusted friends, family members, professionals or social networks they can draw on for social distraction or support when experiencing SI or SB.	None.	Without additional interventions (see adjacent recommendation), service users will not be able to add members of their social network to their safety plan for support. Service users may see their safety plans as deficient due to their inability to use this mechanism.	Support service users to build new relationships or consider old ones; once the individual's social context is shifted, the social support mechanisms in safety planning can be more easily accessed.
Lack of support for friends or family members to help implement safety plan				
At times, family members or friends felt unable to implement a plan due to lack of information, resources, time, capacity or feeling safe enough to do so (context).	Friends and family members lack information, resources, time or capacity to fulfill their roles in the SPI.	None.	Service users will not be able to fully benefit from the support of family members. Mechanisms involving friends, family members and social networks will not be available or will be deficient in some way.	Involve family members in SPI processes with adequate information about the service user's situation and warning signs, offer mental health psychoeducation sessions, construct separate safety plans tailored to support person needs or add support person information to the service user's safety plan.
Pillar 3: Bridging the gap between evidence and experience in implementation				
Creating personalized, tailored safety plans in a preferred format helps with their use				

Table A2. *Cont.*

Theme	Context	Mechanism	Outcome	Recommendation
The extent to which the plan is personalized and accessible impacts willingness and ability to use the plan.	Access to a collaborative co-creation process wherein a safety plan is constructed by a service user and clinician working together. Access to ongoing outpatient SPI support from a skilled clinician for ongoing safety plan review.	Through the original co-creation process and in follow-up outpatient SPI practices, ensure the safety plan is up to date, formatted according to an individual's preference (e.g., flowchart or list) accessible and/or portable according to individual preference (e.g., printed card, sheet of paper or electronic). Ensure the safety plan is located in an accessible format or location.	Individuals will be more likely to use and implement their safety plan.	Formatting plans flexibly with photographs, images or drawings to bridge language barriers, using targeted language and layouts for youth and children and modified or supplemental templates for family members are further proposed in the literature to personalize plans and optimize use.
Rating systems contribute to the implementation of safety plans				
Add a rating system established in comparison to a personalized 'baseline' to an SPI to identify 'warning signs' of an increase in emotional distress such that steps can be taken prior to encountering a crisis situation. and/or: Link warning signs to strategies in safety plans.	Access to clinical support or templates to create a safety rating scale with linked strategies (and/or to link warning signs and strategies). Access to positive support from friends, family members, professionals or members of social support network who can be contacted for social distraction or support around SI and SB.	Construct a safety rating scale with linked strategies (and/or warning signs with linked strategies) with a clinician or using a template. Share completed rating scales with linked strategies (and/or SPIs with warning signs and linked strategies) to chosen friends, family members, professionals or members of social support network. Update safety rating scale and linked strategies (and/or warning signs and linked strategies) as needed through ongoing outpatient SPI practices. Service users will communicate emotional states to chosen support persons using ratings (and/or will directly discuss 'warning signs'), as needed, or will reflect upon ratings (and/or 'warning signs') and linked strategies for self-regulation.	Use of the safety rating scale and linked strategies (and/or 'warning signs with linked strategies) within the SPI may prevent escalation to crisis situations. The safety rating scale (and/or an SPI with linked warning signs and strategies) may improve communication to support persons about emotional states and result in reminders about, or implementation of, strategies associated with each rating (and/or warning sign). Pre-determined strategies related to certain ratings (and/or linked to warning sign) may result in preventing SB, with or without additional social network support. Increased awareness of ratings and/or warning signs may increase the ability to use suicide coping skills. These techniques may reduce cognitive load during a crisis and facilitate implementation of safety plan strategies that may not normally be possible due to difficulties with problem-solving and behavioural self-regulation at this time.	Create templates or draw upon existing ones to add safety rating scales with linked strategies (and/or warning signs with linked strategies) to SPIs. See content in the adjacent context and mechanism columns for additional recommendations for this theme.

References

1. World Health Organization. Preventing Suicide: A Global Imperative. Available online: https://www.who.int/publications/i/item/9789241564779 (accessed on 9 May 2025).
2. World Health Organization. Suicide Worldwide in 2019. Available online: https://www.who.int/publications/i/item/9789240026643 (accessed on 9 May 2025).
3. Government of Canada. Injuries in Canada: Insights from the Canadian Community Health Survey/by Jean-Michel Billette and Teresa Janz: CS82-624/2011001-2E-PDF—Government of Canada Publications—Canada. Available online: https://publications.gc.ca/site/eng/427102/publication.html (accessed on 9 May 2025).
4. Chartier, M.; Bolton, J.; Mota, N.; MacWilliam, L.; Ekuma, O.; Nie, Y.; McDougall, C.; Srisakuldee, W.; McCulloch, S. *Mental Illness Among Adult Manitobans*; Manitoba Centre for Health Policy: Winnipeg, MB, Canada, 2018.
5. Nuij, C.; van Ballegooijen, W.; de Beurs, D.; Juniar, D.; Erlangsen, A.; Portzky, G.; O'Connor, R.C.; Smit, J.H.; Kerkhof, A.; Riper, H. Safety Planning-Type Interventions for Suicide Prevention: Meta-Analysis. *Br. J. Psychiatry* **2021**, *219*, 419–426. [CrossRef] [PubMed]
6. Ferguson, M.; Rhodes, K.; Loughhead, M.; McIntyre, H.; Procter, N. The Effectiveness of the Safety Planning Intervention for Adults Experiencing Suicide-Related Distress: A Systematic Review. *Arch. Suicide Res.* **2021**, *26*, 1022–1045. [CrossRef] [PubMed]
7. Marshall, C.A.; Crowley, P.; Carmichael, D.; Goldszmidt, R.; Aryobi, S.; Holmes, J.; Easton, C.; Isard, R.; Murphy, S. Effectiveness of Suicide Safety Planning Interventions: A Systematic Review Informing Occupational Therapy. *Can. J. Occup. Ther.* **2023**, *90*, 208–236. [CrossRef]
8. Stanley, B.; Brown, G.K. Safety Planning Intervention: A Brief Intervention to Mitigate Suicide Risk. *Cogn. Behav. Pract.* **2012**, *19*, 256–264. [CrossRef]
9. Stanley, B.; Brown, G.K.; Brenner, L.A.; Galfalvy, H.C.; Currier, G.W.; Knox, K.L.; Chaudhury, S.R.; Bush, A.L.; Green, K.L. Comparison of the Safety Planning Intervention with Follow-up vs. Usual Care of Suicidal Patients Treated in the Emergency Department. *JAMA Psychiatry* **2018**, *75*, 894–900. [CrossRef]
10. O'Connor, E.; Rhodes, K.; Procter, N.; Loughhead, M.; Procter, A.; Reilly, J.-A.; Pettit, S.; Ferguson, M. The Experiences of Consumers, Clinicians and Support Persons Involved in the Safety Planning Intervention for Suicide Prevention: A Qualitative Systematic Review and Meta-Synthesis. *Front. Psychiatry* **2024**, *15*, 1482924. [CrossRef]
11. Shah, N.; O'Keeffe, S.; Hayward, S.; Suzuki, M.; McCabe, R. Re-Imagining Crisis Care: Experiences of Delivering and Receiving the Assured Brief Psychological Intervention for People Presenting to Emergency Departments with Self-Harm. *Front. Psychiatry* **2024**, *15*, 1271674. [CrossRef]
12. Chesin, M.S.; Stanley, B.; Haigh, E.A.P.; Chaudhury, S.R.; Pontoski, K.; Knox, K.L.; Brown, G.K. Staff Views of an Emergency Department Intervention Using Safety Planning and Structured Follow-Up with Suicidal Veterans. *Arch. Suicide Res.* **2017**, *21*, 127–137. [CrossRef] [PubMed]
13. Stanley, B.; Chaudhury, S.R.; Chesin, M.; Pontoski, K.; Bush, A.M.; Knox, K.L.; Brown, G.K. An Emergency Department Intervention and Follow-Up to Reduce Suicide Risk in the VA: Acceptability and Effectiveness. *PS Political Sci. Politics* **2016**, *67*, 680–683. [CrossRef]
14. O'Connor, R.C.; Smillie, S.; McClelland, H.; Lundy, J.-M.; Stewart, C.; Syrett, S.; Gavigan, M.; McConnachie, A.; Stanley, B.; Smith, M.; et al. SAFETEL: A Pilot Randomised Controlled Trial to Assess the Feasibility and Acceptability of a Safety Planning and Telephone Follow-up Intervention to Reduce Suicidal Behaviour. *Pilot Feasibility Stud.* **2022**, *8*, 156. [CrossRef]
15. McManama O'Brien, K.H.; Almeida, J.; View, L.; Schofield, M.; Hall, W.; Aguinaldo, L.; Ryan, C.A.; Maneta, E. A Safety and Coping Planning Intervention for Suicidal Adolescents in Acute Psychiatric Care. *Cogn. Behav. Pract.* **2021**, *28*, 22–39. [CrossRef]
16. Levandowski, B.A.; Cass, C.M.; Miller, S.N.; Kemp, J.E.; Conner, K.R. An Intervention with Meaning: Perceptions of Safety Planning among Veteran Health Administration Providers. *Crisis J. Crisis Interv. Suicide Prev.* **2017**, *38*, 376–383. [CrossRef] [PubMed]
17. Patel, S.R.; Sullivan, S.R.; Mitchell, E.L.; Jager-Hyman, S.; Stanley, B.; Goodman, M. Qualitative Study of Telehealth Delivery of Suicide-Specific Group Treatment "Project Life Force". *J. Technol. Behav. Sci.* **2023**, *8*, 272–281. [CrossRef]
18. Buus, N.; Erlangsen, A.; River, J.; Andreasson, K.; Frandsen, H.; Larsen, J.L.S.; Nordentoft, M.; Juel, A. Stakeholder Perspectives on Using and Developing the MYPLAN Suicide Prevention Mobile Phone Application: A Focus Group Study. *Arch. Suicide Res.* **2020**, *24*, 48–63. [CrossRef]
19. Kayman, D.J.; Goldstein, M.F.; Dixon, L.; Goodman, M. Perspectives of Suicidal Veterans on Safety Planning: Findings from a Pilot Study. *Crisis J. Crisis Interv. Suicide Prev.* **2015**, *36*, 371–383. [CrossRef]
20. DeBeer, B.B.; Matthieu, M.M.; Kittel, J.A.; Degutis, L.C.; Clafferty, S.; Qualls, N.; Morissette, S.B. Quality Improvement Evaluation of the Feasibility and Acceptability of Adding a Concerned Significant Other to Safety Planning for Suicide Prevention with Veterans. *J. Ment. Health Couns.* **2019**, *41*, 4–20. [CrossRef]

21. Matthieu, M.M.; Morissette, S.B.; Clafferty, S.; Degutis, L.; Oliver, C.M.; Adkins, D.A.; DeBeer, B.B. Veteran Experiences with Suicide Ideation, Suicide Attempt, and Social Support in Safety Planning Within the Department of Veterans Affairs. *Mil. Med.* **2023**, *188*, e3289–e3294. [CrossRef]
22. Ferguson, M.; Posselt, M.; McIntyre, H.; Loughhead, M.; Kenny, M.-A.; Mau, V.; Procter, N. Staff Perspectives of Safety Planning as a Suicide Prevention Intervention for People of Refugee and Asylum-Seeker Background. *Crisis J. Crisis Interv. Suicide Prev.* **2022**, *43*, 331–338. [CrossRef] [PubMed]
23. Woodward, E.N.; Lunsford, A.; Brown, R.; Downing, D.; Ball, I.; Gan-Kemp, J.M.; Smith, A.; Atkinson, O.; Graham, T. Pre-Implementation Adaptation of Suicide Safety Planning Intervention Using Peer Support in Rural Areas. *Front. Health Serv.* **2023**, *3*, 1225171. [CrossRef]
24. Wilson, M.P.; Moutier, C.; Wolf, L.; Nordstrom, K.; Schulz, T.; Betz, M.E. Emergency Department Recommendations for Suicide Prevention in Adults: The ICARE Mnemonic and a Systematic Review of the Literature. *Am. J. Emerg. Med.* **2019**, *38*, 571–581. [CrossRef]
25. Nabi, Z.; Stansfeld, J.; Plöderl, M.; Wood, L.; Moncrieff, J. Effects of Lithium on Suicide and Suicidal Behaviour: A Systematic Review and Meta-Analysis of Randomised Trials. *Epidemiol. Psychiatr. Sci.* **2022**, *31*, e65. [CrossRef] [PubMed]
26. Maina, G.; Adami, M.; Ascione, G.; Bondi, E.; De Berardis, D.; Delmonte, D.; Maffezzoli, S.; Martinotti, G.; Nivoli, A.; Ottavianelli, E.; et al. Nationwide Consensus on the Clinical Management of Treatment-Resistant Depression in Italy: A Delphi Panel. *Ann. Gen. Psychiatry* **2023**, *22*, 48. [CrossRef] [PubMed]
27. Shafiq, S.; Ronksley, P.E.; Scory, T.D.; Elliott, M.J.; Bulloch, A.G.M.; Patten, S.B. Ten-Year Trends in Lithium Prescribing in Alberta, Canada. *Can. J. Psychiatry* **2024**, *69*, 13–20. [CrossRef] [PubMed]
28. Zisook, S.; Domingues, I.; Compton, J. Pharmacologic Approaches to Suicide Prevention. *Focus* **2023**, *21*, 137–144. [CrossRef]
29. Schmutte, T.; Costa, M.; Hammer, P.; Davidson, L. Comparisons between Suicide in Persons with Serious Mental Illness, Other Mental Disorders, or No Known Mental Illness: Results from 37 U.S. States, 2003–2017. *Schizophr. Res.* **2021**, *228*, 74–82. [CrossRef]
30. Pawson, R.; Tilley, N.; Tilley, N. *Realistic Evaluation*; SAGE Publications Ltd.: London, UK, 1997; ISBN 0-7619-5009-5.
31. Rogers, P.J. Using Programme Theory to Evaluate Complicated and Complex Aspects of Interventions. *Evaluation* **2008**, *14*, 29–48. [CrossRef]
32. Wong, G.; Westhorp, G.; Manzano, A.; Greenhalgh, J.; Jagosh, J.; Greenhalgh, T. RAMESES II Reporting Standards for Realist Evaluations. *BMC Med.* **2016**, *14*, 96. [CrossRef]
33. Tong, A.; Sainsbury, P.; Craig, J. Consolidated Criteria for Reporting Qualitative Research (COREQ): A 32-Item Checklist for Interviews and Focus Groups. *Int. J. Qual. Health Care* **2007**, *19*, 349–357. [CrossRef]
34. Dalkin, S.M.; Greenhalgh, J.; Jones, D.; Cunningham, B.; Lhussier, M. What's in a Mechanism? Development of a Key Concept in Realist Evaluation. *Implement. Sci.* **2015**, *10*, 49. [CrossRef]
35. Jagosh, J.; Bush, P.L.; Salsberg, J.; Macaulay, A.C.; Greenhalgh, T.; Wong, G.; Cargo, M.; Green, L.W.; Herbert, C.P.; Pluye, P. A Realist Evaluation of Community-Based Participatory Research: Partnership Synergy, Trust Building and Related Ripple Effects. *BMC Public Health* **2015**, *15*, 725. [CrossRef]
36. Malterud, K.; Siersma, V.D.; Guassora, A.D. Sample Size in Qualitative Interview Studies: Guided by Information Power. *Qual. Health Res.* **2016**, *26*, 1753–1760. [CrossRef] [PubMed]
37. Sebele-Mpofu, F.Y. Saturation Controversy in Qualitative Research: Complexities and Underlying Assumptions. A Literature Review. *Cogent Soc. Sci.* **2020**, *6*, 1838706. [CrossRef]
38. Braun, V.; Clarke, V. Thematic analysis. In *APA Handbook of Research Methods in Psychology, Vol. 2: Research Designs: Quantitative, Qualitative, Neuropsychological, and Biological*; Cooper, H., Camic, P.M., Long, D.L., Panter, A.T., Rindskopf, D., Sher, K.J., Eds.; American Psychological Association: Washington, DC, USA, 2012; pp. 57–71. [CrossRef]
39. Rahimi, S.; Khatooni, M. Saturation in Qualitative Research: An Evolutionary Concept Analysis. *Int. J. Nurs. Stud. Adv.* **2024**, *6*, 100174. [CrossRef]
40. Downey, J.; Harris, N.; Rybczynska-Bunt, S.; Golder, E.; Shearn, K.; Bradley, N. Reflecting on Reflexivity in Realist Evaluation: A Call to Action. *Int. J. Qual. Methods* **2024**, *23*, 16094069241284206. [CrossRef]
41. Na; P.J.; Shin, J.; Kwak, H.R.; Lee, J.; Jester, D.J.; Bandara, P.; Kim, J.Y.; Moutier, C.Y.; Pietrzak, R.H.; Oquendo, M.A.; et al. Social Determinants of Health and Suicide-Related Outcomes: A Review of Meta-Analyses. *JAMA Psychiatry* **2025**, *82*, 337–346. [CrossRef] [PubMed]
42. Chia, A.Y.Y.; Hartanto, A.; Wan, T.S.; Teo, S.S.M.; Sim, L.; Kasturiratna, K.T.A.S. The Impact of Childhood Sexual, Physical and Emotional Abuse and Neglect on Suicidal Behavior and Non-Suicidal Self-Injury: A Systematic Review of Meta-Analyses. *Psychiatry Res. Commun.* **2025**, *5*, 100202. [CrossRef]
43. Buus, N.; Juel, A.; Haskelberg, H.; Frandsen, H.; Larsen, J.L.S.; River, J.; Andreasson, K.; Nordentoft, M.; Davenport, T.; Erlangsen, A. User Involvement in Developing the MYPLAN Mobile Phone Safety Plan App for People in Suicidal Crisis: Case Study. *JMIR Ment. Health* **2019**, *6*, e11965. [CrossRef]

44. Lesage, A.; Fortin, G.; Ligier, F.; Van Haaster, I.; Doyon, C.; Brouillard, C.; Daneau, D.; Rassy, J. Implementing a Suicide Audit in Montreal: Taking Suicide Review Further to Make Concrete Recommendations for Suicide Prevention. *Arch. Suicide Res.* **2023**, *27*, 29–42. [CrossRef]
45. Shin, H.D.; Zaheer, J.; Torous, J.; Strudwick, G. Designing Implementation Strategies for a Digital Suicide Safety Planning Intervention in a Psychiatric Emergency Department: Protocol for a Multimethod Research Project. *JMIR Res. Protoc.* **2023**, *12*, e50643. [CrossRef]
46. Stahl, N.A.; King, J.R. Expanding Approaches for Research: Understanding and Using Trustworthiness in Qualitative Research. *J. Dev. Educ.* **2020**, *44*, 26–28.

MDPI AG
Grosspeteranlage 5
4052 Basel
Switzerland
Tel.: +41 61 683 77 34

Journal of Clinical Medicine Editorial Office
E-mail: jcm@mdpi.com
www.mdpi.com/journal/jcm

www.ingramcontent.com/pod-product-compliance
Lightning Source LLC
Chambersburg PA
CBHW061558210926
51850CB00009B/2144